OB/GYN
SECRETS

Third Edition

OB/GYN SECRETS

Third Edition

Thomas J. Bader, MD
Assistant Professor
Department of Obstetrics and Gynecology
University of Pennsylvania School of Medicine
Philadelphia, Pennsylvania

HANLEY & BELFUS, INC. / Philadelphia

Publisher: HANLEY & BELFUS, INC.
      Medical Publishers
      210 South 13th Street
      Philadelphia, PA 19107
      (215) 546-7293; 800-962-1892
      FAX (215) 790-9330
      Web site: http://www.hanleyandbelfus.com

Note to the reader: Although the information in this book has been carefully reviewed for correctness of dosage and indications, neither the authors nor the editor nor the publisher can accept any legal responsibility for any errors or omissions that may be made. Neither the publisher nor the editor makes any warranty, expressed or implied, with respect to the material contained herein. Before prescribing any drug, the reader must review the manufacturer's current product information (package inserts) for accepted indications, absolute dosage recommendations, and other information pertinent to the safe and effective use of the product described.

Library of Congress Cataloging-in-Publication Data

Ob/gyn secrets / edited by Thomas J. Bader.—3rd ed.
  p. ; cm. — (The secrets series®)
 Includes bibliographical references and index.
 ISBN 1-56053-475-3 (alk. paper)
  1. Obstetrics—Miscellanea. 2. Gynecology—Miscellanea. I. Title: Ob gyn secrets.
II. Bader, Thomas J. III. Series.
 [DNLM: 1. Genital Diseases, Female—Examination Questions. 2. Pregnancy
Complications—Examination Questions. WP 18.2 O12 2001]
 RG112.O33 2003
 618'.076—dc21

                 2001039726

OB/GYN SECRETS, 3RD ED.   ISBN 1-56053-475-3

Last digit is the print number: 9 8 7 6 5 4 3 2 1

CONTENTS

CONTRIBUTORS

Richard Allen, MD
Adjunct Professor, Department of Obstetrics and Gynecology, Oregon Health Sciences University, Portland; Active Staff, University Hospital, Portland, Oregon

Peter Argenta, MD
Assistant Professor, Division of Gynecologic Oncology, University of Minnesota, Minneapolis, Minnesota

Lily A. Arya, MD, MS
Assistant Professor, Department of Obstetrics and Gynecology, Division of Urogynecology and Reconstructive Pelvic Surgery, University of Pennsylvania Medical Center, Philadelphia, Pennsylvania

Janice B. Asher, MD
Assistant Clinical Professor, Department of Obstetrics and Gynecology, Hospital of the University of Pennsylvania, Philadelphia, Pennsylvania

Kevin Bachus, MD
Private Practice, Rocky Mountain Center for Reproductive Medicine, Fort Collins, Colorado

Thomas J. Bader, MD
Assistant Professor, Department of Obstetrics and Gynecology, University of Pennsylvania School of Medicine, Philadelphia, Pennsylvania

Christina Ann Bandera, MD
Assistant Professor, Department of Obstetrics and Gynecology, Harvard Medical School, Boston; Physician, Division of Gynecologic Oncology, Dana Farber Cancer Institute, Boston, Massachusetts

Lisa B. Baute, MD
Assistant Clinical Professor, Department of Obstetrics and Gynecology, University of Pennsylvania School of Medicine, Philadelphia; Attending Physician, University of Pennsylvania Medical Center, Philadelphia, Pennsylvania

Nina M. Boe, MD
Associate Professor, Department of Obstetrics and Gynecology, Division of Maternal-Fetal Medicine, University of California School of Medicine-Davis, Sacramento, California

Catherine S. Bradley, MD, MSCE
Assistant Professor, Department of Obstetrics and Gynecology, Division of Urogynecology and Reconstructive Pelvic Surgery, University of Pennsylvania Medical Center, Philadelphia, Pennsylvania

Nadine Burrington, MD
North Cascade Women's Clinic, Mount Vernon, Washington

Arthur J. Castelbaum, MD
Northern Fertility and Reproduction Associates, Meadowbrook; Assistant Professor, Department of Obstetrics and Gynecology, Division of Reproductive Endocrinology and Infertility, Thomas Jefferson School of Medicine, Philadelphia, Pennsylvania

Peter J. Chen, MD
Clinical Assistant Professor, Department of Obstetrics and Gynecology, University of Pennsylvania, Philadelphia, Pennsylvania

Christina S. Chu, MD
Assistant Professor, Department of Obstetrics and Gynecology, Division of Gynecologic Oncology, University of Pennsylvania School of Medicine, Philadelphia, Pennsylvania

L. Dorine Day, MD
Perinatologist, St. Joseph's Hospital, Denver; Assistant Clinical Professor, University of Colorado Health Sciences Center, Denver, Colorado

Molina B. Dayal, MD, MPH
Fellow, Department of Obstetrics and Gynecology, Division of Reproductive Medicine and Surgery, Hospital of the University of Pennsylvania, Philadelphia, Pennsylvania

Deborah A. Driscoll, MD
Associate Professor, Department of Obstetrics and Gynecology, Division of Reproductive Genetics, University of Pennsylvania School of Medicine, Philadelphia, Pennsylvania

Bruce Charles Drummond, MD
Department of Obstetrics and Gynecology, Dean Medical Center, Madison, Wisconsin

Scott E. Edwards, MD
Assistant Clinical Professor, Department of Obstetrics and Gynecology, University of Pennsylvania School of Medicine, Philadelphia, Pennsylvania

Mohammed Adel Elkousy, MD
Clinical Instructor, Division of Maternal-Fetal Medicine, University of Pennsylvania School of Medicine, Philadelphia, Pennsylvania

Ty B. Erickson, MD
Private Practice, Idaho Falls, Idaho

Iraj Forouzan, MD
Associate Professor, Associate Director of Residency Program, Department of Obstetrics and Gynecology, Drexel University College of Medicine, Philadelphia; Attending Physician, Hahnemann University Hospital, Philadelphia, Pennsylvania

Gretchen A. Frey, MD
Assistant Clinical Professor, Department of Family Medicine, University of Colorado, Denver, Colorado

Robert Gaiser, MD
Associate Professor and Director of Obstetric Anesthesia, Department of Anesthesiology, University of Pennsylvania, Philadelphia, Pennsylvania

Alfredo Gil, MD
Clinical Assistant Professor, Department of Obstetrics and Gynecology, University of Pennsylvania, Philadelphia, Pennsylvania

Kent D. Heyborne, MD
Chair, Women and Children's Health, and Director, Maternal-Fetal Medicine, Swedish Medical Center, Denver; Assistant Clinical Professor, University of Colorado Health Sciences Center, Denver, Colorado

Anne Honebrink, MD
Clinical Associate Professor, Department of Obstetrics and Gynecology, University of Pennsylvania School of Medicine, Philadelphia; Medical Director, Penn Health for Women, Radnor, Pennsylvania

Sami I. Jabara, MD
Instructor, Department of Obstetrics and Gynecology, Division of Reproductive Endocrinology and Infertility, University of Pennsylvania School of Medicine, Philadelphia, Pennsylvania

Abike James, MD, MPH
Assistant Professor, Department of Obstetrics and Gynecology, University of Pennsylvania School of Medicine, Philadelphia, Pennsylvania

Sonya Kashyap, MD, FRCS(C)
Clinical Fellow, Center for Reproductive Medicine, New York, New York

David Kaufman, MD
Assistant Professor, Department of Pediatrics, Division of Neonatology, University of Virginia School of Medicine, Charlottesville, Virginia

Kirsten Lawrence, MD
Instructor, Division of Maternal-Fetal Medicine, Department of Obstetrics and Gynecology, University of Pennsylvania School of Medicine, Philadelphia, Pennsylvania

Dee'Ann Lisby, MD
Assistant Professor, Department of Pediatrics, Children's Hospital of Philadelphia, Philadelphia; Associate Director of Neonatology, Hospital of the University of Pennsylvania, Philadelphia, Pennsylvania

Saifuddin T. Mama, MD, MPH
Assistant Clinical Professor, Department of Obstetrics and Gynecology, Hospital of the University of Pennsylvania and Pennsylvania Hospital, Philadelphia; University Associate, Department of General Pediatrics, Division of Adolescent Medicine, Children's Hospital, Philadelphia, Pennsylvania

Dominic A. Marchiano, MD
Maternal-Fetal Medicine Fellow, Hospital of the University of Pennsylvania, Philadelphia; Clinical Instructor, Department of Obstetrics and Gynecology, Division of Maternal-Fetal Medicine, University of Pennsylvania School of Medicine, Philadelphia, Pennsylvania

John G. McFee, MD
Associate Director, Department of Obstetrics and Gynecology, Denver Health Medical Center, Denver; Professor, Department of Obstetrics and Gynecology, University of Colorado Health Sciences Center, Denver, Colorado

Anthony O. Odibo, MD, MRCOG
Assistant Professor, Department of Obstetrics and Gynecology, Division of Maternal-Fetal Medicine, University of Pennsylvania Medical Center, Philadelphia; Attending Physician, Hospital of the University of Pennsylvania, Philadelphia, Pennsylvania

Emmanuelle Paré, MD, FRCSC
Fellow, Department of Obstetrics and Gynecology, Division of Maternal-Fetal Medicine, University of Pennsylvania Health System, Philadelphia; Clinical Instructor, Hospital of the University of Pennsylvania, Philadelphia, Pennsylvania

Samantha M. Pfeifer, MD
Assistant Professor, Department of Obstetrics and Gynecology, Division of Reproductive Endocrinology and Infertility, University of Pennsylvania School of Medicine, Philadelphia, Pennsylvania

Martha E. Rode, MD
Attending Physician, Department of Obstetrics and Gynecology, Division of Maternal-Fetal Medicine, Christiana Care Health System, Newark, Delaware

Stephen W. Sawin, MD
Physician, Private Practice, South Jersey Fertility Center, Marlton, New Jersey

Sally Yaël Segel, MD
Assistant Professor, Department of Obstetrics and Gynecology, Division of Maternal-Fetal Medicine, Emory University School of Medicine, Atlanta, Georgia

Harish M. Sehdev, MD
Assistant Professor, Division of Maternal-Fetal Medicine, University of Pennsylvania, Philadelphia; Director, Labor and Delivery, Pennsylvania Hospital, Philadelphia, Pennsylvania

Hyagriv Nara Simhan, MD, MSCR
Assistant Professor, Department of Obstetrics, Gynecology, and Reproductive Sciences, Division of Maternal-Fetal Medicine, University of Pittsburgh, Magee Women's Hospital, Pittsburgh, Pennsylvania

Steven Sondheimer, MD
Professor, Division of Reproductive Endocrinology and Infertility, Department of Obstetrics and Gynecology, University of Pennsylvania School of Medicine, Philadelphia, Pennsylvania

Steven Spandorfer, MD
Assistant Professor, Department of Obstetrics and Gynecology, Center for Reproductive Medicine and Infertility, Weill Medical College of Cornell University, New York, New York

Richard W. Tureck, MD
Professor, Department of Obstetrics and Gynecology, Division of Reproductive Endocrinology and Infertility, University of Pennsylvania School of Medicine, Philadelphia, Pennsylvania

Serdar H. Ural, MD
Assistant Professor, Department of Obstetrics and Gynecology, Division of Maternal-Fetal Medicine, University of Pennsylvania School of Medicine, Philadelphia; Assistant Professor, Hospital of the University of Pennsylvania, Philadelphia, Pennsylvania

Robert J. Wester, MD
Chair, Department of Obstetrics and Gynecology, St. Joseph's Hospital, Denver, Colorado

Yu-Hsin Wu, MD
Clinical Assistant Professor, Department of Obstetrics and Gynecology, Hospital of the University of Pennsylvania, Philadelphia, Pennsylvania

Sharon Zwillinger, MD
Private Practice, Newark, Delaware

PREFACE TO THE FIRST EDITION

This book continues the tradition of The Secrets Series® by presenting an overview of obstetrics and gynecology in question and answer format. Comprehensive coverage is more properly the domain of the major textbooks in the field. *Ob/Gyn Secrets* is intended to be a handy reference that emphasizes the common problems encountered in gynecologic and obstetric practice and that simplifies a vast amount of information without being overly simplistic.

A wide range of topics in obstetrics and gynecology is addressed, with sections on general gynecology, reproductive endocrinology and infertility, gynecologic oncology, general obstetrics, maternal complications, the fetus, the placenta, and labor and delivery.

Some questions have more than one right answer. Some questions have no right answer. Some answers are controversial. The authors have attempted to ask key questions and provide their best answers based on the current information available.

It is hoped that the reader will find this text enjoyable and practically useful and that the patient will be its ultimate benefactor.

PREFACE TO THE SECOND EDITION

In this second edition, we have tried to incorporate changes in practice management, address new technologies, and provide up to date information and references.

We want to thank the contributing authors for their time and effort. Linda Belfus, our publisher, deserves special thanks for her patience and perseverance, for without her this second edition would never have been finished.

We hope our readers will enjoy this format and that their patients will benefit from our efforts.

Helen L. Frederickson, M.D.
Louise Wilkins-Haug, M.D., Ph.D.

PREFACE TO THE THIRD EDITION

The field of obstetrics and gynecology continues to evolve and develop. Each year, new information allows medical professionals to address more effectively the health of women and their babies. In the 6 years since the last edition of *Ob/Gyn Secrets*, the science related to women's health has advanced significantly, and patient management has changed in response to these discoveries. In addition, medicine in general and the field of obstetrics and gynecology in particular has continued to place greater emphasis on evidence-based medicine than on expert opinion. This third edition of *Ob/Gyn Secrets* is consistent with that trend. The authors have made a point of including the best available evidence in formulating questions and answers. A sounder scientific footing for the practice of obstetrics and gynecology will ultimately benefit our patients.

No single textbook can cover every topic. However, *Ob/Gyn Secrets, 3rd edition* does provide students and clinicians with a readable, accurate source of pertinent information regarding women's health and pathology. The question-and-answer format of The Secrets Series® mirrors what we all experience in medicine: a series of questions. Our teachers pose some questions, and others we develop on our own while seeing patients or learning about the field. The authors and I hope that this book will serve as a helpful tool for topic review, and to prepare for exams and clinical rounds.

Thomas J. Bader, M.D.
EDITOR

Dedication

To Janet, George, Laura, Peter, and Jack for their patience
and support.

Acknowledgment

I wish to acknowledge the tireless work of Jacqueline
Mahon, whose leadership, editorial work, and tenacity made
the completion of this book possible. I also want to thank
Posie Reid for her assistance in the preparation of the chap
ters. Finally, my thanks go to the contributing authors for
their dedication to education and their hard work in prepar-
ing their chapters.

I. General Gynecology and Infertility

1. BENIGN LESIONS OF THE VULVA AND VAGINA

Abike James, M.D., M.P.H.

1. What is the vulva composed of?

The vulva is composed of the labia majora, labia minora, mons pubis, clitoris, vestibule, urinary meatus, vaginal orifice, hymen, Bartholin's glands, Skene's ducts, and vestibulovaginal bulbs.

2. Name the five disorders in which infectious agents cause lesions of the vulva.

- Chancroid (*Haemophilus ducreyi*)
- Syphilis (*Treponema pallidum*)
- Lymphogranuloma venereum (*Chlamydia trachomatis* serovar)
- Human papillomavirus
- Genital herpes

3. Describe the clinical features and treatment of each disorder listed in Question 2.

Chancroid: Sexually transmitted with an incubation period of 3–10 days. Presents as small, tender papules that soon break down to form ragged, tender, nonindurated ulcers usually located on the labia, fourchette, perineum, and perianal areas. May be single, but are more often multiple. • Treatment—current drug of choice is **erythromycin**.

Syphilis: Sexually transmitted with an incubation period of about 2 weeks. The first lesion is a macule, which soon becomes papular, then ulcerates to form a primary chancre. Classic description of the primary chancre is an indurated, painless ulcer with a dull red base. If untreated, primary stage typically lasts 3–8 weeks and then the ulcer spontaneously heals. In **secondary syphilis**, skin rashes may be macular, papular, papulosquamous, or pustular, and any of these may occur on the vulva. *Condyloma lata* are seen in secondary syphilis and are characterized by confluent, spongy, gray masses with flat tops and broad bases located at the periphery of the vulva. In **late syphilis**, vulvar lesions termed *gummas* appear as squamous lesions or subcutaneous nodules that sometimes ulcerate. • Treatment—remains **penicillin** for all stages

Lymphogranuloma venereum (LGV): Rare in temperate climates. Incubation period is between 3 days and 3 weeks. The primary lesion is a small, painless papule, vesicle, or ulcer, typically located on the fourchette but may also occur on the labia or cervix. The secondary stage is characterized by enlargement of the inguinal glands to form a painful mass, which tends to suppurate and form sinuses. • Treatment—early LGV responds to **tetracycline**. Prolonged treatment may be necessary.

Human papillomavirus: Sexually transmitted with incubation periods ranging from 3 weeks to 8 months. Manifest on the vulva as genital warts. Commonly are papular, appearing as small, raised, rounded lesions, usually multiple. However, may present as *condylomata acuminata*, which are irregular, fleshy, vascular tumors affecting any part of the vulva. • Treatment—repeat application of **trichloroacetic acid, podophyllin, topical imiquimod (Aldara), cryotherapy, or laser surgery**.

Genital herpes virus: Sexually transmitted with incubation period of first attack usually 2–10 days. Lesions are initially vesicular, but rupture to form single, multiple, or grouped shallow, tender, ulcers, 1–2 mm in diameter. Lesions are most common on the labia majora and minora, clitoris, perineum, and perianal areas. • Treatment—**acyclovir** is the drug of choice for the treatment of outbreaks. However, it does not influence the rate of recurrence.

4. What are the vulvar, non-neoplastic epithelial disorders (previously called vulvar dystrophies)?

Lichen sclerosis, lichen planus, and lichen simplex chronicus.

5. Describe the clinical characteristics and management of the disorders listed in Question 4.

Lichen sclerosis: Most common in prepubertal and postmenopausal patients. Characterized by epithelial thinning with edema and fibrosis of the dermis and associated shrinkage and agglutination of the labia and introital stenosis. The edematous skin has a white, thin, and paperlike appearance. The labia minora is usually lost. Patients often experience pruritis. Sexually active women may experience dyspareunia. Lesions usually are symmetric. Diagnosis is confirmed by biopsy. • Treatment—includes very high potency topical **corticosteroids**, such as clobetasol or halobetasol 0.05% cream.

Lichen planus: A papulosquamous, chronic, and inflammatory dermatosis of unknown etiology. The vulvar lesions are chronic and painful and commonly involve the inner aspects of the labia minora, vagina, and vestibule. Initial presentation may vary from a severe erosive process to mild inflammatory changes involving the vagina. Stria are often present at the margins of the lesions, and loss of architecture may be extreme. Diagnosis is confirmed by biopsy. • Treatment—vaginal **hydrocortisone** suppositories, with the addition of **estrogen** creams for postmenopausal women.

Lichen simplex chronicus: Usually presents with vulvar pruritis. Thickened, white epithelium, slightly scaly and often unilateral and localized, is identified on exam. Biopsy confirms diagnosis. • Treatment—medium-potency **steroids**. Resolution of symptoms usually occurs rapidly.

6. Describe the benign pigmentary lesions of the vulva.

Melanocytic nevi: Vary in color and size (from 1–2 mm to 1–2 cm). Typically are asymptomatic. Diagnosis confirmed histologically usually with simple excision.

Acanthosis nigricans: Cutaneous disorder affecting the axillae, nipples, umbilical area, and crural region. Appears as a poorly defined, velvety hyperpigmentation. Only symptomatic treatment is available.

Vitiligo: Characterized by complete depigmentation of an area of skin that is otherwise normal. The area involved is usually well defined and symmetrical. No effective treatment is available.

7. List the common cystic lesions of the vulva and vagina.

Cysts of epidermal origin: sebaceous cysts, epidermal inclusion cysts, hidradenoma

Cysts of embryonic origin: Gartner's duct cysts (arise from vestigial remnants of the vaginal portion of the Wolffian ducts)

Duct cysts: Bartholin's gland

Cysts of urethral and paraurethral origin: Skene's duct cysts, urethral or sub-urethral diverticulum

8. List the benign solid tumors of the vulva and vagina.

Tumors of epidermal origin: seborrheic keratosis, hidradenoma

Mesodermal origin: fibroma, lipoma, leiomyoma, hemangioma, vulvo-vaginal polyps

Uretheral origin: caruncle

9. What is vulvadynia? How is it managed?

Vulvadynia is defined as diffuse vulvar pain that occurs with or without provocation and is usually constant and unremitting. Pain is described as dull and burning. On exam, the vulvar skin and architecture are normal, and there are usually no architectural abnormalities. Management includes tricyclic antidepressants, anticonvulsants, and pain management programs.

10. What is vestibulitis? How is it managed?

Vestibulitis is defined as a constellation of symptoms and signs, including entry dyspareunia, vestibular erythema, and vestibular tenderness in the absence of an active dermatosis or disorder that would otherwise explain the findings. Management includes symptomatic relief with 5% lidocaine ointment; tricyclic antidepressants may be helpful. Surgical treatment should only be considered in severe cases that are refractory to medical management.

11. Which lesions in the vagina result from abnormal development? How are they treated?

Imperforate hymen: Usually recognized after puberty when retention of menses leads to hematocolpos. Accumulation of retained secretions may also lead to hematometra and hematosalpinx. Inspection of the introitus reveals an imperforate hymen with a bulging fluid mass in the vagina. • Treatment—cruciate incision of the imperforate hymen.

Septate vagina: May be complete or incomplete, with a soft tissue septum running from the introitus to the cervix. Many patients have two cervices, one on either side of the septum. • Treatment—if asymptomatic, no treatment is necessary.

Transverse vaginal septum: A rare congenital defect in which a septum divides the vagina into upper and lower compartments. May be complete or incomplete; in the latter case, an opening in the septum permits menstrual flow. Pregnancy may occur. Delivery may require cesarean section. • Treatment—resection of the septum.

BIBLIOGRAPHY

1. American College of Obstetricians and Gynecologists Educational Bulletin: Vulvar nonneoplastic epithelial disorders. No. 241, October 1997 (Replaces No. 139, January 1990). Int J Gynaecol Obstet 60(2):181–188, 1998.
2. Buttram VL: Müllerian anomalies and their management. Fertil Steril 40:159, 1983.
3. Kaufman RH, Faro S: Benign Diseases of the Vulva and Vagina, 4th ed. St. Louis, Mosby, 1994.
4. Ridley CM, Neill SM: The Vulva, 2nd ed. Oxford, Blackwell Science Ltd, 1999.
5. Schroeder B: Vulvar disorders in adolescents. Obstet Gynecol Clin North Am 27(1):35–48, 2000.
6. Tovell HMM, Young AW: Diseases of the Vulva in Clinical Practice. New York, Elsevier Science Publishing Co., Inc., 1991

2. LOWER GENITAL TRACT INFECTIONS

Thomas J. Bader, M.D.

1. What are the characteristics of normal vaginal fluid?

Vaginal fluid can be described in terms of its microscopic and chemical features and its normal microbial flora. Normal vaginal fluid is white and generally not malodorous. The normal pH is around 4.0. Microscopically it contains squamous epithelial cells and bacteria, but no white blood cells or red blood cells. The principal organisms are lactobacilli. Lactobacilli (also called Döderlein's bacilli) are aerobic gram-variable rods. The vagina also contains gram-negative bacteria as well as anaerobes. Vaginitis is caused by alterations in the normal flora (bacterial vaginosis, candidiasis) or by an outside organism (trichomoniasis).

2. What are the most common forms of vaginitis? What are their symptoms?

Candida vaginitis is caused by an overgrowth of one of many *Candida* species. **Bacterial vaginosis** is caused by an imbalance in the normal flora. **Trichomoniasis** is due to infection with a parasite, *Trichomonas vaginalis*. It is a sexually transmitted disease. **Atrophic vaginitis** is irritation and inflammation secondary to atrophy of the vaginal tissue.

All of these conditions can present with one or more of the following symptoms: increased vaginal discharge, malodorous discharge, vaginal or vulvar pruritus, dyspareunia, vaginal or vulvar burning, vulvar edema and erythema. The characteristics of the symptoms and the gross description of the discharge are *not* sufficient to establish the diagnosis.

3. How are the common causes of vaginitis distinguished from one another?

These various conditions are most easily distinguished by performing four simple tests: physical exam of the vulva and vagina, determination of vaginal fluid pH, microscopic evaluation of vaginal fluid mixed with saline and potassium hydoxide (KOH), and the "whiff test," whereby vaginal fluid is mixed with KOH and the examiner smells the effluent for an amide odor.

Distinguishing Characteristics of the Common Forms of Vaginitis

	NORMAL	CANDIDIASIS	BACTERIAL VAGINOSIS	TRICHOMONIASIS
Gross appearance	White, thin	White, thick	Thin, grey-white	Thick, milky; grey-white or green
pH	4.0	4.0	> 4.5	> 4.5
Microscopic	Epithelial cells only	Budding hyphae on KOH prep	Clue cells; few WBCs	Motile trichomonads
'Whiff' test	−	−	+	−

4. List some important points to keep in mind when making the diagnosis.

- If the pH is normal (< 4.5) the diagnosis is limited to candidiasis, atrophic vaginitis, or normal vaginal fluid.
- Only Candida has the thick, white, "cottage cheese" appearance on gross exam.
- The positive "whiff" test is specific for bacterial vaginosis.
- In candidiasis and trichomoniasis, the organism is visible under the microscope.
- In bacterial vaginosis, the diagnosis is inferred based on the alterations in the characteristics of the vaginal flora: elevated pH; abnormal odor; and the clumping of bacteria onto epithelial cells, leading to the microscopic appearance of "clue cells" (see also Question 7).

5. Describe Candida infection.

Candida causes vulvar and vaginal itching and burning. The most common species is *Candida albicans*. Other species are *C. glabrata* and *C. tropicalis*. Women may have bladder symptoms, and yeast vaginitis may be misdiagnosed as cystitis. There is usually a thick, white discharge. The diagnosis is made by the appearance of budding hyphae (*C. albicans*, *C. tropicalis*) or spores (*C. glabrata*) seen in a KOH preparation under medium power (100×). This test is only about 80% sensitive, however.

Treatment is with either a single dose of an oral agent, such as fluconazole (Diflucan), or a short course (1–7 days) of a vaginal preparation, such as miconazole (Monistat), clotrimazole (Mycelex, Lotrimin), tioconazole (Vagistat), terconazole (Terazol), or butoconazole (Femstat).

6. How is the diagnosis of recurrent yeast established? How is it treated?

There is no precise definition of what constitutes recurrent yeast infections. Most clinicians initiate a work-up for a woman who has multiple infections over the course of a year. It is important to definitively establish the cause of the symptoms. Because different forms of vaginitis can have similar symptoms, patient history and a pattern of self-treatment with over-the-counter anti-fungals are insufficient to establish the diagnosis of recurrent yeast. Confirm the diagnosis through office evaluation, and also evaluate patients for diabetes and HIV infection, both of which can lead to recurrent yeast infections. Check for pregnancy, since yeast infections are more common in pregnancy.

There are a number of treatment regimens for recurrent yeast. The condition is thought to be caused by colonization of the gastrointestinal tract, which serves as a repository, leading to recurrent vaginal infections. Therefore, treatment is aimed at eradicating the yeast systemically through long courses of oral anti-fungals (fluconazole or ketoconazole). However, vaginal application of agents (boric acid, gentian violet) is also effective.

7. What are the characteristics of bacterial vaginosis (BV)?

Bacterial vaginosis, also sometimes called vaginal bacteriosis or nonspecific vaginitis, is thought to be due to a pathologic alteration in the normal vaginal flora. That is, the causative organisms are normally present in the vagina, but in BV there is overgrowth of anaerobic bacteria. Symptoms include pruritus and odor. Many women report increased odor after intercourse. On exam there is a thin, white-grey discharge. The vaginal pH is elevated; addition of KOH solution to the vaginal fluid leads to a characteristic amide odor (the "whiff test"); and the increased bacteria can be seen in a saline preparation of the vaginal fluid under high power (400×). Clue cells are epithelial cells with spherical bacteria clinging to their edges, obscuring the usually sharp border of the epithelial cells.

8. How is bacterial vaginosis treated?

Treatment is with metronidazole or clindamycin orally or vaginally (Flagyl, Metrogel, Cleocin). There is debate as to whether or not BV is sexually transmitted. Treatment of sexual partners is usually reserved for recurrent infections. Bacterial vaginosis has been linked with some poor pregnancy outcomes, including preterm birth. Both metronidzole and clindamycin can be used safely throughout pregnancy.

9. What are the characteristics of trichomoniasis?

Trichomoniaisis is a sexually transmitted disease caused by a unicellular organism, *Trichomonas vaginalis*. Women present with pruritus and increased discharge. On exam, the discharge can be copious. The pH is elevated. Examination of the vaginal fluid in a saline preparation under high power (400×) shows the organism. Trichomonads are tear-shaped or ovoid, mobile, and flagellated. They are usually identified by their motility and their visible flagella.

Treatment is with a single dose of oral metronidazole (Flagyl). Treatment is usually highly effective, but there can be resistant cases requiring a longer course of therapy. Sexual contacts should also be treated.

10. What is atrophic vaginitis? How is it treated?

Atrophic vaginitis is vulvar irritation and inflammation secondary to atrophy of the vaginal mucosa. This occurs due to inadequate estrogen and is associated with menopause. It can also occur with breastfeeding. Atrophic vaginitis is not an infection and does not require antibiotics. It is treated with supplemental estrogen either locally in the vagina or systemically.

11. What are the most common sexually transmitted diseases?

Syphylis, gonorrhea, chlamydial infection, trichomoniasis, and genital herpes. Although *Neisseria gonorrhoeae* can be isolated from the cervix, it primarily infects the upper genital tract.

12. What causes syphylis? How is it treated?

Syphylis is caused by exposure to *Treponema pallidum*. The disease progresses through well-descibed stages. There is an initial ulcer at the point of infection, usually visible on the vulva. In contrast with genital herpes, the ulcer is painless. Systemic symptoms can appear within a year, with a characteristic rash on the palms and soles of the feet. Finally, there is late syphylis, in which systemic effects involve multiple systems including the heart and the central nervous system.

The diagnosis can be made by observing the organism microscopically using dark-field microscopy. However, the diagnosis is usually made by serologic testing for antibodies. Initial screening is performed using either the rapid plasma reagin (RPR) or the Venereal Disease Research Laboratories (VDRL) test. Either of these tests, if positive, should be confirmed with a more specific test for the organism, either the flourescent-labeled Treponema antibody test (FTA) or the microhemagglutination assay of antibodies to *T. pallidum* (MHA-TP). Treatment is with penicillin. The exact regimen depends on the stage of the disease.

13. How is chlamydial infection diagnosed?

Chlamydia can cause a characteristic discharge, which the patient may notice or which may be noticed on exam. This mucopurulent discharge can be cultured, or the diagnosis can be made by identifying chlamydia mRNA with a genetic probe. Depending on the population studied and the definition, chlamydia is among the most common sexually transmitted diseases. It is often asymptomatic. Undiagnosed chlamydial infections can be a cause of infertility and chronic pelvic pain. Treatment is with doxycycline, azithromycin, or one of several quinolones. Chlamydia can also cause upper genital tract infections (i.e., pelvic inflammatory disease).

14. Why is screening for sexually transmitted diseases (STDs) important?

Many common STDs, including HIV infection, syphilis, chlamydial infection, and hepatitis, can be asymptomatic at some stage in the disease. Screening therefore offers benefit to the individual and can also have societal benefits by identifying infected individuals and preventing the spread of the disease.

There are no ironclad rules for who should undergo screening. Various criteria can be applied using demographics and risk-scoring systems, or based on site of care. Any system other than universal screening will miss some individuals perceived to be at low-risk. One approach is to screen all unmarried women under the age of 25.

15. What are the most important principles in managing and controlling sexually transmitted disease?

Prevention, screening, and treatment of patients and their sexual partners. Discuss prevention of STDs through safe sexual practices with all at-risk women. Perform screening as part of a routine health evaluation or at the time of contraceptive management. Always treat the patient *and* all sexual contacts.

16. What causes genital herpes?

Herpes infection is caused by one of two herpes simplex viruses, HSV-1 and HSV-2. HSV-1 more commonly causes peri-oral infection ("cold sores"), and HSV-2 is more commonly isolated in genital infections. HSV-1 infections of the genitals are less likely to recur. Like other herpesviruses (e.g., herpes zoster), infection with HSV is chronic. After the initial skin outbreak, the virus is dormant and can cause subsequent outbreaks.

17. How does genital herpes present?

Herpes typically causes small vesicles which rapidly progress to characteristic shallow, painful ulcers on the labia, vaginal mucosa, cervix, and/or perineum. There may be clusters of ulcers. Inguinal adenopathy frequently is present, as well as vaginal discharge. The most common complaint is pain. The pain of an initial herpes outbreak can be so severe that narcotics, topical anesthetics and even hospitalization may be necessary. Women can also experience urinary retention requiring bladder catheterization, as urine is extremely irritating to the ulcers. Systemic symptoms, such as fever and malaise, may also be present. Herpes antibodies can be isolated from women with no history of herpes infection, indicating the frequent occurrence of asymptomatic infection.

18. What is the difference between a primary and a recurent herpes outbreak?

A primary herpes outbreak is typically more severe and lasts longer (12–21 days). Recurrent outbreaks typically last 2–5 days, and the symptoms are usually more mild. The frequency of HSV recurrence is quite variable. Some women experience a single outbreak and others have recurrences many times a year.

19. When is genital herpes contagious?

Although the latent virus is always present in an infected individual's body, spread is by direct contact with the virus at the site of an outbreak. Therefore, the virus can only be spread when a woman has a secondary outbreak or in the days just prior to the eruption of an ulcer. During this pre-eruption period, the patient typically experiences a prodrome of tingling or burning in the affected region. She may also have mild systemic symptoms from the virus. If a woman has no active lesions and is not experiencing a prodrome, she is generally not infectious. Once ulcers are completely healed, they are no longer infectious.

20. How is genital herpes treated?

Although HSV cannot be cured, the symptoms and duration of both initial and secondary outbreaks can be reduced with anti-viral treatment. Several anti-viral agents are effective, including acyclovir, valacyclovir, and famciclovir. Initial treatment is for 7 days. Treatment of recurrences is for 3 days. Because secondary outbreaks tend to be more mild, and because treatment of secondary outbreaks only shortens the course by a day or two, many women forgo treatment.

21. Who should receive suppression for recurrent HSV outbreaks?

A single daily dose of one of the anti-virals is effective in reducing the frequency of secondary outbreaks. Whether or not to take a suppressant is the woman's decision, but generally suppression is recommended for women who have outbreaks more than two or three times a year.

22. Besides the discomfort and inconvenience of outbreaks, does HSV infection have any other sequelae?

HSV can be significant in pregnancy. Transmission to the newborn can occur if a woman has an active herpes outbreak or prodrome at the time of vaginal delivery. Neonatal infection is principally a problem for women experiencing an initial outbreak, but can rarely occur even with a secondary outbreak. If a woman has a prodrome or active lesion at the time of labor and delivery, she should be delivered by cesarean section.

To prevent recurrences around the time of delivery and to avoid cesarean section, many obstetricians place women with a history of herpes on anti-viral suppression at 36 weeks.

HSV genital infection, particularly with HSV-2, may be a risk factor for cervical cancer, but the evidence that this is an independent factor is inconsistent.

23. What is a Bartholin's cyst? What causes it?

A Bartholin's cyst is something of a misnomer. It is actually a dilation of the duct of the Bartholin's gland. The gland is a mucin-secreting gland in the vulva. The duct becomes obstructed, dilates, and fills with fluid. This soft-tissue mass in the vulva is referred to as a Bartholin's cyst.

24. Are Bartholin's duct cysts infectious?

Most Bartholin's duct cysts are sterile; the cyst is filled only with the mucinous material produced by the gland. If the cyst contains purulent material, it is termed a Bartholin's abscess. These infections are usually polymicrobial. *Neisseria gonorrhoeae* can sometimes be isolated.

25. Are Bartholin's cysts malignant?

Rarely, a Bartholin's malignancy can present as a cyst. The vast majority, however, are benign, and they do not need to be routinely biopsied or excised. A new Bartholin's duct cyst in a woman over 40 should be examined for possible malignancy.

26. How is a Bartholin's cyst treated?

Not all require treatment. They are usually only treated if they are symptomatic. There are three levels of treatment: incision and drainage, marsupialization, and excision. Most Bartholin's duct cysts respond to **incision and drainage**. The incision is made medially toward the vagina and hymenal ring. After making a 5-mm stab incision, a Ward catheter is placed to keep the cyst wall open and allow for continued drainage. The optimal goal is for the catheter to stay in place for weeks to allow epithelialization of the opening. However, the catheter frequently falls out prior to removal.

For women with recurrent Bartholin's duct cysts, the cyst or duct wall can be opened widely and the edges sutured back to leave an open structure. This procedure is called **marsupialization**.

If problems with the duct cyst persist despite marsupialization, the gland and dilated duct can be **excised** in toto. This involves significant dissection and requires regional or general anesthesia.

BIBLIOGRAPHY

1. American College of Obstetricians and Gynecologists. Vaginitis. Technical Bulletin No. 26, 1996.
2. Baldwin HE. STD update: Screening and therapeutic options Inter J Fertil Womens Med 2001; 46:79–88.
3. Centers for Disease Control and Prevention. 1998 guidelines for treatment of sexually transmitted diseases. MMWR 1998;47:1–111.
4. Eschenbach DA. Vaginal infection. Clin Obstet Gynecol 1983;26:186–202.
5. Lee YH, Rankin JS, Alpert S, et al. Microbiological investigation of Bartholin's gland abscesses and cysts. Am J Obstet Gynecol 1977;129:150–153.
6. Morris M, Nicoll A, Simms I, et al. Bacterial vaginosis: A public health review. Br J Obstet Gynaecol 2001;108:439–50.
7. Murthy NS, Mathew A. Risk factors for pre-cancerous lesions of the cervix. Euro J Cancer Prevent 2000;9:5–14.
8. Ormrod D, Scott LJ, Perry CM. Valaciclovir: A review of its long-term utility in the management of genital herpes simplex virus and cytomegalovirus infections. Drugs 2000;59:839–863.
9. Petrin D, Delgaty K, Bhatt R, Garber G. Clinical and microbiological aspects of Trichomonas vaginalis. Clin Microbiol Rev 1998;11:300–317.
10. Sobel JD. Vaginitis.New Eng J Med 1997;337:1896–903.
11. Sobel JD. Bacterial vaginosis Ann Rev Med 2000;51:349–356.
12. Stanberry L, Cunningham A, Mertz G, et al. New developments in the epidemiology, natural history and management of genital herpes Antiviral Res1999;42:1–14.
13. Stenchever MA, Droegemueller W, Herbst AL, Mishell DR (eds): Comprehensive Gynecology, 4th ed. St. Louis, Mosby, 2001.

3. PELVIC INFLAMMATORY DISEASE

Anne Honebrink, M.D.

1. How is pelvic inflammatory disease (PID) defined?

The term PID describes a spectrum of infection and inflammation involving, in varying degrees depending on the severity of the disease, the upper genital tract (endometrium, tubes, and ovaries) as well as the surrounding peritoneum. In more severe cases, the infection can spread along the upper peritoneum to the liver capsule, causing perihepatic adhesions. When this happens, it is referred to as Fitz-Hugh-Curtis syndrome.

2. What is the cause of PID?

PID comprises, for the most part, sequelae of cervical infection with sexually transmitted organisms, chiefly *Neisseria gonorrhoeae* and *Chlamydia trachomatis*. Cervical infection with these organisms breaks down cervical barriers to ascending infection, allowing endogenous super infection of the upper genital tract by aerobic as well as anaerobic organisms normally inhabiting the lower genital tract. In addition, though less commonly the cause, instrumentation of the cervix and uterus during surgical procedures (such as surgical abortion, dilation and curettage, hysteroscopy, endometrial and cervical biopsy, insertion of intrauterine device, and intrauterine insemination) can cause auto-inoculation of the endometrium with endogenous bacteria and lead to PID.

3. What is the difference in the clinical presentation of PID caused by *N. gonorrhoeae* and *C. trachomatis*?

In general, the onset of PID caused by Neisseria is more acute and severe than that caused by Chlamydia. Many cases of PID caused by Chlamydia are silent and are only diagnosed in retrospect when the patient presents with infertility caused by tubal adhesions.

4. What is the relationship of PID to bacterial vaginosis?

It is believed that similar organisms cause bacterial vaginosis (a vaginal infection) and PID. While studies have shown that the diagnosis of bacterial vaginosis is more common in women with PID, a cause-and-effect relationship has not been proven.

5. How does PID present in the clinical setting?

History: Classic PID presents with a history of acute onset of pelvic pain and fever, frequently beginning during or after a menstrual period in a sexually active woman. However, especially when Chlamydia is the initiating organism, the onset of pelvic pain can be more gradual and less severe. Nausea and vomiting as well as loss of appetite, especially in more severe cases, may accompany these symptoms.

Physical Exam: Fever and mild to severe tachycardia are frequently found on investigation of vital signs. Abdominal exam shows varying degrees of bilateral lower abdominal tenderness and possible rebound and/or guarding in more severe cases. Right upper quadrant tenderness will be found with accompanying Fitz-Hugh Curtis syndrome. On pelvic exam, the classic sign of PID is the **"chandelier sign"**—cervical motion tenderness—which describes severe tenderness and accompanying reaction by the patient on movement of the cervix. Palpation of the uterus and adnexa also elicits tenderness, and frequently an adequate exam is limited by guarding. When a tubo-ovarian abscess is present this can be palpated, either as a unilateral adnexal mass or as a mass in the cul-de-sac. Tubo-ovarian abscesses occasionally will point into the cul-de-sac as well.

On **speculum exam**, mucopurulent discharge is seen originating from the cervix. In advanced cases, this sign may have resolved since as endogenous super infection advances, inciting organisms (e.g., Neisseria and Chlamydia) are frequently eliminated.

Laboratory: Cervical cultures or DNA-based testing is frequently positive, especially early in the disease process. White blood cell (WBC) count is elevated, and erythrocyte sedimentation rate and C-reactive protein (though not usually obtained in the clinical setting) are usually elevated as well. There are no specific ultrasound findings in PID, but complex adnexal masses will be seen on ultrasound when tubo-ovarian abscesses or inflammatory complexes are present. In the presence of Fitz-Hugh Curtis syndrome, liver function tests may be elevated.

6. Why does PID typically present either during or after the menstrual cycle?

PID is rare in women who are postmenopausal or premenopausal but amenorrheic. Menstrual blood is a good culture medium for the organisms causing PID. Also, during the menstrual period, the cervical barrier to ascending infection is broken down.

7. What else is in the differential diagnosis with PID?

Included in the differential diagnosis are: appendicitis, diverticulitis, urinary tract infection, nephrolithiasis, inflammatory bowel disease, ectopic pregnancy, septic abortion, endometriosis, degenerating fibroids, ovarian torsion, and ruptured ovarian cyst.

8. What additional tests or history help include or exclude PID from the differential diagnosis?

- Urine or serum human chorionic gonadotropin (hCG) to rule out early pregnancy complications such as septic abortion or ectopic pregnancy. (Although uncommon, PID can occur early in pregnancy and this should be kept in mind even if the patient has a positive pregnancy test.)
- Cervical Gram stain and/or wet preparation of cervical discharge. Gram-negative diplococci on Gram stain are suggestive (but not diagnostic) of GC infection; numerous WBCs on Gram stain or wet mount are suggestive (but not diagnostic) of GC or Chlamydia infection.
- A history of anorexia preceding onset of periumbilical pain which eventually localizes to the right lower quadrant is more indicative of appendicitis than PID.
- Lower abdominal pain in a woman who is not sexually active or who is only sexually active with women is unlikely to be PID.
- Ultrasound can be a helpful adjunct in diagnosis of early pregnancy or tubo-ovarian abscesses.
- Laparoscopy is considered to be the "gold standard" for the diagnosis of PID. It allows direct culture of the cul-de-sac and endosalpinx. However, it may not detect infection limited to the endometrium (endometritis) or mild salpingitis. Because laparoscopy is an operative procedure, it is used infrequently to make the diagnosis of PID. When employed in a study population, the clinical diagnosis of PID had a positive predictive value of 65–90% when compared with laparoscopy.

9. What are the clinical criteria for the diagnosis of PID?

Minimum criteria:
- Sexually active or history of recent instrumentation of cervix or uterus
- Lower abdominal pain
- Adnexal tenderness
- Cervical motion tenderness

Additional criteria that support the diagnosis of PID:
- Oral temperature > 101°F (> 38.3°C)
- Abnormal cervical or vaginal discharge
- Elevated C-reactive protein and/or erythrocyte sedimentation rate
- Elevation of WBC count
- Laboratory documentation of positive cervical testing for GC or Chlamydia
- Ultrasound with documentation of hydrosalpinx/pyosalpinx and/or tubo-ovarian complex
- Laparoscopic documentation of tubal inflammation and/or pyosalpinx

10. Who is at risk for PID?

PID is more common in younger women and teens; most cases occur in the late teens and early 20s. It is more common among women in lower socioeconomic groups and in the African/Afro-Caribbean population, as well as in women with a history of a prior episode of PID. Recent sexual encounter with a new partner as well as a history of multiple sexual partners are also risk factors. Studies also indicate that a history of douching increases the risk of PID.

11. List the potential long-term consequences of PID.

- Infertility secondary to tubal and ovarian adhesions (20% incidence of infertility with one episode of PID; risk of infertility is further increased with each additional episode of PID)
- Chronic pelvic pain (20% incidence in women with a history of PID)
- Tubo-ovarian abscess
- Increased risk of ectopic pregnancy (occurs in 10% of pregnancies conceived after PID is diagnosed; this rate is 6 to10 times greater than the risk of ectopic pregnancy in women without a history of PID)
- Potential passing of sexually transmitted diseases to other sexual partners
- Death, though rare, can occur in neglected cases, especially after rupture of a tubo-ovarian abscess.

12. How common is PID? What is its economic impact?

PID is the most common reason for gynecologic hospital admission in the U.S. It is estimated that 1 million cases of PID are diagnosed in the U.S. each year, generating 2.5 million outpatient visits and 250,000–300,000 inpatient admissions/year for an estimated direct and indirect cost of more than $4 billion.

13. What can be done to prevent PID?

- Aggressive screening of at-risk populations for sexually transmitted diseases (STDs), particularly gonorrhea and chlamydia
- Treatment of patients with positive results and their partners
- Promotion of **consistent condom use**, especially in patients with multiple sexual partners
- Maintenance of a high index of suspicion for STDs and early PID in sexually active women
- Promotion of monogamy or abstinence, especially in the teenage population

14. What can be done to prevent PID recurrences?

While it is debatable whether or not oral contraceptive (OC) use is associated with a lower risk for the primary development of PID, OC use has been associated with a lower risk of recurrence once the diagnosis of PID has been made. Promotion of consistent condom use as well as abstinence or sexual monogamy also can be helpful.

15. What other tests should be recommended when the diagnosis of PID is made?

When one STD is diagnosed, recommend testing for other STDs. This includes testing for the human immunodeficiency virus (HIV), syphilis, and hepatitis B and C. Hepatitis B vaccination should be considered for patients who test negative for hepatitis B. Hepatitis B is currently the only STD for which a vaccine is available. Wet mount of vaginal discharge should be done to exclude the diagnosis of vaginal trichomoniasis or bacterial vaginosis.

16. List the criteria for hospitalization of a patient with PID.

While there is very little study of optimal treatment (oral vs. parenteral) or optimum duration of treatment, the following are generally agreed-upon criteria for admission once the diagnosis of PID is determined:

- Inability to tolerate oral medication
- Uncertain diagnosis, especially if surgical emergencies such as appendicitis are factors
- Temperature elevation > 38.5°C

- Evidence of tubo-ovarian abscess
- Adolescent
- Pregnancy
- Lack of response to oral therapy after 48 hrs
- Nulliparity
- Coexisting diagnosis of HIV/AIDS
- Expected difficulties with compliance and follow-up
- Signs of peritoneal irritation (rebound) on physical exam
- Intrauterine device in place

17. Are intrauterine devices (IUDs) associated with PID?

In the past, some IUD designs (in particular the Dalkon Shield) clearly promoted ascension of bacteria into the upper genital tract and subsequent PID. While some controversy remains with today's copper-containing IUDs, most studies suggest that the IUD itself does not cause pelvic infection. Some studies show an increase in PID after insertion. In addition, studies of tubal infertility in prior IUD users show an association between Chlamydia infection and future diagnosis of tubal infertility, but not an independent association between IUD use and subsequent infertility, supporting the theory that STD exposure and not the IUD causes PID and subsequent tubal damage.

A 60-month study comparing the newer levonorgestrel-containing IUD to a copper-containing IUD showed a removal rate for PID of 2.2 per 100 women in the copper-containing IUD group versus 0.8 in the levonorgestrel-containing IUD group.

18. When the diagnosis of PID is made and an IUD is in place, how should the patient be managed?

Once antibiotics have been administered, standard of care dictates that the IUD should be removed since its presence as a foreign body in the uterus may make treatment of PID more difficult. However, results of a small randomized study show that response to antibiotic treatment was similar whether or not the IUD was removed or left in situ.

19. What principles are involved in the choice of antibiotics for the treatment of PID?

Regimens are designed to cover Neisseria and Chlamydia as well as anaerobes (such as *Bacteroides fragilis*), gram-negative aerobes, and streptococci (endogenous vaginal and lower gastrointestinal flora).

20. What are the oral treatment options for PID?

In 1998 the Centers for Disease Control and Prevention published recommendations for the treatment of PID. Although there is no data comparing different regimens, each regimen listed below has been shown to be effective in treatment.
- Ofloxacin 400 mg plus metronidazole 500 mg orally twice a day for 14 days
- Cefoxitin 2 g with probenecid 1 g × 1 dose orally concurrently or ceftriaxone 250 mg IM × 1 or (or other third-generation cephalosporin such as ceftizoxime or cefotaxime)
  plus
  doxycycline 100 mg orally BID for 14 days

21. What are the parenteral treatment options for PID?
- Cefotetan 2 g IV q 12 hours or cefoxitin 2g IV q 6 hours
  plus
  doxycycline 100 mg IV or orally every 12 hours
- Clindamycin 900 mg IV q 8 hours *plus* gentamicin IV or IM loading dose of 2 mg/kg body weight followed by a maintenance does of 1.5 mg/kg q 8 hours (assuming normal renal function)
- Ofloxacin 400 mg IV q 12 hours *plus* metronidazole 500 mg IV q 8 hrs
- Ampicillin/sulbactam 3 g IV q 6 hours *plus* doxycycline 100 mg IV or orally q 12 hours
- Ciprofloxacin 200 mg IV q 12 hours *plus* doxycycline 100 mg IV; or orally q 12 hours *plus* metronidazole 200mg IV q 8 hours

All of these regimens should be continued until patient improvement is noted, and then doxycycline 100 mg orally twice a day should be continued for a total of 14 days of antibiotic treatment.

22. What are the testing methods for Neisseria and Chlamydia?

Since Chlamydia grows intracellularly, culture of the organism is technically more difficult than Neisseria. Development of nucleic acid amplification testing for Chlamydia since the 1990s has led to higher sensitivity (85% and higher) (though similar specificity, 97–99.5%) when compared to older culture and antigen testing (sensitivity 65–85%, specificity > 97%).

In addition to culture on Thayer Martin media, similar nucleic acid amplification testing is now widely available for the diagnosis of Neisseria. Advantages of nucleic acid amplification testing include performance on urine specimens as well as testing of endocervical (women) and urethral (men) sources.

23. Summarize the principles for diagnosis and treatment and prevention of PID.
- Consider the diagnosis in all sexually active women of reproductive age who present with lower abdominal pain.
- Rule out pregnancy.
- Err on the side of over-diagnosis to help prevent the sequelae of PID.
- Initiate treatment with recommended regimens as soon as possible once the diagnosis is established.
- Reassess the patient in 48–72 hours if oral treatment is chosen to assure response.
- Refer or directly treat all sexual partners.
- Screen for asymptomatic gonorrhea and chlamydia in sexually active men and women.
- Encourage barrier methods and spermicide use to help prevent infection.
- When PID is diagnosed, recommend testing for other STDs such as syphilis, HIV, and hepatitis B

BIBLIOGRAPHY

1. Andersson K, Odlind V, Rybo G. Levonorgestrel-releasing and copper-releasing (Nova T) IUDs during 5 years of use: A randomized comparative trial. Contraception. 1994;49:56–72.
2. Baeten J, Nyange P, Richardson B, et al. Hormonal contraception and risk of sexually transmitted disease acquisition: Results from a prospective study. Am J Obstet Gynecol 2001;185:380–385.
3. Berg AO. Screening for Chlamydia infection. Recommendations and rationale. Am J Prev Med. 2001;20(3suppl):90–94.
4. Black CM. Current methods of laboratory diagnosis of *Chlamydia trachomatis* infections. Clin Microbiol Rev 1997;10:160–184.
5. Centers for Disease Control and Prevention. 1998 Guidelines for treatment of sexually transmitted diseases. MMWR 1998;47(RR):1–11.
6. Grimes D. Intrauterine devices and infertility: Sifting through the evidence. Lancet 2001; 358:6–7.
7. Hemsel D, Ledger W, Martens M, Monif G, et al. Concerns regarding the Centers for Disease Control's published guidelines for pelvic inflammatory disease. Clin Infect Dis 2001;32:103–107.
8. Hubacher D, Lara-Ricalde R, Taylor D, et al. Use of copper intrauterine devices and the risk of tubal infertility among nulligravid women. N Engl J Med 2001;345(8):561–567.
9. Morris M, Nicoll A, Simms I, et al. Bacterial vaginosis: A public health review. Br J Obstet Gynaecol 2001;108:439–450.
10. Ness R, Soper D, Holley R, Peipert J, Randall H, et al. Hormonal and barrier contraception and risk of upper genital tract disease in the PID evaluation and clinical health (PEACH) study. Am J Obstet Gynecol 2001;185:121–127.
11. Risser WL, Risser JM, Cromwell PT. Pelvic inflammatory disease in adolescents: A review. Tex Med 2002;98(2):36–40.
12. Ross J. Pelvic inflammatory disease. Clinical Evidence, 2000. (BMJ Publishing group)
13. Shafer MA, Sweet RL. Pelvic inflammatory disease in adolescent females. Adolescent Med State Art Rev 1990; 1:545–546.
14. Sodeberg G, Lindgren S. Influence of an intrauterine device on the course of acute salpingitis. Contraception 1981;24:137–143.
15. Sweet RL. Sexually transmitted diseases: Pelvic inflammatory disease and infertility in women. Infect Dis Clin North Am 1987;1:199–215.

4. THE MENSTRUAL CYCLE

Kevin Bachus, M.D.

GENERAL QUESTIONS

1. What is the mean age of menarche and menopause?
The mean age of menarche is 12.7 years; the mean age of menopause is 51.4 years.

2. What is the mean duration and interval for menses?
Mean duration 5.2 days (3–8 day range); normal interval 28 days (range 21–35 days). Only 15% of women have a "typical" 28-day cycle.

3. In a woman's lifetime, when is the greatest variability in the menstrual cycle?
In the first 2 years after menarche and 3 years before menopause. Anovulatory cycles occur in up to 6 and 34% of these cycles, respectively.

4. What are the differences between the basal and functional layers of the endometrium with regard to hormonal responsiveness and presence throughout the menstrual cycle?
The basal layer is relatively unresponsive to hormonal stimulation and remains intact throughout the menstrual cycle. The functional layer is very responsive to hormonal stimulation, and most of this layer (subdivided into the compacta and spongiosa) is lost during menstruation.

5. How are prostaglandins involved in the process of menstruation?
Prostaglandins are maximal just prior to menses and appear to be important in initiating menstrual blood flow by causing constriction of the spiral arterioles and stimulating myometrial contractions.

6. How many germ cells are in the prenatal, neonatal, and pubertal ovary?
At 20 weeks' gestation, 6–7 million germ cells are present, which declines to 2 million by birth and 300,000 by puberty.

FOLLICULAR PHASE

7. What is a primordial follicle?
An oocyte arrested in the diplotene stage of the first meiotic prophase surrounded by a single layer of granulosa cells. Its growth is independent of gonadotropin stimulation.

8. What is the preantral follicle?
An oocyte surrounded by the zona pellucida with several layers of granulosa cells and a theca layer. Growth of the follicle in this stage becomes dependent on gonadotropins.

9. Which hormones are necessary for accumulation of granulosa cells and progressive follicular growth?
Follicle-stimulating hormone (FSH) is responsible for induction of luteinizing hormone (LH) receptors and aromatase enzyme, which are responsible for conversion of androgens to estrogens within the developing follicle. Estrogen acts synergistically with FSH to increase the

number of FSH receptors on the cells as well as to increase mitotic activity of the granulosa cell, which leads to proliferation of the granulosa cell layer.

10. Which hormone signals follicular recruitment and when in the menstrual cycle does it begin?

FSH, which is the signal of follicular recruitment, begins its increase in the late luteal phase of the preceding cycle.

11. What function does LH have in the follicular phase?

LH interacts with theca cells, which results in androgen production. These androgens serve as a substrate for aromatization to estrogen within the developing dominant follicle. These androgens, however, produce follicular atresia within nondominant follicles.

12. What is the two-cell, two-gonadotropin concept of ovarian steroidogenesis?

In response to LH, theca cells produce androgens (primarily androstenedione), which diffuse to the adjacent granulosa cells where they become aromatized to estrogen. This aromatization is facilitated in an estrogen microenvironment, which in turn is dependent on FSH stimulation of granulosa cells.

13. Which hormones are detrimental to progressive follicular maturation?

Androgens in high enough concentrations undergo 5α reduction to more potent androgens. Premature increases in LH also decrease mitogenic activity of granulosa cells. In both cases, degenerative changes occur.

ANTRAL FOLLICLE

14. What mechanisms promote the atresia of a nondominant follicle?

Selection of the dominant follicle occurs by days 5–7 of the menstrual cycle. As estrogen concentrations from the dominant follicle increase, FSH is inhibited centrally by negative feedback inhibition. This causes withdrawal of gonadotropin support of less developed follicles. The dominant follicle escapes the atretic consequences of falling FSH levels by having a greater number of FSH receptors via an increased mass of granulosa cells. Additionally, increased vascular development within the theca layer may offer preferential delivery of FSH to the dominant follicle. By altering the gonadotropin secretion by its own production of estrogen, the dominant follicle optimizes its own environment to the detriment of other follicles.

PERIOVULATORY FOLLICLE

15. What is the most reliable predictor of impending ovulation?

Ovulation occurs approximately 34–36 hours after the start of the LH surge or 10–12 hours after the peak of the LH surge.

16. What are the primary hormonal signals necessary for an adequate LH surge that will trigger ovulation?

Estradiol is necessary in threshold concentrations of > 200 pg/ml for approximately 50 hours and must be present until after the actual LH surge begins. This positive feedback response of estrogen upon the pituitary resulting in an LH surge is facilitated by low levels of progesterone.

17. What does an LH surge do?

It initiates resumption of meiosis in the oocyte, causes luteinization of granulosa cells, and synthesizes prostaglandins and progesterone essential for follicular rupture. Although antral fluid volume increases at the time of ovulation, the rupture of the follicle is not felt to be secondary to

increased hydrostatic pressure. More likely, degenerative changes in the follicular wall result
with destruction of collagen, which allows passive expansion and ultimate rupture of the follicle.

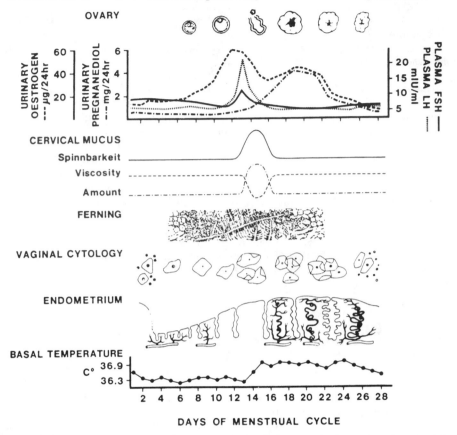

The cyclical biological consequences of the hypothalamic–pituitary–ovarian interactions. The physiologic
and morphological events in the uterus, cervix and vagina are largely determined by the fluctuating levels of
ovarian hormones. (From MacKay EV, et al (eds): Illustrated Textbook of Gynaecology. Artarmon, Australia,
Holt-Saunders, 1983, with permission.)

OVULATION

18. When is the first polar body extruded from the oocyte?

Ovulation is accompanied by the completion of the first meiotic division with extrusion of
the first polar body.

19. What causes the extrusion of the oocyte from the follicle?

The physical act of ovulation likely involves prostaglandins and lysosomal enzymes, which
cause degenerative changes in the follicular wall. Contrary to what is believed by many, this process
does not seem to involve a significant increase in hydrostatic pressure from within the follicle.

LUTEAL PHASE

20. Which hormone is necessary for normal corpus luteum function?

The lifespan and steroidogenic capacity of the corpus luteum are dependent on continued
tonic LH secretion, which results in sustained progesterone output. Normal luteal function

requires optimal preovulatory follicular development (i.e., adequate FSH stimulation) and continued tonic LH support. If human chorionic gonadotropin (hCG) is present in adequate concentrations, the corpus luteum of pregnancy can be maintained.

21. When in the luteal phase does progesterone peak?
Progesterone peaks approximately day 8 after the LH surge, mediates maturity of secretory endometrium, and suppresses new follicular growth. Light microscopic changes are so uniform that each of the luteal phase days can be identified by characteristic findings within the glands and stroma.

22. When is implantation likely to occur?
The most likely day of implantation is day 22–23, which coincides with peak intracellular apocrine secretory activity.

23. What is a luteal phase defect?
Corpus luteal insufficiency produces luteal phase defects. The role of luteal phase defect in causing infertility is unclear because of difficulty in diagnosis.

BIBLIOGRAPHY

1. Carpenter SE: Psychosocial menstrual disorders: Stress exercise and diet's effect on the menstrual cycle. Curr Opin Obstet Gynecol 6:121, 1994.
2. MacKay EV, et al (eds): Illustrated Textbook of Gynaecology. Artarmon, Australia, Holt-Saunders, 1983.
3. Mishell DR: Reproductive endocrinology. In Droegemueller W, et al (eds): Comprehensive Gynecology St. Louis, Mosby, 1992, pp 79–140.
4. Seibel MM: Oocyte maturation and follicular genesis. In Seibel MM (ed): Infertility: A Comprehensive Text. Norwalk, CT, Appleton & Lange, 1990, pp 37–49.
5. Speroff L, Glass LRH, Kase NG: Regulation of the menstrual cycle. In Clinical Gynecologic Endocrinology and Infertility, 5th ed. Baltimore, Williams & Wilkins, 1994, pp 93–107.
6. Yen SSC: The human menstrual cycle. In Yen SSC, Jaffe RB (eds): Reproductive Endocrinology: Physiology, Pathophysiology, and Clinical Management, 3rd ed. Philadelphia, W.B. Saunders, 1991, pp 181–237.

5. PUBERTY

Stephen W. Sawin, M.D.

1. What is the definition of puberty?

Puberty is the developmental process by which fully competent adult reproductive capacity is established. It is characterized by marked neuroendocrine and physiologic changes in the reproductive system, culminating in mature secondary sexual characteristics and, in girls, the ability to ovulate and menstruate. Significant increases in somatic growth as well as dramatic psychosocial changes also characterize puberty. Of note, changes in growth and psychosocial development do not always parallel the reproductive changes, and this can lead to misunderstanding regarding an individual's "maturity."

2. What are the physical signs of puberty, when do they occur, and in what order?

The first sign of puberty is often said to be breast budding (thelarche) around age 10. In fact, an increase in linear growth velocity can be appreciated 1–2 years prior to breast budding, heralding the onset of puberty. Thelarche is followed by pubic hair development (pubarche) at age 11, attainment of peak growth velocity (9 cm/year) at age 12, and menses (menarche) at age 13. The average age of menarche for U.S. girls has trended downward over the last century, presumably due to better nutrition and less stringent working conditions for minors. On average it takes 2.5 years from the onset of breast budding to the first period (see table).

Average Timing of Pubertal Events in U.S. Girls[2]

PUBERTAL EVENT	MEAN AGE ± SD
Breast budding	10.8 ± 1.1 years
Pubic hair	11.0 ± 1.2 years
Maximum growth rate	12.1 ± 0.88 years
Menarche	12.9 ± 1.2 years

3. Describe the hormonal changes that occur with puberty.

The first sign of puberty is an increase in luteinizing hormone (LH) pulsatility at night. This pulsatility is followed by LH and follicle-stimulating hormone (FSH) pulses throughout the day, leading to increasing estrogen levels from the growing ovarian follicle, and finally positive feedback of estradiol to initiate an LH surge capable of inducing ovulation. Elevated progesterone levels in the luteal phase follow ovulation. Ovulation is often inconsistent for 1–2 years after menarche, leading to irregular menstrual periods. After this time, most teenagers should have established normal cycles, and a failure to do so may indicate a reproductive disorder. Estrogen also stimulates growth hormone, which in turn stimulates insulin-like growth factor I leading to increased somatic growth. The adrenal gland starts to produce increased quantities of the androgens DHEA, DHEAS, and androstenedione at 6–8 years of age, but this is not thought to be part of the pubertal process.

4. What effects does estrogen have on bone?

Estrogen increases bone growth, especially in the axial skeleton. Growth hormone has more effect on the long bones. As a result of this, hypogonadal patients often have a short trunk as compared to their arm span and lower extremity length (eunichoid habitus). Growth hormone–deficient subjects often have the opposite appearance. Estrogen also promotes fusion of the epiphyseal plates. Patients with precocious puberty have an early growth advantage, but ultimately have short stature due to premature epiphyseal closure if left untreated.

5. List the factors that determine when puberty starts.

Puberty occurs earlier in patients who have a family history of early puberty; are African American; live closer to the equator, at lower altitudes, or in urban settings; are obese; or are blind. Patients with diabetes, extreme obesity, poor nutrition, or excessive stress and those who over-exercise tend to have more delayed puberty. The critical body fat theory of Frisch proposed that 17–22% body fat is necessary to initiate puberty. While this theory is attractive in explaining early puberty in more obese adolescents and regression to pre-pubertal physiology in patients with anorexia nervosa, it is not inclusive enough to explain the timing of puberty in all patients. Pathologic conditions that affect pubertal onset are discussed in Questions 9–19.

6. Does puberty simply represent the final, complete development of the hypothalamic-pituitary-gonadal (HPG) axis?

No. It appears that the HPG axis is intact as early as 20 weeks of life. Pituitary gonadotrophs have been found to produce LH and FSH at this gestational age, and in boys testicular testosterone is essential for normal internal and external genital development. In female fetuses, functional ovarian cysts are occasionally seen. These findings indicate a functional HPG axis in fetal life. LH and FSH levels peak at 20 weeks of gestation and then are suppressed by maternal estrogen. Immediately postpartum, LH and FSH levels flare for 1–2 years and then are suppressed until puberty either by exquisite sensitivity to very low levels of estrogen or by a central inhibiting factor.

7. What is Tanner staging?

Dr. J.M. Tanner proposed a five-stage system to grade breast and pubic hair development in girls and genital and pubic hair development in boys (see table).

Tanner Stages of Pubertal Development

BREAST DEVELOPMENT	PUBIC HAIR DEVELOPMENT
Elevation of papilla only	No pubic hair
Breast budding	Scattered labial hair
Enlargement of breasts without areola separation	Hair spreading to mons pubis
Secondary mound formed by areola	Slight lateral spread
Mature breast with single contour of breast and areola	Hair on medial thighs

8. What are the age limits for the normal onset of puberty?

The onset of puberty is said to be normal if it occurs within 2.5 standard deviations from the mean. The range that is generally accepted is between ages 8 and 14 years. Girls with no secondary sexual characteristics by age 14 years should have a work-up, as should girls with normal secondary sexual characteristics but no period by age 16 years. African-American girls may start puberty before age 8 years; this is normal in this group. Isolated breast or pubic hair development without other signs of puberty may occur and does not require extensive evaluation, but does warrant observation to exclude the possibility of precocious puberty. Premature thelarche usually occurs in the first several years of life, and premature adrenarche has been considered a possible early sign of polycystic ovary syndrome later in life.

9. Is precocious puberty more common in boys or girls? What about delayed puberty?

Precocious puberty is more common in girls (five times more frequent than in boys), and delayed puberty is more common in boys. Girls also progress through puberty faster than boys. On average, girls complete puberty within 3 years, as opposed to 5 years for boys.

10. What is meant by isosexual and heterosexual precocious puberty?

Isosexual precocious puberty is premature pubertal development compatible with the individual's genetic sex. **Heterosexual** precocious puberty refers to pubertal changes occurring opposite to the patient's genetic sex, and in girls this denotes excessive androgen production from the adrenal glands or ovaries. Isosexual problems are far more common than heterosexual ones.

11. What is the difference between gonadotropin releasing hormone (GnRH)-dependent versus GnRH-independent precocious puberty?

Older terms for GnRH-**dependent** precocious puberty are "true," "complete," or "central." These terms refer to premature activation of the HPG axis. The term "GnRH-dependent" is meant to convey that these cases are the result of early activation of the hypothalamic GnRH pulse generator. GnRH-**independent** precocious puberty has also been called precocious pseudo-puberty or "incomplete or peripheral" precocious puberty. In these cases, sex steroid production occurs independent of the HPG axis. In some cases peripheral hormone production can activate the HPG axis, leading to a mixed picture.

12. In what percent of cases of precocious puberty is no specific cause identified?

In girls 75% of precocious puberty is idiopathic, as opposed to only 40% for boys. Newer, more sensitive intracranial imaging techniques such as magnetic resonance imaging may detect subtle abnormalities in cases otherwise thought to be idiopathic.

13. What are the causes of GnRH-*dependent* precocious puberty? How are they treated?

GnRH-dependent precocious puberty is usually **idiopathic** and is treated with GnRH agonists (e.g., luprelide acetate) to suppress premature activation of GnRH pulsatility. Tumors of the central nervous system (CNS) are the most serious cause of GnRH-dependent precocious puberty, with **hamartomas** being the most common. These tumors are treated with surgery, radiation, and GnRH agonists.

14. What are the causes of GnRH-*independent* precocious puberty? How are they treated?

The most common cause of GnRH-independent precocious puberty is a **functional ovarian cyst**. Granulosa cell tumors can secrete estrogen and should be removed surgically. McCune-Albright syndrome (polyostotic fibrous dysplasia) is characterized by multiple cystic bone lesions, café-au-lait spots, and precocious puberty. Autonomous estrogen production from the ovary, due to a genetic mutation in the gonadotropin receptor that renders it constitutively activated, results in precocious puberty. This syndrome is treated with testolactone, an aromatase inhibitor. Hypothyroidism can cause precocious puberty and is treated with thyroid replacement. Exogenous hormonal drug ingestion should be revealed in the history and stopped. Adrenal steroid–producing tumors are rarely encountered and are treated surgically.

15. What is the only form of precocious puberty in which the bone age is delayed instead of advanced?

Primary hypothyroidism.

16. Describe the essential parts of the history and physical exam in a patient with precocious puberty.

The patient or her parents should be asked about growth and pubertal milestones, family history of reproductive abnormalities, the possibility of exogenous hormonal drug ingestion, symptoms of thyroid disease, and neurological symptoms or a history of CNS insults. On physical exam, height, weight and the percentile for age should be assessed. Conduct Tanner staging, a neurological and thyroid exam, a skin exam looking for café-au-lait spots, and an abdominal exam and pelvic and/or rectal exam looking for masses.

17. What laboratory and radiographic studies are ordered?

Pertinent laboratory studies include serum estradiol, LH, FSH, thyroid-stimulating hormone, and hCG. For heterosexual cases, DHEAS, 17 hydroxyprogesterone, and testosterone should be measured. The most important radiographic test is a left wrist bone age to assess skeletal maturation.

Other tests may include a pelvic ultrasound or CT looking for ovarian or adrenal masses, or an MRI of the CNS looking for tumors. A skull radiograph will detect multiple cystic lesions characteristic of McCune-Albright syndrome.

18. Describe the work-up of a patient with primary amenorrhea and delayed puberty.

Patients with delayed puberty are classified by the presence or absence of breast development (a sign of estrogen production) and by the presence or absence of a uterus (absent when anti-müllerian hormone from testicular tissue is produced). If breast development is absent, an FSH level distinguishes ovarian failure from hypothalamic-pituitary failure. If uterine development is absent, a testosterone level and karyotype will distinguish uterovaginal agenesis from androgen insensitivity syndrome. The absence of both breasts and a uterus is extremely rare. In the presence of both breast and uterine development, the work-up is identical to secondary amenorrhea (see figure).

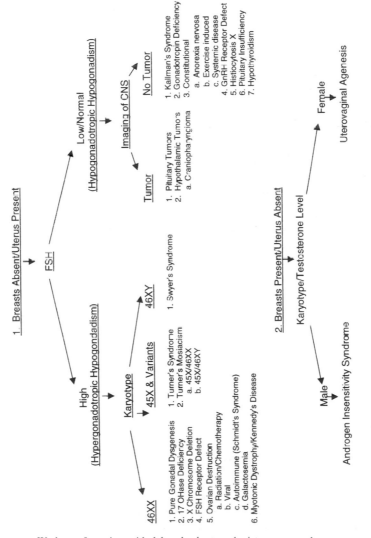

Work-up of a patient with delayed puberty and primary amenorrhea.

19. What are the most common causes of primary amenorrhea/delayed puberty?

The most common cause of primary amenorrhea and delayed puberty is gonadal dysgenesis (usually Turner's syndrome). This is followed by uterovaginal agenesis and androgen insensitivity syndrome. Anorexia nervosa and extreme exercise are also common causes of delayed puberty.

CONTROVERSIES

20. Is adrenarche the same as pubarche?

This is debatable. Technically "adrenarche" (*adren* = adrenal; arch from Greek *arkhein* = to begin, rule, command) refers to increased adrenal androgen production, and "pubarche" (from Greek *puber* = adult; *pubes* = pubic hair) is the appearance of pubic hair. These terms are commonly used synonymously. Adrenarche is not essential for normal ovarian function (gonadarche), as evidenced by the fact that patients with hypoadrenalism can undergo normal puberty, and gonadal function can precede adrenarche in precocious puberty. Gonadal function is not necessary for proper adrenal function, as patients with gonadal dysgenesis have normal adrenarche.

BIBLIOGRAPHY

1. Clark PA, Rogol AD: Growth hormones and sex steroid interactions at puberty. Endocrinol Metab Clin North Am 25:665–681, 1996.
2. Frisch R, Revelle R: Height and weight at menarche and a hypothesis of menarche. Arch Dis Child 46:695–701, 1971.
3. Harlan WR, Harlan EA, Gillo GP: Secondary sex characteristics of girls 12 to 17 years of age: The U.S. Health Examination Survey. J Pediatr 96:1074, 1980.
4. Marshall WA, Tanner JM: Variations in pattern of pubertal changes in girls. Arch Dis Child 44:291, 1969.
5. Mishell DR, Stenchever MA, Droegenmueller W, Herbst AL (eds): Comprehensive Gynecology, 3rd ed. St. Louis, Mosby, 1997.
6. Morris W (ed): American Heritage Dictionary of the English Language. Boston, Houghton Mifflin, 1978.
7. Reindollar RH, Byrd JR, McDonough PG: Delayed sexual development: A study of 252 patients. Am J Obstet Gynecol 140:371, 1981.
8. Rosenfield RL: Puberty and its disorders in girls. Endocrinol Metab Clin North Am 20:15–42, 1991.
9. Speroff L, Glass RH, Kase NG (eds): Clinical Gynecologic Endocrinology and Infertility, 6th ed. Baltimore, MD, Lippincott Williams & Wilkins, 1999.

6. AMENORRHEA

Nadine Burrington, M.D.

1. What is amenorrhea?

Amenorrhea is the complete absence of menstruation in a woman of reproductive age.

2. Differentiate primary and secondary amenorrhea. What is the incidence of each?

Primary amenorrhea:
- No period by age 14 in the absence of growth and secondary developmental characteristics (breasts and pubic hair), *or*
- No period by age 16 regardless of the extent of secondary development
- The incidence of primary amenorrhea is < 1%.

Secondary amenorrhea:
- The absence of menses for longer than 6 months, *or*
- The absence of menses for a total of three previous cycle intervals
- The incidence of secondary amenorrhea is approximately 0.7%.

3. What is the first step in determining the cause of amenorrhea?

A thorough history and physical examination can usually lead you to the correct diagnosis or determine the additional testing to be performed. Consider these questions:
- Is there a history of coital exposure? (**Pregnancy is the most common cause of amenorrhea.**)
- In primary amenorrhea, what was the nature and sequence of other pubertal events?
- Is there any history of severe systemic illnesses or stress (emotional, physical, or nutritional) that could affect normal hypothalamic function?
- Any changes in sleep, thirst, appetite, or smell, and presence of headaches, vomiting, visual field defects, fatigue, or galactorrhea? These could suggest hypothalamic or pituitary problems.
- Is the patient taking medications or has she received chemotherapy or radiation?
- Is the patient of normal height and weight? Does she have normal pulse and blood pressure?
- Is there evidence of low estrogen or hirsuitism?
- Is a normal reproductive tract evident on physical examination?

4. List the initial blood tests that should be performed on a patient with amenorrhea.

Thyroid function tests to confirm suspected or rule out asymptomatic hypothyroidism. Patients with hypothyriodism return to normal menses with thyroid replacement.

Prolactin level to rule out hyperprolactinemia, which is the cause of amenorrhea in 10–20% of patients. Hyperprolactinemia may occur even without galactorrhea. Patients with galactorrhea should have an MRI or thin-section coronal CT scan with IV contrast. A coned-down view of the sella turcica is an older, less sensitive test.

5. What is a progesterone challenge test?

A progesterone challenge test is 200 mg of parenteral progesterone in oil, 300 mg of oral micronized progesterone, or 10 mg of oral medroxyprogesterone acetate for 5 days. A **positive test** is any bleeding (even spotting) within 2–7 days of the test. This result means the serum estrogen level is > 40 pg/ml; thus the anterior pituitary is producing luteinizing hormone (LH) and follicle-stimulating hormone (FSH), and the endometrium and outflow tract are functioning. In such a scenario, if the thyroid function tests and prolactin level are normal, the patient is anovulatory.

A **negative test** suggests an outflow tract defect such as complete destruction of the endometrial lining by Asherman's syndrome, fibrosis after severe endometritis, cervical stenosis, uterine agenesis, imperforate hymen, or transverse vaginal septum; or a hypoestrogen state.

6. What tests should be performed on a patient with amenorrhea, normal thyroid function and prolactin levels, and no bleeding on a progesterone challenge test?

FSH and LH levels. This test determines if the low estrogen levels are due to failure of the CNS-pituitary axis or of the ovarian follicles.

• Low levels of FSH suggest hypothalamic causes of amenorrhea.

• High levels of FSH suggest ovarian failure.

7. What are the most common causes of primary amenorrhea?

Gonadal failure, such as Turner's syndrome. Gonadal agenesis accounts for one-third of all patients with primary amenorrhea.

Müllerian anomalies, such as uterovaginal agenesis (Mayer-Rokitanski-Kuster-Hauser syndrome), account for 20% of primary amenorrhea. They occur in 1 per 4000 female births. (See table.)

Causes of Primary Amenorrhea

Breast Development Absent and Uterus Present
Constitutional delay of puberty
Hypothalamic dysfunction
Extreme physical, psychological, and/or nutritional stress
Chronic illness
Pituitary failure
Gonadal dysgenesis
Gonadal failure
Gonadotropin deficiency
Kallmann's syndrome

Breast Development Present and Uterus Present
Hyperandrogenic amenorrhea (PCOS)
Hypothalamic dysfunction
Hypothyroidism
Hyperprolactinemia
Obstruction (imperforate hymen/transverse vaginal septum)

Breast Development Present and Uterus Absent
Androgen insensitivity
Agenesis (Mayer-Rokitanski-Kuster-Hauser syndrome)

8. In what two syndromes do you find breast development but no uterus present?

Patients with **androgen insensitivity** or **testicular feminization** are XY genotype, but phenotypically are females because an androgen intracellular receptor is not functioning (maternal X-linked recessive gene). Androgen induction of the wolffian duct system does not occur despite normal male levels of testosterone. Because müllerian-inhibiting factor is still present, the müllerian system does not develop. Patients typically have large breasts with immature nipples, but no axillary or pubic hair. Incomplete testicular feminization with some pubic and axillary hair and phallic development also occurs. These patients should be allowed to finish normal sexual maturity, and then the gonads should be removed, because 20% of patients develop gonadoblastoma or dysgerminoma.

Patients with **müllerian agenesis** have sexual hair and mature nipples. Because 40% have associated renal anomalies, intravenous pyelography or renal ultrasound should be performed. Serum testosterone levels are in the normal female range in patients with müllerian agenesis and in the normal male range in testicular feminization. Only patients with testosterone levels in the normal male range need karyotyping.

9. A 15-year-old girl complains of amenorrhea. She is in the 25th percentile for height and weight. She is not an athlete and eats an appropriate diet. On physical examination,

there is no evidence of breast growth or pubic hair, but a vagina and uterus are present. **What work-up will help to determine the cause of amenorrhea?**

The patient has no evidence of estrogenation. **Serum gonadotropin levels** can help determine the cause of amenorrhea.

An *elevated* serum gonadotropin level indicates gonadal failure. A karyotype usually shows an X-chromosome abnormality, causing gonadal dysgenesis. One-third of all patients with gonadal failure have cardiovascular or renal abnormalities, so these patients should have a chest radiograph, electrocardiogram, intravenous pyelogram, and thyroid function tests to rule out the common problems associated with gonadal dysgenesis. If the patient has a Y-chromosome, the gonads must be removed.

Low gonadotropin levels indicate unstimulated gonads. This can be seen in constitutional delay, severe stress (although not apparent in this patient), or hypothalamic or pituitary dysfunction. Patients must be evaluated for intracranial tumors by checking thyroid function and growth hormone, prolactin, and cortisol levels. Pituitary stimulation tests may also be appropriate. MRI or thin-section coronal CT scan with IV contrast are also recommended.

Normal levels of **FSH and LH** in a patient with a negative progesterone challenge test are consistent with pituitary-CNS failure. This is probably due to glycoprotein hormones that are immunologically active , but biologically inactive. Further evaluation in these patients is similar to recommendations for low gonadotropins.

10. What are the pituitary causes of amenorrhea?
- Damaged cells—lack of FSH and LH secretion due to anorexia, thrombosis, or hemorrhage (as seen in Sheehan's syndrome, which is related to hypotension in pregnancy, and in Simmonds' syndrome, which is unrelated to pregnancy).
- Neoplasms—most secrete prolactin, but are not always associated with galactorrhea.
- Amenorrhea is also associated with acromegaly and Cushing's syndrome.

11. What are the hypothalamic causes of amenorrhea?
- Congenital GnRH deficiency (as seen in Kallmann's syndrome, which is associated with anosmia and midline craniofacial defects) and isolated gonadotropin deficiency
- CNS neoplasms or infiltrating diseases such as tuberculosis and sarcoid
- Stress
- Anorexia or bulimia

12. Name the disease that causes a high level of FSH in secondary amenorrhea.
Premature ovarian failure. In amenorrhea due to ovarian failure *before age 40*, patients have symptoms of hypoestrogenism, increased FSH, and generalized sclerosis or only primordial follicles with no progression past the antrum stage on ovarian biopsy. Many of these patients have an autoimmune disease, such as Hashimoto's, Addison's, diabetes or hypoparathyriodism.

If the patient is *younger than 30*, a karyotype should be performed to detect 46XX/XY mosaicism. If this is present, the gonads must be removed to prevent malignancy. Chromosomes should also be checked in patients < 63 inches (or < 60 inches tall in young women) to rule out mosaic Turner's syndrome. Also, check antithyroid antibodies, antinuclear antibodies, and 24-hour cortisol levels to rule out other autoimmune illnesses.

Ovarian failure can result from irradiation or chemotherapy. Other rare causes include: rare tumors (usually lung cancer), single gonadotropin deficiency (likely due to mutations of gonadotropin genes), resistant or insensitive ovary syndrome (likely absent or defective gonadotropin receptors), and galactosemia (rare autosomal recessive disorder of galactose metabolism resulting in toxic effects on the germ cell migration).

13. In which scenarios should I order chromosome analysis?
- Gonadal failure. Patients with a uterus but no breasts and a high FSH level.
- Androgen insensitivity. Patients with no uterus and normal male testosterone levels.

• Premature ovarian failure if less than 30 years old
• Patients with short stature (< 60 inches), especially with any Turner stigmata to check for mosaic Turners.

14. Which drugs cause amenorrhea?
• Drugs that stimulate prolactin excretion
• Antipsychotics, such as phenothiazine derivatives, haloperidol, and droperidol
• Tricyclic antidepressants
• Antihypertensives, such as reserpine and methyldopa
• Anti-anxiety agents, such as benzodiazepines
• Other drugs, such as metoclopramide, opiates, barbituates, and estrogens

15. What psychiatric disorder is a major cause of amenorrhea in adolescents?
Anorexia nervosa is a major cause of amenorrhea. The incidence of anorexia is 1 per 1000 white female adolescents. Besides amenorrhea, these patients have severe weight loss, often with bradycardia, hypotension, constipation, dry skin, hypothermia, and low levels of tri-iodothyronine (T3) due to impaired peripheral conversion of thyroxine to T3. The bone response to estrogen replacement is impaired as long as abnormal weight is maintained; therefore, initial treatment is counseling to help maintain an adequate weight rather than hormone therapy. Mortality rate is 5–15%.

16. What causes athletic amenorrhea? Should it be treated?
The cause of amenorrhea in athletes may be due to high stress levels, energy deficit, as well as eating disorders. Stress and exercise cause an increase in catechol estrogens and beta endorphins; this influences the release of GnRH by acting on the neurotransmitters. Without appropriate GnRH release, FSH and LH are not released appropriately. Many patients are hypoestrogenic, with significant loss of bone density that may lead to osteoporosis and stress fractures.

Yes, athletic amenorrhea should be treated. Encourage patients to improve their diet, to decrease stress levels, to decrease the amount of strenuous exercise, if possible, and to replace estrogen and progesterone, if other changes do not increase estrogen levels.

17. What rare enzyme defect can cause amenorrhea?
Deficiency of 17-alpha-hydroxylase affects both ovarian and adrenal gland hormone production. Since it prevents the formation of sex hormones, this leads to the absence of breast development, although the uterus is present. These patientsalso have hypernatremia, hypokalemia, and hypertension because of increased mineralocorticoid production. Sodium retention and potassium excretion are excessive, while cortisol production is decreased. Therefore, patients require cortisol as well as sex hormones to attain breast development and to prevent osteoporosis.

18. What is a major cause of anovulatory amenorrhea?
Polycystic ovarian syndrome (PCOS) also called Stein-Leventhal syndrome. PCOS is now thought to be a complex interaction of systemic hormones with a common pathway, involving abnormalities in ovarian and androgen metabolism and leading to widespread systemic influences on ovulation, glycemic control, and cholesterol metabolism. Five percent of reproductive-age women are affected by PCOS.

19. What are the criteria for diagnosing polycystic ovarian syndrome?
There is no consensus, but criteria are likely to include:
   • Hyperandrogenism with or without skin manifestations
   • Chronic anovulation
   • Polycystic ovaries on ultrasound
   • Absence of other androgen disorders and hyperprolactinemia

20. Which syndromes may be confused with PCOS?
Hyperprolacinemia
Late-onset adrenal hyperplasia
Ovarian and adrenal neoplasia
Cushing's syndrome
These conditions can be excluded by physical examination and the following tests:
Serum prolactin
17-OH progesterone level
Serum testosterone (elevated in both adrenal hyperplasia and neoplasms)
Dehydroepiandrosterone sulfate (DHEA-S)
1-mg overnight dexamethasone suppression test

21. What are the most common presenting symptoms of PCOS?

Symptoms	Frequency (%)
Infertility	74
Hirsuitism	69
Amenorrhea	51
Obesity	41
Dysfunctional uterine bleeding	29

22. Which laboratory values may be abnormal in patients with PCOS?
Elevated levels may be found for:

Testosterone and androstenedione—caused by LH-stimulated stromal and thecal production and decreased FSH-induced granulosa cell aromatization of androgens to estrogens

Estrone—fat cells metabolize androstenedione to estrone (which leads to feedback augmentation of LH and suppression of FSH)

Dehydroepiandrosterone (DHEA)

Dehydroepiandrosterone sulfate (DHEA-S)—seen in 50% of PCOS patients (95% comes from the adrenal gland)

Luteinizing hormone—often seen in a 3:1 ratio with FSH

Hyperinsulinemia—seen more frequently in obese PCOS patients. Diagnosed by fasting-insulin-to-glucose ratio of < 4.5 and/or abnormal oral glucose tolerance test. Hyperinsulinemia may also contribute to increased ovarian production of androgens and reduced sex hormone–binding globulin.

Low levels may be found for:

Follicle stimulating hormone—may be normal or low

Sex hormone-binding globulin—caused by hyperandrogenism and obesity

Estradiol

23. What are the clinical implications of PCOS?

Hirsuitism—increased androgen secretion and decreased sex hormone–binding globulin lead to increased free testosterone, which readily enters target cells.

Acanthosis nigricans—a gray-brown, velvety area of hyperpigmentated skin found in skin folds and on the back of the neck and in the axillae; frequently associated with hyperinsulinemia (HAIR-AN syndrome)

Anovulation—causes infertility and an increased risk of endometrial cancer (3–5%)

Cardiovascular disease—increases due to adverse changes in lipids (hypertriglyceridemia and decreased HDL cholesterol), with an increased risk of heart attack (two to seven times greater) and stroke (three times greater). Women with PCOS should have a lipid profile tested at age 35 and every 3–5 years thereafter if normal.

Abnormal glucose metabolism—increases the risk of obesity and diabetes mellitus (25–35% risk of type II DM by age 30). Women with PCOS should be screened for impaired glucose tolerance and diabetes if obese, before attempting pregnancy, and after age 40.

24. If PCOS is inherited, what is the pattern of inheritance?

Some studies suggest X-linked dominant, but others imply an autosomal dominant mode of inheritance. There is a theoretical 50% inheritance, but actual expression is approximately 40% due to modification by both genetic and environmental factors.

25. What treatments are available for PCOS?

If fertility is desired:

- Clomiphene achieves an 80% ovulation rate and a 50–60% pregnancy rate.
- Human menopausal gonadotropin is a second-line therapy and may significantly increase the risks of multiple gestations and ovarian hyperstimulation syndrome.
- Wedge resection or laparoscopic ovarian drilling are also successful treatments.
- Anti-diabetic drugs have been shown to improve ovulation, but safety and teratogenicity questions have not been answered.

If fertility is not desired:

- Oral contraceptives are the best first-line drugs for PCOS. They lower serum androgen levels by 40–50%; increase sex hormone–binding globulin, thereby decreasing hirsuitism by 80%; and control menses, thereby preventing endometrial hyperplasia.
- Spironolactone lowers ovarian (but not adrenal) androgen production and competes with androgen receptors in the hair follicle, thereby decreasing hirsuitism. It is often used in addition to oral contraceptives.
- In obese patients, diet and weight loss are the gold standard, but are very difficult for most patients to continue long term.
- Anti-diabetic drugs (metformin, thiazolidinediones, d-chiro-insitol) improve serum androgen levels, but long-term use has not been thoroughly studied.

Treatments for PCOS Symptoms

Obesity	**Hirsutism**
Diet	Oral contraceptives
Exercise	Progestins
Anti-obesity drugs	Spironolactone
Metformin	Cimetidine
	Electrolysis
	Laser vaporization
	Traditional acne treatments
Infertility	**Recurrent Abortion**
Clomiphene citrate	hCG
hMG	Progesterone supplementation
Wedge resection/	
ovarian drilling	
Metformin	
Dysfunctional Uterine Bleeding	
Oral contraceptives	
Progestins	
Dilation and curettage	

CONTROVERSIES

26. What is the best treatment for PCOS?

Some researchers believe that insulin-lowering drugs may be the best treatment for PCOS. However, no long-term studies have been performed; teratogenicity questions have not been answered; and not all patients are insulin resistant by current testing.

27. Is there still a need for progesterone challenge testing?

History, pelvic exam, and ultrasound should rule out outflow tract agenesis or obstruction. Although this is a test that some think checks for adequate serum estrogen levels, there may not be a good correlation.

BIBLIOGRAPHY

1. American Academy of Pediatrics Committee on Sports Medicine and Fitness: Medical concerns in the female athlete. Pediatrics 106(3):610–613, 2000.
2. Biller B: Diagnostic evaluation of hyperprolactinemia. J Repro Med 44(12;supplement): 1095–1099, 1999.
3. Copeland L: Textbook of Gynecology, 2nd ed. Philadelphia, W. B. Saunders, 2000.
4. Iglesias E, Coupey S: Menstrual cycle abnormalities: Diagnosis and management. Adolesc Med 10(2):255–273, 1999.
5. Kreipe R, Mou S: Eating disorders in adolescents and young adults. Obstet Gynecol Clin North Am 27(1):101–124, 2000.
6. Legro R: Polycystic ovary syndrome: Current and future treatment paradigms. Am J Obstet Gynecol 179(6; part 2):S101–S108, 1998.
7. Speroff L, Glass R, Kase N: Clinical Gynecologic Endocrinology and Infertility, 6th ed. Baltimore, Lippincott Williams and Wilkins, 1999.
8. Taylor A: Insulin-lowering medications in polycystic ovary syndrome. Obstet Gynecol Clin North Am 27(3):583–595, 2000.

7. PREMENSTRUAL SYNDROME AND DYSMENORRHEA

Thomas J. Bader, M.D., and Richard Allen, M.D.

1. What is premenstrual syndrome (PMS)?

The first published description was in 1931, and the syndrome was given the name PMS by Dalton in 1953. Speroff defines it as "a constellation of symptoms that occurs in a cycling pattern, always in the same phase of the menstrual cycle, interfering with work or lifestyle and followed by a period entirely free of symptoms."

2. What symptoms are associated with PMS?

Symptoms may be both physical and emotional. Physical symptoms include weight gain, breast swelling and tenderness, skin changes such as acne, hot flashes, diarrhea or constipation, headache, craving of sweets, and pelvic pain. Emotional symptoms include irritability, insomnia, depression, confusion or forgetfulness, anxiety, fatigue, and a feeling of being "out of control."

3. Do we know what causes PMS?

The short answer is no, but we do know that PMS is real. Numerous theories have been postulated, virtually all of which have to do with various hormonal alterations: ovarian hormones (estrogen and progesterone), fluids and electrolytes (prolactin, aldosterone, renin/angiotensin, and vasopressin), neurotransmittters (monoamines, acetylcholine), and other hormones (endorphins, androgens, glucocorticoids, melatonin, and insulin). Recent experience with the selective serotonin reuptake inhibitors (SSRIs) suggests that serotonin may play a significant role in the disease either as a primary cause or as a secondary effect. It is likely that there is no single cause.

4. What is the theory behind progesterone as a cause and treatment for PMS?

This theory was first proposed by Dalton in England as a defense in a murder trial! It was postulated that a decrease in progesterone levels, perhaps with an inadequate luteal phase, triggered depression and other emotional symptoms. If that were so, then treatment with progesterone (usually given as a natural intravaginal suppository) would "cure" PMS. Unfortunately, this treatment works only in a small group of patients, and the benefits may be due to a placebo effect. In fact, progesterone actually worsens symptoms in most patients. Progesterone increases monoamine oxidase (MAO) levels in the plasma during the luteal phase. One theory relates levels of MAO to depression as a result of deficiency in catecholamines.

5. What is the role of an aldosterone antagonist?

The physical symptoms of fluid retention (i.e., weight gain and breast tenderness) and some of the emotional symptoms may be related to elevations in renin/angiotensin and aldosterone. Therefore, a specific antagonist, such as spironolactone, would be a treatment of choice. Spironolactone also has antiandrogenic effects and offers excellent symptomatic relief to many women.

6. Will changes in diet help?

Carbohydrate craving, especially for chocolate and sweets, is a common symptom. This is thought to be related to serotonin levels. By ingesting sugars the body attempts to increase serotonin, which in turn increases levels of L-tryptophan in the brain. In normal metabolism, serotonin levels rise and fall throughout the day. A rise in serotonin accompanies the ingestion of protein, which then lowers serotonin to begin a new cycle. In PMS, serotonin levels do not reach a level high enough to trigger protein ingestion, even after ingestion of carbohydrates. Therefore, the patient with PMS continues to crave and overeat carbohydrates. Thus, a healthy diet that is low in fat, salt, and sugar but more moderate in proteins and complex carbohydrates (whole grains, vegetables, and fruit) is most beneficial to the patient with PMS. Vitamin and mineral supplements have been studied without definitive results.

7. Do prostaglandins help?

Prostaglandin PGE_1 may be low in some women with PMS, particularly those women whose symptoms are associated with alterations in carbohydrate metabolism. Prostaglandins also contribute to dysmenorrhea; thus an inhibitor such as a non-steroidal anti-inflammatory drug (NSAID; ibuprofen and others) can be beneficial.

8. Can sterilization reduce PMS?

No. Sterilization (via tubal ligation) alone has not been shown to reduce PMS symptoms. In extraordinary circumstances, for women with severe, debilitating disease, total hysterectomy with bilateral salpingo-oophorectomy can be effective therapy.

9. What is the role of psychogenic medications in the treatment of PMS?

Premenstrual syndrome has a significant psychological component. Women with severe depressive disorders that require medication, such as lithium, MAO inhibitors, and sedatives, probably should be referred for appropriate psychiatric counseling. Double-blind, placebo-controlled studies have shown marked reductions of PMS symptoms in patients receiving the serotonin reuptake inhibitor fluoxetine at a dosage of 20 mg a day throughout the menstrual cycle. Recent research has shown that other SSRIs (i.e., sertraline) may be helpful. Alprazolam also has been used successfully.

10. How is PMS treated?

First, the physician must reassure the patient that her symptoms are real and can be treated. She should then be encouraged to chart her symptoms for several cycles to see if it is indeed premenstrual. While she is doing so, the importance of a healthy diet, exercise, and sleep should be stressed. A plan of management should be formulated with the patient depending on her symptoms and their specific treatment. Specific simple medical treatments such as SSRIs, spironolactone, and prostaglandin inhibitors can then be prescribed. Progesterone therapy should be reserved for a small subgroup that does not respond to the above. If the patient also needs contraception, oral contraceptives are a good option. The vast majority of women who are troubled with PMS *can* be helped.

11. What therapy is suggested for the breast tenderness associated with PMS?

Bromocriptine, 5 mg/day during the luteal phase.

12. What is dysmenorrhea?

Dysmenorrhea is pelvic pain associated with menstrual periods. The pain is usually described as cramping in nature. Pain can also be felt outside of the pelvis; women can experience backache, headache, and extremity pain. Dysmenorrhea can also be accompanied by many other systemic symptoms, including lightheadedness, insomnia, and gastrointestinal symptoms such as nausea, vomiting, and diarrhea.

13. What is the difference between primary and secondary amenorrhea?

Primary, or intrinsic, dysmenorrhea is dysmenorrhea that is not associated with identifiable pathology. *Secondary* dysmenorrhea can be caused by a number of gynecologic conditions. The most common conditions associated with secondary dysmenorrhea are uterine myomas, adenomyosis, endometriosis, and pelvic infection.

14. What is the incidence of dysmenorrhea?

Depending on the population and the definition, a very high percentage of women (as high as 72%) experience some discomfort associated with their menses. A smaller, but still significant, percentage of women experience dysmenorrhea to a point that it interferes with their activities or causes them to miss work or school. Dysmenorrhea is less common and less severe in women who have given birth.

15. Is dysmenorrhea a form of chronic pelvic pain?

No. The characteristics of dysmenorrhea obtained in the history distinguish this condition from chronic pelvic pain. Women with dysmenorrhea, particularly those with secondary dysmenorrhea, can have pelvic symptoms between menstrual periods. But dysmenorrhea is characterized by the onset or the exacerbation of symptoms in association with the menses.

16. How is dysmenorrhea evaluated?

The history and physical exam are the major tools in the evaluation of this symptom. History is essential to rule out other gynecologic or non-gynecologic (i.e., urologic or gastrointestinal) causes of pain. The nature of the symptoms should be consistent with dysmenorrhea, and the timing of the onset or exacerbation should be directly tied to menstrual bleeding.

17. What is the mechanism that causes pain in primary dysmenorrhea?

The principal cause seems to be increased production of prostaglanin $F_{2\alpha}$. This substance causes uterine cramping and is the mechanism for the systemic symptoms (i.e., nausea, diarrhea, headache) associated with dysmenorrhea.

18. How is dysmenorrhea managed?

Both primary and secondary dysmenorrhea can be managed medically, at least initially. The two mainstays of medical treatment are NSAIDs and oral contraceptives (OCPs). NSAIDs decrease prostaglandin production, which helps improve symptoms. OCPs cause atrophy of the endometrium, the principal site of prostaglandin production. They also can reduce the amount and duration of bleeding, which can improve a woman's experience. Finally, OCPs also provide contraception.

The COX-2 inhibitors (rofecoxib and others) are a new class of oral analgesics originally developed to treat arthritis. They have been shown effective in the management of dysmenorrhea.

In secondary dysmenorrhea, when associated pathology has been identified, treatment may be directed at the underlying pathology. So in the case of uterine myomas or endometriosis, surgical management should be considered. Usually, however, medical therapy is tried first before resorting to surgery—even in cases where there is known uterine pathology.

19. What non-medical options exist for treating dysmenorrhea?

Massage, exercise, and the direct application of a heating pad applied to the lower abdomen may help some women. Alternative medical therapies such as accupuncture and hypnosis have also been tried.

20. What should be done when the response to medical therapy is inadequate?

Women with *secondary* dysmenorrhea who have an inadequate response to medical therapy should be offered treatment of the underlying pathology, and this usually means surgery. Women who are thought to have *primary* dysmenorrhea who respond poorly should be offered a more extensive work-up looking for a pathological cause for their symptoms. This work-up could include pelvic ultrasound or sonohysterography, laparoscopy, and/or MRI (specifically to look for adenomyosis).

In women with no underlying pathology or when surgical management is unacceptable (such as hysterectomy for adenomyosis), short-term therapy with oral narcotics (e.g., codeine, oxycodone) can be used for the few days of severe, debilitating symptoms. Side effects, particularly the sedation, make this therapy unattractive to many healthy women.

BIBLIOGRAPHY

1. American College of Obstetricians and Gynecologists: Premenstrual Syndrome. ACOG Committee Opinion 155, 1995.

2. Andersch B, Milsom I: An epidemiologic study of young women with dysmenorrhea, Am J Obstet Gynecol 144:655–660, 1982.
3. Brandenburg S, Tuynman Qua H, Verheij R, Pepplinkhuizen L: Treatment of premenstrual syndrome with fluoxetine: An open study. Int Clin Psychopharmacol 8:315, 1993.
4. Casper RF, Hearn MT: The effect of hysterectomy and bilateral oophorectomy in women with severe premenstrual syndrome. Am J Obstet Gynecol 162:105–109, 1990.
5. Frank RT: The hormonal causes of premenstrual tension. Arch Neurol Psychiatry 26:1052, 1931.
6. Freeman E, Rickles K, Sondheimer S, Polanski M: Ineffectiveness of progesterone suppository treatment for premenstrual syndrome. JAMA 264:349, 1990.
7. Freeman E, et al: Treatment of severe PMS. JAMA 274:51, 1995.
8. Ginsburg KA: Some practical approaches to treating PMS. Contemp Obstet Gynecol 40:24, 1995.
9. Green R, Dalton K: The premenstrual syndrome. BMJ 1:1007, 1953.
10. Mark AS, Hricak H, Heinrichs LW, et al: Adenomyosis and leiomyoma: Differential diagnosis with MR imaging. Radiology 163(2):527–529, 1987.
11. Morrison BW, Daniels SE, Kotey P, et al: Rofecoxib, a specific cyclooxygenase-2 inhibitor, in primary dysmenorrhea: A randomized controlled trial. Obstet Gynecol 94(4):504–508, 1999.
12. Smith S, Rinehart JS, Ruddock VE, Schiff I: Treatment of premenstrual syndrome with alprazolam: Results of a double-blind, placebo-controlled, randomized crossover clinical trial. Obstet Gynecol 70:37–42, 1987.
13. Speroff L, Glass RH, Kase NG (eds): Clinical Gynecologic Endocrinology and Infertility, 6th ed. Baltimore, Lippincott Williams & Wilkins, 1999.
14. Sundell G, Milsom I, Andersch B: Factors influencing the prevalence and severity of dysmenorrhea in young women. Br J Obstet Gynaecol 97:588–594, 1990.

8. ABNORMAL UTERINE BLEEDING

Lisa B. Baute, M.D.

1. What are the characteristics of a normal menstrual cycle?
A normal cycle has an average length of 28 days, but can range from 21 to 35 days. The average duration is 4 days, with a range of 1–8 days. Blood loss is usually about 35 ml, and is considered abnormal when it is greater than 80 ml.

2. Define abnormal uterine bleeding.
Bleeding at irregular time intervals, or bleeding that is excessive but at the time of expected menses.

3. List the terms used to describe the patterns associated with abnormal uterine bleeding.
Menorrhagia: excessive bleeding at regular intervals
Metrorrhagia: irregular menstrual bleeding
Menometrorrhagia: excessive, prolonged, and irregular bleeding
Intermenstrual bleeding: bleeding between normal cycles
Polymenorrhea: frequent, regular bleeding that occurs at intervals < 21 days
Oligomenorrhea: infrequent, irregular bleeding that occurs at intervals > 45 days
Postmenopausal bleeding: bleeding that occurs > 1 yr after menopause, or at irregular intervals while on hormone replacement therapy

4. List the causes of abnormal uterine bleeding.
Pregnancy related
 Miscarriage
 Ectopic pregnancy
 Gestational trophoblastic disease

Infection
 Cervicitis
 Endometritis

Neoplasm
 Cervical dysplasia/carcinoma
 Endometrial hyperplasia/polyps/carcinoma
 Submucous leiomyomas
 Estrogen-producing ovarian tumors

Systemic
 Thyroid disease
 Liver disease
 Coagulation disorders
 Sepsis

Iatrogenic
 Oral contraceptives
 Progestin-only contraceptives
 Intrauterine devices
 Hormone replacement therapy
 Steroids

5. What should you ask about when taking a history from a patient reporting abnormal uterine bleeding?
- Detailed menstrual history:
  Number of days of flow
  Number of pads/tampons used per day
  Impact on daily living
- History of any unusual bleeding from gums, easy bruising, and prolonged bleeding after minor cuts
- Symptoms of weight gain, constipation, hair loss, fatigue, and edema
- Galactorrhea
- Sexual history and use of contraception

6. What should be noted when performing a physical exam?
- Tanner stage of breast and pubic hair development
- Height
- Weight
- Excessive hair growth (hirsutism)

7. What laboratory tests should be ordered during the evaluation of abnormal uterine bleeding?
- ß-hcg
- Complete blood count
- Coagulation profile
- Thyroid-stimulating hormone
- Prolactin
- Follicle-stimulating hormone, luteinizing hormone (LH), testosterone, DHEA-S (if suspicion of polycystic ovarian disease)

8. What is dysfunctional uterine bleeding (DUB)?
DUB is a diagnosis of exclusion after pregnancy-related; infectious, neoplastic, systemic, and iatrogenic causes have been ruled out. DUB is bleeding as a result of anovulation or oligoovulation. The ovary produces estrogen, but a corpus luteum is not formed, and progesterone is not secreted. This results in continuous endometrial proliferation without progesterone-induced desquamation and bleeding.

9. What are the major causes of anovulation?

Physiologic	Pathologic
Adolescence	Hyperandrogenic states
Perimenopause	Hyperprolactinemia
Lactation	Hypothyroidism
Pregnancy	Premature ovarian failure

10. How is age related to anovulation?
Anovulation is common in the **perimenarchal** adolescent, due to immaturity of the hypothalamic-pituitary axis. The axis is unable to respond to estrogen with an LH surge. Anovulation is also common in the **perimenopausal** woman. However, it is then related to declining ovarian function.

11. When is an endometrial biopsy appropriate as part of the evaluation of abnormal uterine bleeding?
Evaluate the endometrium when hyperplasia or endometrial cancer is suspected. The incidence of endometrial cancer increases with age: it doubles by the age of 35 (6.1/100,000 in 1995), and is as high as 36.2 per 100,000 in women ages 40–49. Therefore, based on age alone,

all women over age 35 should have an endometrial biopsy if they are experiencing abnormal uterine bleeding. In addition, because obesity is associated with the peripheral conversion of androgens to estrogens and anovulation, consider a biopsy in any obese female under age 35 who has experienced a prolonged period of anovuation/unopposed estrogen, or who did not respond to medical therapy.

12. When is an ultrasound indicated in the evaluation of abnormal uterine bleeding?
An ultrasound is appropriate when organic causes of abnormal uterine bleeding have been ruled out, and a structural abnormality (e.g., fibroids, polyps) is suspected.

13. What medical management is available for the treatment of abnormal uterine bleeding?
Obviously, if a cause such as hypothyroidism was noted during the work-up, then management is aimed at treating that problem. However, approximately one-third of patients do not have an obvious organic or structural cause. In these patients, medical management is aimed at stabilization of bleeding and treatment of any hormonal abnormality.

In an *adolescent*, bleeding is often associated with anovulation, which can be treated with cyclic medroxyprogesterone acetate (Provera) or a monophasic oral contraceptive. Iron is sometimes necessary if the patient is anemic. An adolescent suffering from acute menorrhagia/hemorrhage can be treated with intravenous conjugated estrogen, 25 mg every 4 hours until bleeding abates. Alternatively, oral contraceptives can be used for stabilization. A monophasic pill containing 35–50 mcg of estradiol can be given three times a day for 3 days, then twice a day for 2 days, then once a day until the pack is finished. The pill should then be continued in the standard fashion for at least 2 months before discontinuing. If abnormal bleeding recurs and a coagulation disorder is not found, then birth-control pills offer an effective treatment.

In a *woman of reproductive age*, therapy with oral contraceptives can also be considered. In Europe, a levonorgestrel-releasing intrauterine device (IUD) has been used to successfully control menorrhagia. This IUD is now available in the United States ("Mirena," Berlex Laboratories, Inc., Montville, NJ) and can be used similarly. However, if the patient desires pregnancy, consider ovulation induction with clomiphene citrate or gonadotropin therapy.

A *perimenopausal patient* with irregular bleeding can be treated with a low-dose oral contraceptive if she does not smoke. Once the patient is menopausal, she can be treated with hormone replacement therapy (assuming endometrial hyperplasia/cancer has been ruled out).

14. Is there any medical therapy that is non-hormonal?
Women with menorrhagia have higher levels of prostacyclin (PGI_2) than women with normal periods. In addition, the ratios of PGE_2 to PGF_2-alpha are elevated in women with menorrhagia. Normally, PGF_2-alpha predominates in the late luteal and menstrual phases and is thought to act as a potent vasocontrictor in conjunction with endothelin-1 (EN-1) to cause spiral artery vasospasm. Nonsteroidal anti-inflammatory agents (NSAIDs) can be used to reduce endometrial prostaglandin levels. Although the exact mechanism is unknown, it is thought that NSAIDs cause a disproportionate decrease in endometrial PGE_2 and PGI_2 (vasodilatory), allowing PGF_2 and EN-1 to act more efficiently. In a review of studies using NSAIDs, five of seven randomized, controlled trials found that blood loss was less with NSAIDs than with placebos. Some of the more commonly used NSAIDs include ibuprofen, naproxen, and mefenamic acid.

15. What treatment is available for abnormal uterine bleeding caused by uterine fibroids?
Medically, bleeding related to uterine fibroids can be treated with a gonadotropin-releasing hormone (GnRH) agonist such as leuprolide acetate (Lupron). GnRH agonists cause amenorrhea in association with shrinkage of both myomas and total uterine volume. A decrease in blood flow to myomas is thought to be part of the mechanism, but the entire mechanism is not clearly understood.

The benefit of leuprolide is temporary. When therapy is stopped, the myomas and the uterus return to their pretreatment size. This temporary effect can be helpful in preparation for surgery, specifically prior to vaginal hysterectomy. In addition leuprolide can canuse significant side effects due to the hypoestrogenic state the medication induces. These side effects and long-term effects of decreased estrogen (e.g., bone loss) further limit long-term use.

If a patient declines or fails medical therapy, several surgical options are available. The most definitive is a hysterectomy. Surgery can also be performed to remove only the myomas (myomectomy). This procedure preserves the uterus. A less-invasive procedure can be performed using the hysteroscope to resect submucous fibroids that may be causing bleeding.

16. What types of surgical therapy are available should medical therapy fail?

Endometrial ablation can be performed to selectively destroy the basalis layer of the endometrium. The original method involved hysteroscopically directed thermal ablation using a rollerball or resectoscope. However, newer modalities avoid the complications of operative hysteroscopy such as fluid overload, hyponatremia, uterine perforation, and hemorrhage.

17. Describe some of the newer ablation devices.
- Thermal balloon ablation: a latex balloon is inserted into the uterus and filled with 5% dextrose, which is then heated to 87°C and circulated for 8 minutes.
- Hydrothermal ablation: normal saline that has been superheated to 80–90°C flows into the uterus through an insulated sheath under direct hysteroscopic visualization; intrauterine pressure never exceeds 55 mmHg—well below the 70–75 mmHg opening pressure of the fallopian tubes—to ensure that fluid does not pass into the peritoneal cavity.
- Microwave endometrial ablation: microwave energy is delivered through an 8-mm intrauterine applicator; once the tip is activated, a temperature of 95°C is achieved, and the temperature display is used to monitor the ablation process as the surgeon moves the probe laterally from one cornua to another and then to the midline. The average treatment time is 1–4 minutes and is determined by the size of the uterus and the thickness of the endometrium.

18. How successful is endometrial ablation?

Studies of the resectoscope and rollerball have shown a success rate of 70–97%. More than 85% of patients have long-term success and do not require further treatment. Studies comparing the thermal balloon to rollerball ablation have shown similar rates of success controlling menorrhagia (89% vs. 90%, respectively).

19. What is available for the patient who fails medical therapy and endometrial ablation?

Hysterectomy continues to be the definitive therapy for patients who are not assisted by other methods.

BIBLIOGRAPHY

1. American College of Obstetricians and Gynecologists: Dysfunctional Uterine Bleeding. ACOG Prac Bull 14, 2000.
2. Cooper JM, Erickson ML: Global endometrial ablation technologies. Obstet Gynecol Clin North Am 27(2):385–396, 2000.
3. Minjarez DA, Bradshaw KD: Abnormal uterine bleeding in adolescents. Obstet Gynecol Clin North Am 27(2):63–78, 2000.
4. Munro MG: Medical management of abnormal uterine bleeding. Obstet Gynecol Clin North Am 27(2):287–304, 2000.
5. Shwayder JM: Pathophysiology of abnormal uterine bleeding. Obstet Gynecol Clin North Am 27(2):219–234, 2000.
6. Stabinsky SA, Einstein M, Breen JL: Modern treatments of menorrhagia attributable to dysfunctional uterine bleeding. Obstet Gynecol Surv 54(1):61–72, 1999.

9. HIRSUTISM

Samantha M. Pfeifer, M.D.

1. What is the definition of hirsutism?
Hirsutism is excessive growth of body hair in anatomic sites where growth is considered a male sex characteristic. Normal pattern of hair distribution is age and race dependent.

2. List the three types of body hair.
- Lanugo hair follicles: lightly pigmented, thin in diameter, found in neonates
- Vellous hair follicles: fine, non-pigmented hair found in most body regions in adults
- Terminal hair follicles: pigmented, coarse hair found in scalp, axilla, and pubic area of adult men and women, and face and chest of men

3. What are the three phases of the growth cycle of the hair follicle?
- Anagen: growth phase
- Catagen: involution; hair stops growing and moves up in the follicle
- Telogen: resting phase, prior to hair loss

4. What are the causes of hirsutism?
- Increased exposure to androgens due to:
  Exogenous androgens
  Increased adrenal androgen production
  Increased ovarian androgen production
  Alterations in binding globulins
- Increased end-organ sensitivity due to increased 5α-reductase activity in skin

5. List the androgens produced by the body and their sites of production.
Ovary: testosterone, androstenedione
Adrenal gland: dehydroepiandrosterone (DHEA), dehydroepiandrosterone sulfate (DHEAS)
Peripheral tissue: testosterone and dihydrotestosterone (DHT)

6. What are the modulators of androgen action?
- Sex hormone–binding globulin (SHBG)
  SHBG binds to circulating androgens, decreases free circulating androgens
  Only free androgens, not bound, act on target tissue.
- 5α-reductase
  Enzyme that converts androgens to DHT
  For androgen to exert its effect on hair follicle, it has to be converted to DHT.

7. What is the Ferriman and Gallwey Scoring system?
It is a standardized grading system for scoring hirsutism depending on body site. Less than 8 is normal; greater than 15 is severe.

8. Give the differential diagnosis of hirsutism in women.
Polycystic ovary syndrome (PCOS)
Non-classic adrenal hyperplasia
Cushing syndrome
Androgenic tumors (ovary, adrenal gland)
Hyperprolactinemia

Exogenous androgens
Idiopathic

9. What medications are considered to have androgenic activity?
Anabolic steroids, danazol, testosterone

10. What is the significance of an abrupt onset of symptoms?
An abrupt onset of hirsutism is more likely to be associated with androgen-producing tumors or exogenous hormone use.

11. What testing should be considered in a patient with hirsutism?
- Total testosterone (level > 200 ng/dl suggests tumor)
- DHEAS (level > 700 µg/dl suggests tumor)
- 17-hydroxyprogesterone (should be drawn in the early morning, during the follicular phase of cycle)
- Prolactin
- Cortisol 24-hour urine collection, or overnight dexamethasone suppression test

12. Describe the medical treatments available for hirsutism. What is their mechanism of action?
- Combined oral contraceptive pill (OCP)
  Increases sex hormone–binding globulin
  Decreases production of androgens from ovary
- Cyproterone acetate
  Strong progestin used in combination with estrogen in oral contraceptive pill with anti-androgenic activity. Not available in the US.
- Spironolactone
  Competitive inhibition of binding at androgen receptor
- Flutamide
  Inhibits binding at androgen receptor
- Finasteride
  5α-reductase inhibitor, targeted to type 2 isoenzyme
- GnRH analogs
  Used to suppress hypothalamic-pituitary-ovarian axis and decrease androgen production. Used in combination with estrogen and progestin "add-back" regimen.
- Glucocorticoids
  Suppresses adrenal androgen production in adrenal hyperplasia
- Insulin-sensitizing agents
  Improved insulin sensitivity in women with PCOS

13. Are some OCPs better than others for treating hirsutism?
No. Though some progestins contained in OCPs are more androgenic in laboratory testing, all are equally effective clinically.

14. What adjuvant therapies are available?
Weight loss (obese patients)	Shaving
Bleaching	Electrolysis
Waxing	Laser
Depilatories	Eflornithine HCL cream (Vaniqa)
Plucking	

15. Of the mechanical methods of hair removal listed in Question 14, which is recommended?
Shaving. Shaving does not increase the rate of growth, and there is less risk of folliculitis and scarring.

16. Which drugs are FDA-approved for the treatment of hirsutism?
Combined oral contraceptives
Eflornithine HCL cream (Vaniqa)

17. How soon is an effect on hirsutism seen once treatment has begun?
A treatment effect is not seen for 3–6 months.

18. What is the best treatment approach?
A combined approach using medications to suppress androgen production and block its action to slow new hair growth, and adjuvant therapy to remove existing hair.

POLYCYSTIC OVARY SYNDROME

19. List the common synonyms for PCOS.
Stein-Leventhal syndrome
Chronic ovarian hyperandrogenism

20. What are the criteria for diagnosing PCOS?
Hyperandrogenism, either clinical or biochemical
Menstrual dysfunction associated with oligo- or anovulation

21. What findings are commonly associated with PCOS?
Elevated LH/FSH ratio ($\geq 2{:}1$)
Perimenarchal onset of symptoms
Polycystic ovaries on ultrasound
Obesity
Insulin resistance (seen in both lean and obese patients)

22. Which syndromes may be confused with PCOS? What is the appropriate test for evaluation?
- Late-onset congenital adrenal hyperplasia (21-hydroxylase deficiency)
    17-OH progesterone (draw in early morning, during follicular phase)
- Cushing's syndrome
    1-mg overnight dexamethasone suppression test
    24-hour urine for free cortisol
- Ovarian and Adrenal neoplasms
    Serum testosterone (elevated with both ovarian and adrenal tumors)
    Dehydroepiandrosterone sulfate (DHEAS)
- Hyperprolactinemia
    Serum prolactin

23. What is the proposed pattern of inheritance of PCOS?
Autosomal dominant

24. What are two mechanisms leading to excess production of androgens by ovarian theca cells in PCOS?
Increased LH pulse frequency and amplitude
Insulin acting on the ovary either directly or through mediators

25. How is the concentration of sex hormone–binding globulin (SHBG) affected by levels of sex steroids?
SHBG levels decrease in the presence of high testosterone levels, and increase in response to estrogens.

26. What are the most common clinical manifestations of PCOS?

Symptoms	Frequency (%)
Infertility	74
Hirsutism	69
Amenorrhea	51
Obesity	41

27. How does PCOS present in the adolescent female?
Premature adrenarche
Persistent oligomenorrhea
Hirsutism
Acne
Weight gain

28. What laboratory values may be abnormal in patients with PCOS?
↑ Testosterone (total and/or free)
↑ LH : FSH ratio (≥ 2:1)
↑ Androstenedione
↑ DHEAS
↓ Fasting glucose/insulin ratio (< 4.5)

29. What are health consequences of PCOS?
Hyperlipidemia
Adult-onset diabetes mellitus
Endometrial hyperplasia
Infertility
Obesity

30. How can the extent of hirsutism be quantitated?
Ferriman and Gallwey scoring system

31. Describe acanthosis nigricans.
A gray-brown, velvety area of hyperpigmented skin found in skin folds and on the back of the neck and axilla. It is a marker of insulin resistance.

32. What percentage of women with PCOS are obese?
50–75%

33. What are the "cysts" in PCOS?
Atretic follicles, usually 3–5 mm in diameter.

34. What therapy is useful for hirsutism associated with PCOS?
Combined oral contraceptive
Spironolactone (anti-androgen)
Flutamide (anti-androgen)
Finasteride (5α-reductase inhibitor)
GnRH analog
Metformin (insulin-sensitizing agent) in women with insulin resistance
Eflornithine HCl cream (Vaniqa)

35. What percentage of women with PCOS have impaired glucose tolerance? Diabetes?
Impaired glucose tolerance 35%
Diabetes 10%

36. List some surgical treatments for PCOS.
Wedge resection of the ovary
Laparoscopic drilling
Laparoscopic needle cautery

37. What can be done to prevent the development of endometrial hyperplasia in patients with PCOS?
Combined oral contraceptives
Cyclic progestin therapy

38. What are treatments for infertility due to anovulation in patients with PCOS?
Weight loss
Clomiphene citrate
Metformin (in obese women and/or those with insulin resistance)
Ovarian drilling
Human menopausal gonadotropins
In-vitro fertilization

39. What are the expected ovulation and pregnancy rates with clomiphene citrate therapy in women with PCOS?
Ovulation rate: 80%
Pregnancy rate: 50%

BIBLIOGRAPHY

1. Barbieri RL: Induction of ovulation in infertile women with hyperandrogenism and insulin resistance. Am J Obstet Gynecol 183:1412–1418, 2000.
2. Dunaif A, Thomas A: Current concepts in the polycystic ovary syndrome. Annu Rev Med 52:401–419, 2001
3. Ferriman D, Gallwey JD: Clinical assessment of body hair growth in women. J Clin Endo Metab 21:1440–1447, 1961.
4. Heiner JS, Greendale GA, Kawakami AK, et al: Comparison of a gonadotropin-releasing hormone agonist and a low-dose oral contraceptive given alone or together in the treatment of hirsutism. J Clin Endo Metab 80:3412–3418, 1995.
5. Hock DL, Seifer DB: New treatments of hyperandrogenism and hirsutism. Obstet Gynecol Clin North Am 27:567–581, 2000.
6. Moghetti P, Tosi F, Tosti A, et al: Comparison of spironolactone, flutamide, and finasteride efficacy in the treatment of hirsutism: A randomized, double-blind, placebo-controlled trial. J Clin Endo Metab 85:89–94, 2000.
7. Rittmaster RS: Hirsutism. Lancet 349:191–195, 1997.
8. Zacur HA: Polycystic ovary syndrome, hyperandrogenism, and insulin resistance. Obstet Gynecol Clin North Am 28:21–33, 2001.

10. LEIOMYOMATOUS UTERUS

Sonya Kashyap, M.D., and Steven Spandorfer, M.D.

1. What is a leiomyoma?

A leiomyoma is also called a fibroid, fibromyoma, or myoma. It is a growth of the muscular wall of the uterus, and is benign > 99% of the time. It may also contain various amounts of fibrous tissue.

2. How common are myomas?

Uterine myomas are the most common pelvic tumor. They are found incidentally in 25% of white women and 50% of black women. They account for 25–30% of all hysterectomies, but 77% of women who have hysterectomies are found to have incidental myomas on pathology. They are most common in the fourth and fifth decades of life.

3. What is the etiology of myomas?

Myomas are thought to arise from a somatic mutation of a monoclonal myometrial cell line. They probably have a genetic presdisposition since they often occur in clusters and are likely to reoccur. However, myomas have not been documented to occur more frequently in mothers, daughters, or siblings of affected individuals.

4. Do leiomyomas ever grow in response to estrogen therapy?

Myomas are sensitive to estrogen levels. They contain both progesterone and estrogen receptors, and the environment within and around the myoma is hyperestrogenic. Myomas grow during a woman's menstrual life and frequently shrink after menopause. Nevertheless, studies suggest most myomas do not grow in pregnancy—a hyperestrogenic state. If growth during pregnancy does occur, it is most likely to occur in the first trimester. Myomas also generally do not grow in response to oral contraceptives or hormone replacement therapy. If myomas grow after menopause, the possibility of malignancy should be considered.

5. How common is malignancy in a leiomyoma?

Between 0.3 and 0.7% of myomas are malignant. It is not known if these tumors originate as a malignancy or if they degenerate into malignancy.

6. What are the most common locations of myomas?

- Subserosal: just beneath the serosa of the uterus, on the external surface
- Intramural: in the uterine wall
- Submucosal: protruding into the endometrial lining

7. What symptoms are associated with myomas?

The most common symptoms are dysmenorrhea, abnormal uterine bleeding, and pressure. Large myomas may cause pelvic pressure and urinary frequency. Submucosal myomas are often associated with dysfunctional uterine bleeding, most commonly menorrhagia. Intramural myomas may also be associated with abnormal bleeding. All myomas can cause pain, either associated with menses (dysmenorrhea) or with degeneration of the myoma.

8. How do myomas lead to dysfunctional uterine bleeding?

There are several possible mechanisms:
- Increased surface area of the endometrium
- Ulceration of the endometrium overlying the myoma

• Endometrial hyperplasia at the junction of the myoma and normal endometrium
• Inability of the uterine wall to contract and close spiral arteries during menses due to distortion by the myoma
• Abnormal microvascular pattern with stasis and change in the venous drainage

9. When do myomas require removal?
• Any myoma that is rapidly growing or any growth occurring after menopause should be removed. Rapid growth after menopause is a classic symptom of leiomyosarcoma.
• Persistent abnormal bleeding unresponsive to medical therapy
• Excessive pain or pressure
• Consider removal when there is growth beyond 8 cm in a woman who has not completed her childbearing.

10. What are potential therapies for myomas?
Surgical: hysterectomy or myomectomy, depending on the patient's age, reproductive status, and general health. Myomectomy can be accomplished via laparotomy, laparoscopy, or using a hysteroscope for submucosal myomas.

Medical therapy: with gonadotropin-releasing hormone (GnRH) agonists. These agents induce a menopausal state, reducing estrogen levels and leading to shrinkage of the myoma. Maximum reduction in size (30–64%) should occur by 3–6 months. Medical therapy is also very useful prior to myomectomy to reduce blood loss. GnRH agonists are only effective for a short time. To sustain the effect, the medications must be given chronically. Discontinuation of GnRH agonists before menopause will cause regrowth of the myomas. Because of the hypoestrogenic state induced by GnRH agonists and the importance of estrogen to the health and well-being of young women, low-dose estrogen replacement is usually provided in addition to the GnRH agonist. This is called "add-back" therapy. Progesterone is also given, to avoid endometrial hyperplasia. The easiest way to administer estrogen add-back therapy is with combination hormone replacement therapy, containing estrogen and progesterone in one pill.

Interventional radiology: uterine artery embolization can be accomplished by introducing catheters into the vascular supply of the uterus. The blood supply is embolized, leading to an improvement in symptoms related to myomas. Evaluation of this technology is ongoing.

11. List the types of degeneration that myomas undergo.
• Hyaline degeneration (65%)
• Myxomatous degeneration (15%)
• Calcific degeneration (10%)
• Carneous degeneration (the most acute form of degeneration; complicates 5–10% pregnancies in women with myomas)
• Cystic degeneration
• Fatty degeneration

12. Do myomas cause infertility?
Generally myomas are not thought to be a major cause of infertility. If myomas have an impact on reproduction, it may be through distortion of the uterine cavity leading to recurrent miscarriage.

Myomas can cause mechanical obstruction at the level of the cervix or tubal ostia, which may result in infertility. Myomas on the posterior uterine wall might theoretically inhibit implantation. When no other cause for infertility is found and myomas are removed, a 70% pregnancy rate results.

BIBLIOGRAPHY
1. Aharoni A, Reiter A, Golan D, et al. Patterns of growth of uterine leiomyomas during pregnancy: A prospective longitudinal study. Br J Obstet Gynaecol 1988;95:510–513.

2. Candiani GB, Fedele L, Parazzini F, Villa L. Risk of recurrence after myomectomy. Br J Obstet Gynaecol 1991;98:385–389.
3. Friedman AJ, Haas ST. Should uterine size be an indication for surgical intervention in women with myomas? Am J Obstet Gynecol 1993;168:751–755.
4. Leibsohn S, d'Ablaing G, Mishell DR Jr, Schlaerth JB. Leiomyosarcoma in a series of hysterectomies performed for presumed uterine leiomyomas. Am J Obstet Gynecol 1990;162:968–974.
5. Stenchever MA, Droegemueller W, Herbst AL, Mishell DR (eds): Comprehensive gynecology, 4th ed., St. Louis, Mosby, 2001.

11. ENDOMETRIOSIS AND ADENOMYOSIS

Saifuddin T. Mama, M.D., M.P.H.

1. What is endometriosis?

Endometriosis is a disorder in which hormonally responsive endometrial tissue is found outside the uterus. Histology reveals endometrial glands and stroma, macrophages laden with hemofuscin and hemosiderin, as well as fibrosis.

2. What is adenomyosis?

In this disorder, endometrial tissue is found within the uterine myometrium.

3. Why are these disease entities important?

The high prevalence of endometriosis, its progressive nature, its impact on quality of life as it relates to both pelvic pain and infertility, and the difficulty in controlling the symptoms and course of the disease make this a frustrating disease entity. Adenomyosis is important because of the severe menorrhagia and disabling dysmenorrhea that accompany this disease.

4. How prevalent is endometriosis?

The true extent in the general female population is controversial. It is thought to occur in 5–15% of pre-menopausal women, with > 50% prevalence noted in chronic pelvic pain patients and 20–50% prevalence in infertile women. There is an increased incidence in first-degree family members of women with endometriosis. It also affects teenagers, and there is no racial preponderance.

5. How prevalent is adenomyosis?

It is detected in 15–20% of uteri, mainly in peri-menopausal women. There are reports of an association between tamoxifen administration and adenomyosis.

6. What are the anatomical sites for endometriosis?

The main sites are the posterior cul-de-sac, including the surface peritoneum on the uterosacral ligaments, bilateral ovarian fossa, broad ligament, ovarian surfaces, fallopian tubes, and anterior cul-de-sac. Peritoneal defects are often seen, usually lateral to the uterosacral ligaments. Endometriosis has been reported in diverse tissue, including lung, nasal mucosa, bladder, kidney, and incisional sites.

7. Describe the etiology of endometriosis.

Theories for histiogenesis include:

Metastatic theory—This theory ascribes endometriosis to implantation following retrograde menstruation into the peritoneal cavity, lymphatic dissemination or hematogenous spread of endometrial tissue, or iatrogenic dissemination due to procedures. Supporting this theory are the location of endometriosis in dependent portions of the body, the ability of endometrial cells to implant, an increased incidence of endometriosis in patients with uterine or vaginal outlet obstruction, and the identification of endometriosis at distant sites outside the abdominal cavity.

Embryonic cell rest and coelomic metaplasia theory—This theory attempts to explain endometriosis as the de novo development of endometrial tissue outside the uterus. However, there is no evidence for this despite common embryonic tissue for ovarian germinal epithelium, mullerian epithelium, and peritoneal mesothelium.

While evidence suggests that the metastatic theory may facilitate pathogenesis, it appears that altered macrophage capacity to induce cytolysis of ectopic endometrial cells, along with increased ability of this tissue to survive, proliferate, invade, and induce angiogenesis, along with impaired cell apoptosis may be the etiology. There is an overall increase in the number of macrophages in endometriosis. Contributing to this are increased synthesis of growth factors, cytokines, and angiogenic factors by peritoneal macrophages with impaired cytotoxic ability. The cause of the altered macrophage and ectopic endometrial cell changes is unknown.

8. **What is the clinical presentation of endometriosis?**
   Significant symptoms are:
   - Pelvic pain—usually occurring cyclically just prior to, or with, menses and located unilaterally or bilaterally in the lower quadrants. With progression of disease, there is increased pain specifically in the week before menses. With severe disease, pain is present throughout the month. The pain is believed to be secondary to tissue edema and blood extravasation stimulating mechanoreceptors innervated by A-delta and C primary afferent fibers. There is no relationship between the extent of disease and the severity of pain.
   - Infertility—the effect of scarring and adhesions distorts pelvic architecture and affects oocyte transport from the ovary to the tube. The peritoneal environment affects the oocytes and sperm. In the presence of endometriosis, peritoneal fluid inhibits sperm function. This affects 30–40% of women with endometriosis.
   - Dyspareunia—noted with an immobile, fixed uterus. This is usually present with severe disease. There is an association between endometriosis and pain in specific coital positions.
   - Rectal discomfort and tenesmus—related to posterior cul-de-sac scarring and immobility
   - Abnormal uterine bleeding

9. **How does adenomyosis present?**
   The symptoms are abnormal uterine bleeding, usually prolonged, along with severe dysmenorrhea.

10. **What are the physical findings with endometriosis and adenomyosis?**
    If present, they are quite variable. With *endometriosis* there can be diffuse lower abdominal pain in different locations; nodularity and tenderness along the uterosacral ligaments; immobility of pelvic viscera leading to pain with manipulation; a fixed, retroverted uterus; narrowing of the posterior vaginal fornix; and adnexal tenderness and immobility.
    With *adenomyosis* the mobile uterus is often top-normal size or enlarged, with no evidence for leiomyomas.

11. **How is endometriosis diagnosed?**
    By laparoscopy or laparotomy. The wide spectrum of the disease has to be appreciated, not only the macroscopic black and blue-black lesions, but also the red, red-pink, yellow-brown, white, and clear vesicular lesions along with peritoneal defects, fibrosis, and scarring. There can also be microscopic implants, which can only be appreciated after histologic diagnosis of biopsies of normal-appearing surface peritoneum.
    Endometriomas which are ovarian "chocolate" cysts arise from endometriosis within the ovary and can often be diagnosed by ultrasound, MRI, or CT. Surface endometriosis cannot be visualized by imaging. Serum markers such as CA-125 or anti-endometrial antibodies lack specificity and reproducibility. Peritoneal fluid markers such as cytokines, growth factors, and angiogenic factors present a possible future means for diagnosis.

12. **How is adenomyosis diagnosed?**
    A thickened junctional zone present on MRI is highly suggestive; however, the definitive diagnosis is by pathology. Adenomyosis is usually more extensive in the posterior wall, with trabeculated myometrium.

13. How is endometriosis staged?

The staging system is the Revised American Society for Reproductive Medicine Classification of Endometriosis (see Bibliography). This staging is done postoperatively, documenting the extent and location of the endometrial implants and adhesions.

14. Describe medical management options for endometriosis.

Medical management involves suppression of ovarian estradiol production, thereby decreasing the stimulus for endometriotic growth and proliferation. Ectopic endometrial tissue growth is retarded, and, with decreased hormonal activity, atrophy and/or decidualization occurs.

Combined oral contraceptives containing estrogen and a progestin may be used.

Danazol, a synthetic derivative of 17-alpha-ethinyl testosterone, inhibits multiple enzymes in steroidogenesis as well as cytosolic hormone receptors. This leads to a high-androgen, low-estrogen environment that reduces activity of all endometrial tissue and endometriosis. Although it is effective, it is used less frequently than other agents due to its side effects.

Progestins, such as medroxyprogestrone, induce endometrial atrophy and act as gonadotropin inhibitors.

Gonadotropin-releasing hormone (GnRH) agonists severely reduce circulating estrogen levels (to < 20 pg/mL) and are very effective in resolution of active disease and reduction of pain. Long-term use is associated with trabecular bone loss, and beyond a 6-month period, hormone add-back therapy with estrogen and progestins is necessary.

Anti-inflammatory agents (e.g., nonsteroidal anti-inflammatory drugs [NSAIDs]) are used in conjunction with hormonal therapy.

Antidepressants, such as amitriptyline, have proved helpful in low doses as adjunctive therapy to all of the above.

15. Describe surgical treatment options for endometriosis.

Surgical procedures include excision or destruction with laser vaporization, electrocoagulation or thermacoagulation, and lysis of adhesions. Occasional adjunctive pain management procedures, such as presacral neurectomy, and uterosacral ablation can also be employed. Definitive surgery involves total abdominal hysterectomy, bilateral salpingo-oophorectomy, excision of all peritoneal surface lesions or endometriomas, and lysis of adhesions.

There is clear evidence that **combined surgical and medical therapy** results in better long-term symptom improvement. Future treatment modalities under evaluation include: anti-estrogens, aromatase inhibitors, and angiogenic inhibitors.

16. How is adenomyosis treated?

Oral contraceptives, in conjunction with NSAIDs and GnRH agonists, can provide symptomatic relief. Definitive surgery with hysterectomy is eventually needed for symptomatic patients who fail medical therapy.

BIBLIOGRAPHY

1. American College of Obstetricians and Gynecologists. Medical management of endometriosis. ACOG Practice Bulletin 11:1–13. Washington DC, ACOG, 1999.
2. American Society for Reproductive Medicine. Revised American Society for Reproductive Medicine classification of endometriosis, 1996. Fertil Steril 1997;67:817–821.
3. Braun DP, Gebel H, Rana N, Dmowski WP. Cytolysis of eutopic and ectopic endometrial cells by peripheral monocytes and peritoneal macrophages in women with endometriosis. Fertil Steril 1998;69:1103–1108.
4. Bulun SE, Zeitoun KM, Takayama K, et al. Aromatase as a therapeutic target in endometriosis. Trends Endocrinol Metab 2000;11:22–27.
5. Burns WN, Schenken RS. Pathophysiology of endometriosis-associated infertility. Clin Obstet Gynecol 1999;42:586–610.
6. Dokras A, Olive DL. Endometriosis and assisted reproductive technologies. Clin Obstet Gynecol 1999;42:687–697.

7. Gebel HM, Braun DP, Tambur A, et al. Spontaneous apoptosis of endometrial tissue is impaired in women with endometriosis. Fertil Steril 1998; 69:1042–1047.
8. Neven P. Tamoxifen and endometrial lesions. Lancet 1993;342–452.
9. Nezhat CR, Berger GS, Nezhat FR, et al. Endometriosis. New York, Springer-Verlag, 1995.
10. Speroff L, et al (eds): Clinical Gynecologic Endocrinology and Infertility, 6th ed. Philadelphia, Lippincott Williams & Wilkins, 1999.

12. ACUTE AND CHRONIC PELVIC PAIN

Sami I. Jabara, M.D., and Richard W. Tureck, M.D.

1. What is the definition of chronic pelvic pain in women?

Chronic pelvic pain in women may be defined as nonspecific pelvic pain of more than 6-month duration that may or may not be relieved by analgesics (narcotics and nonsteroidals). It is a nonspecific term that involves pain associated with laparoscopically evident pathology, occult somatic pathology, and nonsomatic disorders.

2. How common is chronic pelvic pain in women?

Chronic pelvic pain prompts up to 10% of outpatient gynecology consultations and is responsible for approximately 10–35% of laparoscopies and 12% of hysterectomies performed in the U.S. There are no reliable data about disability and lost workdays attributable to chronic pelvic pain, but the total direct and indirect cost in the U.S. may be conservatively estimated to exceed 2 billion dollars annually.

3. What is the major difference between acute and chronic pelvic pain?

Acute pain is of short duration and generally is associated with tissue damage appropriate to the degree of symptoms. *Chronic pain* often has an indefinite beginning, and the structural damage alone usually is not enough to account for the degree of pain that the patient reports.

4. Describe the innervation of the individual pelvic organs.

The pelvic organs receive their innervation from the autonomic nervous system, which comprises both sympathetic and parasympathetic fibers. Most afferent stimuli are transmitted by sympathetic nerves though cell bodies that lie in the thoracolumbar distribution. Parasympathetic nerve fibers are also involved to a lesser extent in the transition of painful stimuli. The organs that are müllerian in embryonic origin, such as the uterus, fallopian tubes, and upper vagina, transmit impulses via sympathetic fibers into the spinal cord at the level of T-10, T-11, T-12, and L-1. Impulses from the uterus travel through the uterosacral ligaments to the uterine inferior plexus. From the uterus, they join other pelvic afferents to form the hypogastric plexus at the level of the rectum and vagina. Impulses from the upper vagina, cervix, and lower uterine segment travel through the parasympathetic system to the sacral roots S2–S4.

The ovaries and distal fallopian tubes derive their nerve supply independently and enter the spinal cord at T-9 and T-10. The bladder, rectum, perineum, and anus are derived from the urogenital sinus and are innervated by both sympathetic and parasympathetic systems. Fibers from the perineum and anus combine to form branches of the pudendal nerve, eventually terminating in sacral roots S2 and S4.

5. What is visceral pain?

The perception of pain arises as an integration of multiple stimuli through a network of neuronal pathways. Visceral pain is more diffuse than pain of somatic origin. A variety of mechanisms can induce visceral pain, such as distention of the hollow viscera, sudden stretching of the capsule of solid organs, hypoxia or necrosis of viscera, production of prostanoids, chemical irritation of visceral nerve endings, and inflammation. Pelvic pain is visceral and may be either referred or splanchnic. *Splanchnic pain* occurs when an irritable stimulus is appreciated in a specific organ secondary to tension (stretching, distension, or pulling) or peritoneal irritation/inflammation. *Referred pain* occurs when autonomic impulses arise from a diseased visceral organ, eliciting an irritable response within the spinal cord. Pain is sensed in the dermatomes corresponding to cells receiving those impulses.

6. **What is the differential diagnosis of chronic pelvic pain?**

Gynecologic causes	Orthopedic musculo-skeletal causes	Gastrointestinal causes
Pelvic inflammatory disease	Psoas muscle pain	Irritable bowel syndrome
Endometriosis	Stress fracture of pelvis	Constipation
Pelvic adhesions	Abdominal wall pain	Inflammatory bowel disease
Pelvic relaxation	**Urinary tract causes**	
Ovarian cysts	Interstitial cystitis	
Mittelschmerz	Bladder spasms	
Adenomyosis		

7. **What are the most common causes of acute pain related to the reproductive organs?**
Eleven causes are most common:

Mittelschmerz is a dull pressure or aching sensation during mid-cycle in either the right or left lower quadrant secondary to ovulation, distention of the ovarian capsule, or mild bleeding associated with the process of ovulation.

Functional ovarian cysts may be follicular or corpus luteum. *Follicular cysts* result from failure of egg release from a mature follicle during ovulation. Symptoms include an aching sensation in the right or left lower quadrant. Findings include an enlarged cystic ovary on exam or ultrasound. Clinical course may include spontaneous resolution, torsion with pain, rupture with pain, and rupture with hemorrhage possibly requiring surgical evaluation. *Corpus luteum cysts* may persist in the center of the corpus luteum. The lutein cysts may be functional or nonfunctional; therefore, menstruation may be delayed. Cyst persistence is rare except in cases of pregnancy, and can be treated by oral contraceptive pills or laparoscopy. Complications include torsion, rupture, and hemorrhage.

Intrauterine pregnancy may cause abdominal pain by possible stretching of the visceral peritoneum by the enlarging uterus, early uterine contractions, stretching of the ovarian capsule from the corpus luteum cyst, rupture of the corpus luteum, and threatened miscarriage. The diagnosis of pregnancy is based on historical information of amenorrhea, nausea, breast tenderness, fatigue, and urinary frequency and on the physical findings of a softening isthmus and enlarging fundus.

Ectopic pregnancy (Fig. 1) may cause pelvic pain before and after rupture secondary to stretching of the hollow viscus of the fallopian tube or peritoneal irritation from a hemoperitoneum. Ectopic pregnancies occur in 1–2 % of all gestations. Location of the gestation may be tubal, cervical, ovarian, intramural, or abdominal. The most common location of an ectopic pregnancy is the ampullary portion of the fallopian tube.

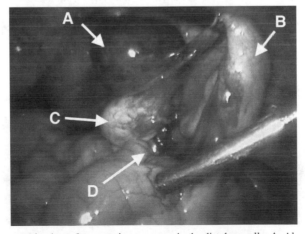

FIGURE 1. Laparoscopic view of an ectopic pregnancy in the distal ampulla, **A**. Also evident are **B**, the proximal portion of the tube; **C**, an ovary; **D**, bowel adhered to the ovary.

Pelvic infections are a common cause of both acute and chronic pelvic pain. The infection (gonorrhea or chlamydia or other) commonly involves the fallopian tubes and ovaries, parametrial and pelvic wall tissue, uterus, and other organs of the pelvic and abdominal cavity.

Uterine tumors (i.e., leiomyomas or leiomyosarcomas) can cause pain secondary to torsion necrosis, stretching of the visceral peritoneum of the uterus, or pressure against surrounding intra-abdominal structures.

Adnexal neoplasia may cause abdominal or pelvic pain when associated with hemorrhage, necrosis, torsion, or rupture. Symptoms may include gradual onset of abdominal pain, intermittent or acute severe pain, abdominal distention, nausea, vomiting, anorexia, or unilateral lower extremity edema.

Ovarian torsion (Fig. 2) may involve a normal or cystic ovary, tube, or uterine mass. Symptoms may be constant and severe or intermittent. Associated symptoms include nausea, vomiting, diaphoresis, and severe pelvic pain. Venous blood flow ceases first, resulting in enlargement. Arterial obstruction causes necrosis. The patient most commonly presents with an acute abdomen requiring immediate surgical exploration.

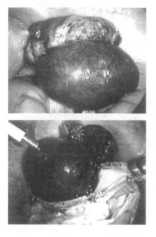

FIGURE 2. Ovarian torsion. Notice the large, swollen, bluish hue of the ovary due to venous obstruction.

Endometriosis is defined as the presence of endometrial glands and stroma at sites other than the uterine cavity. These endometriotic implants on the peritoneal surfaces of the intra-abdominal structures can result in hemorrhage and pelvic adhesion formation (Fig 3). Approximately 25–40% of patients undergoing laparoscopy for chronic pelvic pain have evidence of endometriosis. The pain is characteristically present several days before the period and ends with menstruation; however, it may be constant throughout the cycle. Dyspareunia and infertility are also common presenting complaints.

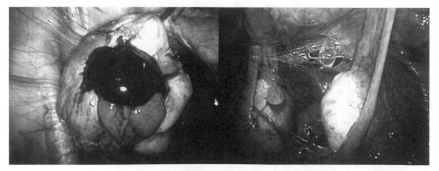

FIGURE 3. *Left*, a ruptured endometrioma. *Right*, filmy adhesions between the right ovary and the posterior uterus.

Adenomyosis, characterized by the presence of endometrial glands within the myometrium, typically causes dysmenorrhea that starts 1 week prior to the menstrual cycle and continues until the last day of the cycle. The uterus is usually enlarged, and diagnosis is performed clinically. MRI is helpful in differentiating adenomyosis from a well-circumscribed fibroid.

Dysmenorrhea is lower abdominal or pelvic pain associated with the immediate premenstrual phase and menstruation.

8. How do pelvic adhesions cause pelvic pain?

Adhesion formation (Fig. 4) occurs after trauma to the visceral or parietal peritoneum, inflicted via an operative procedure, endometriosis, or infection. Surgical intervention accounts for approximately 70% of all adhesion formation. In cases in which ischemic damage to peritoneum occurs, lysis of fibrin does not take place due to reduced fibrinolytic activity, and fibrous adhesions occur. Foreign-body granulomas due to talc and/or gauze or suture material are also involved in the creation of adhesions.

Mechanical components have been proposed as the underlying cause of pain sensation in patients with pelvic or abdominal adhesions. Patients experience pain via mechanical stimulation (stretching) of visceral nociceptors.

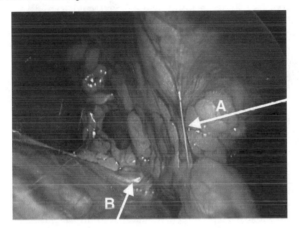

FIGURE 4. **A**, Dense adhesions between bowel and anterior abdominal wall, and **B**, between the anterior uterus and anterior abdominal wall.

9. What is the treatment for pelvic adhesions?

Laparoscopic lysis of adhesions in patients with chronic pelvic pain results in improvement of symptomatology in 65–85% of patients. This improvement is maintained in approximately 75% of patients 6–12 months following surgery.

10. Which diseases of the urinary tract cause pelvic pain?

Urinary tract infection, cystitis, and pyelonephritis may present with lower abdominal and/or right flank pain, dysuria, hematuria, and frequency of urination. The patient is usually febrile. White blood cells and bacteria are noted on urinalysis. Treatment is antibiotics.

Ureteral obstruction secondary to a stone, tumor, or blood clot may cause severe, sudden pain beginning in the flank and radiating into the groin and ipsilateral labia. Symptoms include restlessness, sweats, nausea, vomiting, frequency of urination, and colicky pain. Findings include hematuria, flank tenderness, and tachycardia.

Perinephric abscess is usually unilateral and caused most commonly by staphylococci. Symptoms include flank tenderness—more pronounced than in pyelonephritis—and fever.

Interstitial cystitis and urethral syndrome, which entail frequency, urgency, and dysuria in the absence of bacteriuria.

11. What are the most common gastrointestinal causes of pelvic and lower abdominal pain?

Appendicitis is the most common surgical condition in the abdomen, although it is less common in women than in men. Pain is secondary to luminal distention and necrosis. The symptoms vary, depending on the anatomic location of the appendix and the status of the infection. A dull aching is initially reported in the periumbilical area, advancing to a more severe pain at McBurney's point. Right hip extension may cause an increase in pain.

Diverticulitis is most commonly seen in elderly women and may present with peritonitis similar to appendicitis or as a pelvic mass. Pain may be acute and severe, or there may be a history of chronic bouts of pain.

Bowel obstructions secondary to postoperative adhesion, neoplastic lesions, hernias, foreign bodies, gallstones, parasites, enteritis, or traumatic hematoma of the bowel wall may cause colicky abdominal pain with associated distention, dehydration, hypovolemia, vomiting, and constipation.

Strangulated hernias and hernias in general are commonly symptomatic. Pain occurs when the intraperitoneal contents are trapped in the hernia sac and the blood supply is compromised. The most common forms associated with abdominal pain are inguinal, femoral, umbilical, and obturator hernias. Presenting symptoms are obstructive. Treatment is surgical with restoration of a patent bowel lumen.

Cholecystitis, cholangitis, gastroduodenal ulcers, and pancreatitis most commonly cause upper abdominal pain, but rarely are associated with lower abdominal symptoms.

Irritable bowel syndrome is usually associated with bowel spasms and diarrhea. Irritable bowel syndrome may be confused with pain of gynecologic origin, which can result in unwarranted hysterectomy.

12. What are the causes of deep vaginal pain?

Tender trigger points in the paracervical region or margins of the vaginal cuff after hysterectomy. These points are reproducible. Injection with 1% procaine or 0.25% bupivacaine requires minimal penetration (3–5 mm) of vaginal mucosa to reproduce the painful sensation. The treatment may need to be repeated weekly, up to three times.

Trigger point pain is aggravated by coitus, menses, and examination. Trigger points are hard to identify because the pain is diffuse. Blocks result in temporary improvement, lasting only until the anesthesia wears off. Diagnostic laparoscopy is indicated to rule out pelvic adhesions and endometriosis. Laser therapy is available for fulguration of endometriosis, lysis of adhesions, and uterosacral ligament transection.

13. Differentiate myofascial trigger points and abdominal wall trigger points.

Myofascial trigger points are hyperirritable spots usually within a taut band of skeletal muscle or muscle fascia. Abdominal wall trigger points have been identified in fat or fascial planes above the aponeurosis on needle localization.

14. How are myofascial trigger points detected and treated?

The points are painful on compression (**jump sign**) and may give rise to characteristic referred pain (to the arm, leg, or back), tenderness, and autonomic phenomenon (tearing, coryza, visual disturbances, tinnitus). Treatment involves hyperstimulation, analgesia (such as stretch and cold spray), needling with local injection, transcutaneous electrical nerve stimulation (TENS), and acupuncture, all of which act as counterirritants that alter the central gate or threshold control and result in a prolonged response.

15. What diagnostic method can be used to distinguish visceral pathologic conditions from chronic abdominal pelvic pain of neurologic origin?

The tissue source of pain can be identified by a careful neurologic assessment with palpation of small areas of tissue; by placement of a needle into the tissues either abdominally or vaginally;

or by injection of saline or anesthetic into the local tissue and reproduction of the same pain with the needle tip.

16. True or false: Sexual abuse is associated with chronic pelvic pain.

True. Women with chronic pelvic pain have a high incidence of sexual abuse history (48%, compared with 6.5% of pain-free controls).

17. What is the best approach to the patient with chronic pelvic pain?
- Conduct a complete and careful medical, social, and sexual history and physical examination.
- Establish a diagnosis. Differentiate between somatic and visceral foci for pain, using trigger-point identification and analgesia for these foci to improve accuracy of pelvic examination.
- Consider helpful adjunctive diagnostic tools: pelvic ultrasound, CT scan, MRI, and abdominal and renal radiographic procedures.
- Use minimal medication. Analgesics can be taken continuously, but limited if addicting. Antidepressants may potentiate analgesics. Anxiolytics also may potentiate analgesics, but have a high addiction potential. Hormonal treatment of endometriosis (e.g., gonadotropin-releasing hormone agonists) is effective, but cannot be used for a prolonged time due to undesireable side effects.
- Limit surgical therapy to severe, refractory cases, and avoid removal of normal pelvic tissues. Laparoscopic conservative surgery in women with endometriosis-associated chronic pelvic pain provides relief > 6 months in only 40–70% of women. The success rate for surgical treatment of pain with hysterectomy, even without uterine pathology, is up to 78%. Presacral neurectomy can be considered in difficult, nonresponsive cases (effective in 50–75% of patients). However, the recurrence rate is very high (> 50%).
- Offer psychological consultation, based on history and response to evaluation and treatment. Multidisciplinary therapy is successful in chronic pelvic pain. This approach incorporates skills of a gynecologist, a psychiatrist, and an anesthesiologist.

18. What is the role of laparoscopy in chronic pelvic pain?

Forty percent of all laparoscopy is done for chronic pelvic pain. Although 40% of patients have diagnosable abnormalities, 50% may be helped with diagnostic and operative laparoscopies.

19. Is one nonsteroidal anti-inflammatory drug (NSAID) better than the others in the treatment of dysmenorrhea?

All NSAIDs are equally potent in the treatment of dysmenorrhea. However, the newer Cox II inhibitors, unlike the nonselective cyclo-oxygenase inhibitors, have less-significant gastrointestinal side effects.

BIBLIOGRAPHY

1. Droegemueller W, et al (eds): Comprehensive Gynecology. St. Louis, Mosby, 2001.
2. Berek J, Adashi E, Hillard P (eds): Novak's Gynecology. Baltimore, WIlliams & Wilkins, 1996.
3. Esposito M, Tureck R, Mastroianni L: Understanding endometriosis. The Female Patient 24:79–85,1999.
4. Howard FM: An evidence-based medicine approach to the treatment of endometriosis-associated chronic pelvic pain: Placebo-controlled studies. J Am Assoc Gynecol Laparoscop 7(4):477–488, 2000.
5. Lampe A, Solder E, Ennemoser A, et al: Chronic pelvic pain and previous sexual abuse. Obstet Gynecol 96(6):929–933, 2000.
6. Lescomb GH, Ling FW: Chronic pelvic pain. Med Clin North Am 79:1411, 1995.
7. Mathias SD, Kupperman M, et al: Chronic pelvic pain: Prevalence, health-related quality of life, and economic correlates. Obstet Gynecol 87:321, 1996.
8. McDonald JS: Management of chronic pelvic pain. Obstet Gynecol Clin North Am 20:817, 1995.
9. Rapkin AJ: Neuroanatomy, neurophysiology, and neuropharmacology of pelvic pain. Clin Obstet Gynecol 119–128, 1990.

10. Reiter RC, Gambone JC: Demographic and historic variables in women with idiopathic chronic pelvic pain. Obstet Gynecol 75:428, 1990.
11. Roseff SJ, Murphy AA: Laparoscopy in the diagnosis and therapy of chronic pelvic pain. Clin Obstet Gynecol 137–143, 1990.
12. Slocumb JC: Chronic somatic myofascial and neurogenic abdominal pelvic pain. Clin Obstet Gynecol 145–152, 1990.

13. ANOVULATION AND INDUCTION OF OVULATION

Sonya Kashyap, M.D., and Steven Spandorfer, M.D.

1. What is anovulation?

Anovulation is the failure of the ovary to produce an ovum (or egg). Technically, anovulation refers to the absence of ovulation; however some women ovulate infrequently.

Anovulation can be primary (associated with primary amenorrhea) or secondary (failure of normal ovulation after a history of ovulatory cycles).

2. How does anovulation present?

Anovulation presents with irregular cycles or a total lack of menstrual cycles. The patient may have primary amenorrhea, secondary amenorrhea, or oligomenorrhea.

3. What are common causes of primary anovulation?

Women can have primary amenorrhea (the absence of menses) without primary anovulation. That is, the ovary can function normally with normal ovulatory function, but a defect in the uterus and/or the outflow tract can prevent normal menstrual function. However, most amenorrhea is due to ovarian dysfunction/anovulation.

The common causes of primary anovulation are:
• Hypothyroidism
• Hypothalamic dysfunction
• Weight-related issues
• Dysgenetic gonads

4. What are possible causes of secondary anovulation?

• Polycystic ovarian syndrome
• Hypo/hyperthyroidism
• Adrenal enzyme disorders
• Hyperprolactinemia
• Stress
• Pregnancy
• Premature ovarian failure
• Hypothalamic causes

5. What is the appropriate therapy for anovulation?

Therapy should be directed to the specific cause.

6. What is polycystic ovarian syndrome (PCOS)?

PCOS is a complex mix of endocrine aberrations and symptoms. Symptoms of the syndrome include: irregular bleeding (due to anovulation), hirsutism, obesity, and infertility. Signs include enlarged ovaries with a polycystic appearance on ultrasound, characteristic skin changes, and multiple endocrine abnormalities involving androgens, sex hormones, and insulin function. Women with PCOS do not need to have all of the elements of the syndrome for the diagnosis to be made.

The anovulation portion of PCOS is treated with ovulation induction, which is frequently combined with androgen suppression and weight loss. Recently there has been increasing interest in treating the aberrant insulin metabolism, as well. This has been found to improve the likelihood of ovulation in selected patients.

7. How does thyroid dysfunction cause anovulation?

Hypothryoidism can cause anovulation, possibly indirectly through an increase in prolactin production. Treatment of the underlying thyroid disease should include thyroid replacement as well as a work-up for thyroid antibodies and other autoimmune disorders. Thyroid replacement should regulate cycles.

8. How does the adrenal function affect ovulation?

Elevated adrenal androgen production can lead to central suppression of ovulation. Treatment is ovulation induction with or without suppression of adrenal androgen production.

9. How does an elevated prolactin level affect ovulation?

Elevated prolactin levels interfere with production of gonadotropin-releasing hormone (GnRH), which leads to poor production of gonadotropins by the pituitary and consequent ovarian dysfunction.

Hyperprolactinemia can result due to **hyperthyroidism** or due to a **prolactin-secreting tumor** (prolactinoma, pituitary adenoma). Patients with hyperprolactinemia should be evaluated for the presence of hypothyroidism, galactorrhea, and visual disturbances or headaches. If hyperthyroidism is the cause, correction of the underlying thyroid disorder should correct the increased prolactin production.

If thyroid function is normal, the presence of pituitary micro- or macroadenoma should be investigated with MRI or CT of the head. Prolactin-secreting tumors are the most common pituitary tumors. These tumors are essentially all benign. They are classified broadly based on size as either *microadenomas* (< 10 mm) or *macroadenomas* (> 10 mm). A microadenoma that is asymptomatic (i.e., no headaches or visual symptoms) can be followed with re-imaging in 1 year to ensure stability. Macroademonas require prompt therapy—either medical or surgical. Treatment with dopamaine agonists reduces prolactin levels and restores ovulation.

10. What is premature ovarian failure?

It is normal for the ovary to cease ovulation and most hormone production. When this occurs *after* the age of 40, it is termed menopause and considered to be physiologic. If it occurs *before* the age of 40, it is termed premature menopause or premature ovarian failure. Women who experience ovarian failure prior to age 30 should have genetic evaluation to ensure a normal karyotype. These women should also have an autoimmune work-up because of possible autoimmune causes of ovarian failure.

11. What hypothalamic problems can interfere with ovulation?

There are a number of events that can interfere with normal hypothalamic secretion of GnRH, leading to ovulatory dysfunction and anovulation. Low or normal levels of gonadotropins (luteinizing hormone [LH] and follicle-stimulating hormone [FSH]) characterize these conditions.

Weight loss: Significant weight loss and loss of body fat in particular are associated with hypothalamic anovulation and amenorrhea. Extreme weight loss such as that associated with eating disorders can also be associated with other endocrine abnormalities. These conditions carry a mortality rate as high as 5–15%. Therefore, this condition requires careful assessment; patients require intensive psychotherapy for both mental and physical health.

Exercise: Increased opioid production from excess exercise, in combination with the loss of weight and body fat that accompany strenuous exercise, may inhibit ovulation through positive effects on norepinephrine and GnRH. Treatment with nalaxone, an opiate antagonist, has been shown to resume normal cycles.

Stress: Extreme stress may induce anovulation by the same opioid pathway.

12. What is Kallman's syndrome?

Kallman's sydrome is characterized by primary amenorrhea and anosmia. It results from failure of neuronal migration of GnRH neurons from the medial olfactory placode to the median basal hypothalamus. It can be inherited in an x-linked or autosomal recessive pattern, and it results in inappropriate GnRH secretion. Women with Kallman's syndrome have normal ovaries and can undergo ovulation induction.

13. What are dysgenetic gonads?

Dysgenetic gonads refer to gonads in individuals with an abnormal karyotype (e.g., 45 XO, phenotypic females with 46 XY karyotype). These individuals require karyotype testing and work-up for other associated abnormalities. Mosaicism may be found with the presence of a Y chromosome. Except for patients with androgen insensitivity, phenotypic females with a Y chromosome require prompt removal of the gonads, which are at risk for the development of gonadoblastomas and then germ cell malignancies.

14. What is ovulation induction?

Ovulation induction is the general term for the use of medication to stimulate the ovary to produce an egg. There are three classes of medication used for induction of ovulation: clomiphene citrate (Clomid), gonadotropins (FSH with or without LH), and GnRH.

15. What is the primary indication for clomiphene citrate?

The primary indication is oligo-ovulation especially due to PCOS. Clomiphene is taken orally once a day, on days 5–9 of the menstrual cycle, at a starting dose of 50 mg a day.

16. When does ovulation occur after clomiphene?

Generally, ovulation occurs 5–12 days after the last pill.

17. What are the side effects of clomiphene?

The most common side effects are vasomotor flushes (10%), abdominal distension (5.5%), bloating, abdominal pain, breast tenderness (2%), nausea and vomiting, headache, and loss of hair. Visual symptoms such as blurring or scotoma require discontinuation of the medication.

18. Are there pregnancy risks associated with clomiphene?

Clomiphene has *not* been associated with an increased rate of anomalies or miscarriage.

19. How does clomiphene work?

Clomiphene is a nonsteroidal agent that is distantly related to diethylstilbesterol and acts as a weak estrogen at the level of the pituitary. It binds estrogen receptors and occupies them for long periods of time, which alters the pituitary's perception of the level of circulating estrogen. Therefore, the negative feedback of estrogen on the pituitary is abolished, which results in increased action on the ovary by FSH.

20. Can clomiphene be used in cases of hypothalamic amenorrhea?

Since clomiphene's primary mechanism of action is to alter the pituitary production of FSH, an intact hypothalamic-pituitary axis should be a prerequisite for clomiphene therapy. Some physicians suggest a trial of clomiphene in a woman with hypothalamic dysfunction who is not also hypoestrogenic. The yield for this therapy is very low.

21. What steps should be taken if a woman fails to ovulate despite therapy with clomiphene?

The dose can be increased in subsequent cycles to a maximum of 250 mg per day for 5 days. If this dose does not produce ovulation, then the next step is therapy with gonadotropins.

22. How do you treat hypothalamic amenorrhea?

The best option is to induce ovulation with gonadotropins. This requires expertise and careful monitoring by a reproductive endocrine specialist since the risks of ovarian hyperstimulation (see Question 24) and multiple pregnancies are significant.

23. How are gonadotropins administered?

Daily injections of FSH or FSH with LH are given. When dominant follicles are evident (by serum estrogen levels and ultrasonography of the ovary), ovulation is induced by injecting human chorionic gonadotropin (hCG).

24. What is ovarian hyperstimulation? What is its incidence with gonadotropin therapy?

In ovarian hyperstimulation, the ovaries are significantly enlarged due to production of an excessive number of follicles. Fluid accumulates in the abdomen, resulting in weight gain, abdominal distension, and possibly severe fluid and electrolyte imbalances. Hospitalization may be required. The incidence is 1–2%.

25. Can hyperstimulation occur with clomiphene?

Yes, but it is extremely rare. In fact, many physicians suggest that back-to-back cycles of clomiphene are acceptable because the ovarian size enlarges only slightly and quickly returns to normal.

26. What is the incidence of multifetal pregnancy after ovarian stimulation with gonadotropins?

The rate varies from 10 to 40%.

27. What are the advantages and disadvantages of GnRH therapy compared with gonadotropin therapy?

Compared to therapy with gonadotropins, GnRH therapy may lead to less frequent ovarian hyperstimulation and may require less intensive monitoring. However, whereas gonadotropin therapy involves daily injections, GnRH therapy requires continuous subcutaneous injections. Women on GnRH therapy must wear a pump for subcutaneous infusion throughout the day.

BIBLIOGRAPHY

1. Adashi EY, Rock JA, Rosenwaks Z (eds): Reproductive Endocrinology, Surgery, and Technology. Vol. 2. Philadelphia, Lippincott Raven, 1996.
2. Barbieri RL. Induction of ovulation in infertile women with hyperandrogenism and insulin resistance. Am J Obstet Gynecol 2000;183:1412–1418.
3. De Moura MD, Ferriani RA, de Sa MF. Effects of clomiphene citrate on pituitary luteinizing hormone and follicle-stimulating hormone release in women before and after treatment with ethinyl estradiol. Fertil Steril 1992;58:504–507.
4. Glueck CJ, Awadalla SG, Phillips H, et al. Polycystic ovary syndrome, infertility, familial thrombophilia, familial hypofibrinolysis, recurrent loss of in vitro fertilized embryos, and miscarriage. Fertil Steril 2000;74:394–397.
5. Glueck CJ, Wang P, Fontaine R. et al. Metformin-induced resumption of normal menses in 39 of 43 (91%) previously amenorrheic women with the polycystic ovary syndrome. Metabolism: Clin Experiment 1999;48:511–519.
6. Gorlitsky GA, Kase NG, Speroff L. Ovulation and pregnancy rates with clomiphene citrate. Obstet Gynecol. 1978;51:265–269.
7. Kessel B, Hsueh AJ. Clomiphene citrate augments follicle-stimulating hormone-induced luteinizing hormone receptor content in cultured rat granulose cells. Fertil Steril 1987;46:334–340.
8. Messinis IE, Milingos SD. Current and future status of ovulation induction in polycystic ovary syndrome. Human Repro Update 1997;3:235–253.
9. Nestler JE. Role of hyperinsulinemia in the pathogenesis of the polycystic ovary syndrome, and its clinical implications. Semin Repro Endo 1997;15:111–122.
10. Nestler JE, Jakubowicz DJ, Evans WS, et al. Effects of metformin on spontaneous and clomiphene-induced ovulation in the polycystic ovary syndrome. New Engl J Med 1998;338:1876–1880.
11. Sozen I, Arici A. Hyperinsulinemia and its interaction with hyperandrogenism in polycystic ovary syndrome. Obstet Gynecol Surv 2000;55:321–328.
12. Speroff L, Glass RH, Kase NG (eds): Clinical Gynecologic Endocrinology and Infertility, 6th ed. Baltimore, Lippincott Williams & Wilkins, 1999.
13. Velazquez E, Acosta A, Mendoza SG. Menstrual cyclicity after metformin therapy in polycystic ovary syndrome. Obstet Gynecol 1997;90:392–395.

14. INFERTILITY

Thomas J. Bader, M.D., and Robert J. Wester, M.D.

1. A couple has sought your opinion concerning infertility? What do you tell them when asked about the chances of becoming pregnant?

The normal fecundability rate—that is, the chance of conception per cycle attempted—is about 0.2 or 20% in normally fertile couples. This figure is particularly useful in trying to understand the success rates (or lack thereof) for treatment modalities offered to infertile couples.

2. Is fecundability in couples related to their age?

Most certainly in women, much less so in men. Studies of pregnancy rates in women (who have azospermic husbands and undergo artificial donor insemination) demonstrate that the success of pregnancy is related to the woman's age. For women under 30 years old, the pregnancy rates were 70–75%, but fell to 60% in women 30–35 years old, and 50% in women over age 36. Other studies of couples having difficulty achieving pregnancy noted infertility rates of 10% in women under age 30, 15% in women 30–35, 30% in women 35–40, and 60% in women over age 40.

3. How is infertility defined? How common is it?

Failure to conceive after 1 year of unprotected intercourse is the general definition of infertility. This problem affects 10–15% of couples of reproductive age (i.e., 15–44 years old).

4. Describe three important goals that a generalist obstetrician-gynecologist may wish to achieve in working with an infertile couple.

Patient education. A couple needs to know the basics of human reproduction, the chances of becoming pregnant, when best to have intercourse, common causes of infertility, investigative tests available, cost and discomfort associated with tests, and therapies available, with expected success rates.

Basic patient evaluation. Essential elements include documentation of ovulation and tubal patency, assessment of peritoneal factors (adhesions and endometriosis), and testing for male factor problems.

Emotional support and guidance. The clinician should counsel the couple on how far to go with tests and procedures, when referral for more elaborate testing and therapy is appropriate, and when to consider adoption.

5. What are the general causes of infertility? How common is each?

Ovulatory dysfunction (10–25%)
Pelvic factors (tubal disease or endometriosis; 30–50%)
Male factor (30–40%)
Cervical factors (5–10%)
Unknown (also called unexplained)

6. What is the difference between primary and secondary infertility?

Primary infertility is a condition in which the woman has never been pregnant despite more than 1 year of unprotected intercourse. A woman with *secondary infertility* has a history of a proven pregnancy (liveborn, ectopic, or abortion), yet is currently unable to conceive after 1 year of unprotected intercourse.

7. What are the characteristics of a normal semen analysis?

Volume > 2 ml
Sperm motility ≥ 50% with active progression

pH of 7.2–7.8
Normal sperm morphology ≥ 30%
Sperm count ≥ 20 million/ml

8. Define unexplained infertility and discuss the treatment options available.

Despite current tests and knowledge, about 10% of couples who have been thoroughly investigated have no demonstrable cause of childlessness. It is appropriate to offer such couples superovulation with gonadotropin therapy and intrauterine insemination after a careful discussion of
the risks, costs, and success rates.

9. A couple has just stopped using birth control and asks for general information about trying to conceive. What information should you provide?

Explain the natural fecundability rate (20% chance per cycle of achieving pregnancy), importance of avoiding smoking and caffeine (both of which may decrease fertility), preconceptional use of folic acid (e.g., prenatal vitamins) to minimize neural tube defects, and information
about the timing of intercourse and when to return if not pregnant.

10. Ovulation dysfunction accounts for 10–15% of infertility. How is the adequacy of ovulation tested?

Presumptive evidence of ovulation can be determined by a biphasic basal body temperature
chart or noted by an elevated progesterone (> 5 ng/ml) in the luteal part of the menstrual cycle.
The basal body temperature is taken first thing in the morning (before getting out of bed). This
temperature is recorded daily. A sustained rise in basal body temperature (> 98°F) in the second
half of the menstrual cycle is consistent with ovulation.

11. Of the causes of infertility, which is most consistently treated with success?

Treatment of ovulation disorders is successful in as many as 80–90% of cases, whereas the
rate of successful treatment for other causes of infertility is closer to 30%.

12. What evidence from a patient's history is suggestive of ovulation?

Menses at regular monthly intervals
Mittelschmerz (localized lower quadrant discomfort during ovulation)
Moliminal symptoms (breast tenderness and pelvic discomfort)
Mild dysmenorrhea

13. Describe the most commonly used ovulation-inducing drug.

Clomiphene citrate is the most commonly used ovulation-inducing drug. It is a weak anti-es-
trogen that works at the hypothalamic level to initiate the changes needed to produce an ovulatory cycle. Complications and side effects include hot flashes, mood swings, multiple pregnancy
(5% twins), ovarian cysts, and, rarely, visual disturbances.

14. Documentation of tubal patency is an important aspect of the infertility work-up. How is this initially done?

A hysterosalpingogram (HSG) is a radiographic procedure performed on an outpatient
basis several days after the onset of menses. A radiopaque dye is injected transcervically into
the uterine cavity. This allows assessment of the endometrial cavity structure, tubal patency, and
tubal architecture.

15. What are the contraindications to an HSG? The possible complications?

Acute pelvic infection is an absolute contraindication. Women with adnexal tenderness
demonstrated on pelvic exam or with a history of pelvic infection may benefit from a course of
antibiotics (e.g., doxycycline) before the procedure. Possible complications include pain (which
can be minimized by premedication with a nonsteroidal agent) and development of acute salpingitis (1–3% of procedures).

16. An HSG can demonstrate various uterine lesions. What are the more common ones?
Intrauterine adhesions
Submucous fibroids
Polyps

17. In choosing a dye for the performance of an HSG, why do most clinicians prefer a water-soluble contrast agent over an oil-based agent?
A water-soluble agent allows ideal visualization of the tubal mucosa, whereas an oil-based media obscures this detail of tubal anatomy.

18. When is it appropriate to offer laparoscopy to an infertile woman?
Laparoscopy allows endoscopic visualization of the internal female anatomy, thereby assessing the pelvis for peritubal or periovarian adhesions, endometriosis, and external structure of the uterus. Generally this test is offered to a woman after male factor and ovulatory functions have been noted to be normal or corrected. If distal tubal occlusion is found, it may be treated laparoscopically. Implants of endometriosis can be diagnosed and treated at the time of laparoscopy.

19. In regards to infertility, what is the best method for removal of a myoma (myomectomy)?
There is no "best" approach. As with all surgical procedures, the surgeon's comfort level and experience are factors in the choice of surgical approach. Myomectomy was originally only performed via an abdominal incision. Now even some large myomas can be removed via the laparoscope. There does not appear to be any difference in future fertility between myomectomy performed via a laparotomy incision and those procedures done via the laparoscope. Submucosal myomas where a significant portion of the tumor projects into the uterine cavity can be removed with the operative hysteroscope. The location of the myoma and the surgeon's assessment will determine which approach is recommended.

20. Do congenital uterine anomalies cause infertility?
There are a variety of congenital uterine anomalies caused by imperfect fusion of the Mullerian duct system. These anomalies range from a muscular septum arising from the uterine fundus and dividing the uterine cavity, to more extreme malformations such as bicornuate uterus where the uterus has two horns. Congenital uterine anomalies are associated with pregnancy loss, but generally are not associated with infertility. However, uterine anomalies may be associated with severe endometriosis, which can impair fertility.

21. How are uterine malformations managed?
The data on management of uterine anomalies is limited due to the fact that there are likely many women with uterine anomalies who never come to medical attention. Even among those women with known uterine anomalies, there is a wide variety of findings and clinical presentations. Treatment is usually reserved for women who have experienced pregnancy loss that is felt to be due to the uterine anomaly.

For women with a **uterine septum**, the accepted therapy is resection of the septum using the hysteroscope. Postoperative treatment of the uterine cavity with high doses of estrogen and/or the insertion of an intrauterine device (IUD) or a foley balloon in hopes of avoiding adhesion formation is sometimes employed. These interventions are probably unnecessary.

The management of a **bicornuate uterus** is controversial. Some advocate reconstruction of the uterus with a procedure such as the Tompkins or Strassman metroplasty. Others feel that prophylactic cerclage is the superior approach. Finally, there are women who have successful pregnancies without either surgical repair or cervical cerclage.

22. Does endometriosis cause infertility?
Although endometriosis is a relatively common gynecologic condition, affecting 5–10% of women, and is a documented cause of pelvic pain and dysmenorrhea, the exact relationship between

endometriosis and infertility is unclear. While mild endometriosis may contribute to infertility in ways that are not entirely understood, severe endometriosis can lead to scarring and distortion of the pelvic anatomy. There is evidence that treatment of even mild endometriosis may enhance fertility.

23. How is endometriosis treated surgically?

When surgery for endometriosis is necessary, it is almost always conducted using the laparoscope. Generally even endometriomas and adhesions can be treated laparoscopically. The method of treatment doesn't seem to impact fertility. Cautery, excision, and laser ablation all have similar effects on fertility.

24. What is the postcoital test?

Within 12 hours of intercourse and at midcycle, a woman's cervical mucus is assessed for quality, quantity, and number of motile sperm. A normal postcoital test demonstrates abundant, clear, watery, and relatively acellular cervical mucus with > 5 motile sperm present per high-powered field.

25. What is the most common cause of an abnormal postcoital test? How helpful is this test in the work-up of an infertile couple?

The most common cause of an abnormal postcoital test is mistiming. The value of the test has been called into question because many normally fertile couples have abnormal tests. Furthermore, the increasing use of intrauterine insemination with ovulation induction makes results of the test of less diagnostic benefit for many couples undergoing investigation of infertility.

26. How does the treatment of proximal and distal tubal disease differ?

In general, the most effective treatment of tubal factor infertility is in-vitro fertilization. However, in some cases surgical repair of tubal disease is possible. It must be noted that tubal surgery places a women at risk for an ectopic pregnancy. Distal tubal disease can be treated with distal salpingostomy, while proximal obstructions can be repaired with hysteroscopic or radiologic tubal canalization. Combination cases of distal and proximal disease should be treated with in vitro fertilization (IVF).

Tubal surgery is most likely to be successful if the tubal mucosa has not undergone significant damage. If the tubal mucosa has been obliterated by tubal disease, IVF is probably the best approach. In addition, if the tubal damage has resulted in the formation of a hydrosalpinx, there is evidence that removal of the tube or tubes improves IVF outcome.

27. What clues in the patient's history should alert the physician to the possibility of tubal factor?

A history of previous ectopic pregnancy, previous tubal surgery, ruptured appendix, tuberculosis, use of an intrauterine device, septic abortion, and sexually transmitted diseases, such as chlamydial infection and gonorrhea. Note that 50% of women with tubal damage and/or pelvic adhesions have no history of these factors.

28. What does the term assisted reproductive technology (ART) mean?

ART refers to any of a variety of procedures involving manipulation of gametes and embryos to treat infertility. Specific procedures include in vitro fertilization, intracytoplasmic sperm injection, gamete intrafallopian transfer, and zygote intrafallopian transfer. It is important to inform patients of the cost, overall success rates (defined as infants delivered), and complications of these procedures.

29. The evaluation of the infertile couple can be divided into three basic or primary tests (for which therapy is available and of proven benefit) and a series of secondary tests, the results of which do not consistently provide evidence of a causal relationship. What are these tests?

In the first group are the tests that should be offered to all couples who fit the definition of infertility: semen analysis to assess male factor, documentation of ovulation, and assessment of tubal patency (HSG). Additional tests that may be appropriate in some women are an assessment of ovarian reserve in women over 35 years of age and laparoscopic evaluation of the pelvis. Depending on the specific abnormality, treatment of these problems may lead to an enhanced pregnancy rate. Alternatively, the information from these tests may direct the couple toward a form of ART.

In the second level of testing are assessment of cervical factor (with the postcoital test), assessment of immunologic factors, luteal phase defects, hamster egg penetration assay, and cultures of the cervix and semen. Treatment of abnormal results of these tests has not proved conclusively to enhance fertility.

BIBLIOGRAPHY

1. Agarwal SKk, Haney AF: Does recommending timed intercourse really help the infertile couple? Obstet Gynecol 84:307, 1994.
2. Al-Inany H: Laparoscopic ablation is not necessary for minimal or mild lesions in endometriosis associated subfertility. Acta Obstet Gynecol Scand 2001;80(7):593–595.
3. Dechaud H, Anahory T, Aligier N, et al: Salpingectomy for repeated embryo nonimplantation after in vitro fertilization in patients with severe tubal factor infertility. J Assist Repro Genet 2000;17(4):200–206.
4. Golan A, Langer R, Neuman M, et al: Obstetric outcome in women with congenital uterine malformations. J Repro Med 1992;37(3):233–236
5. Heinonen PK: Reproductive performance of women with uterine anomalies after abdominal or hysteroscopic metroplasty or no surgical treatment. J Am Assoc Gynecol Laparoscop 1997,4(3).311–317.
6. Homer HA, Li TC, Cooke ID: The septate uterus: A review of management and reproductive outcome. Fert Steril 2000;73(1):1–14.
7. Jones HW Jr, Toner JP: The infertile couple. N Engl J Med 329:1710, 1993.
8. Nawroth F, Schmidt T, Freise C, Foth D, Romer T: Is it possible to recommend an "optimal" postoperative management after hysteroscopic metroplasty? A retrospective study with 52 infertile patients showing a septate uterus. Acta Obstet Gynecol Scand 2002;81(1):55–57.
9. Osuga Y, Koga K, Tsutsumi O, et al: Role of laparoscopy in the treatment of endometriosis-associated infertility. Gynecol Obstet Invest 2002;53 S1:33–39.
10. Rossetti A, Sizzi O, Soranna L, et al: Fertility outcome: Long-term results after laparoscopic myomectomy. Gynecol Endocrin 2001;15(2):129–134.
11. Sammour A, Tulandi T: Laparoscopic fertility-promoting procedures of the fallopian tube and the uterus. Inter J Fert Womens Med 2001;46(3):145–150.
12. Seibel MM: Workup of the infertile couple. In Seibel MM (ed): Infertility: A Comprehensive Text. Norwalk, CT, Appleton & Lange, 1990, pp 1–21.
13. Swerdloff RS, Wang C, Kandee FR: Evaluation of the infertile couple. Endocrinol Metab Clin North Am 17:301, 1988.
14. Tulandi T, al-Took S: Reproductive outcome after treatment of mild endometriosis with laparoscopic excision and electrocoagulation. Fert Steril 1998;69(2):229–231.

15. IN VITRO FERTILIZATION

Arthur J. Castelbaum, M.D.

1. What is in vitro fertilization (IVF)?

IVF is a procedure whereby eggs are fertilized with sperm outside the body. Very few couples undergo other forms of assisted reproductive technologies, such as gamete intrafallopian transfer (GIFT), which involves placement of eggs and sperm in the fallopian tube, or zygote intrafallopian tube transfer (ZIFT), which entails placement of embryos in the fallopian tube.

2. How successful is IVF?

Approximately 25% of couples going through an IVF cycle have a live-born child (Fig. 1). Five percent have a miscarriage or an ectopic (tubal) pregnancy. IVF pregnancies miscarry at rates similar to pregnancies conceived spontaneously.

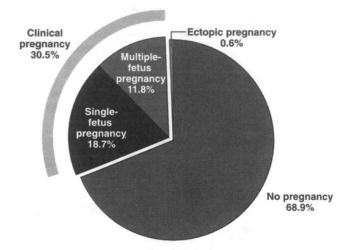

Figure 1. Outcome of assisted reproductive technology cycles. (From Centers for Disease Control and Prevention, et al: 1998 Assisted Reproductive Technology Success Rates. National Summary and Fertility Clinic Reports. Washington DC, U.S. Department of Health and Human Services, 2000. *Note*: All figures in this chapter are from this report.)

3. Is IVF experimental? Is it commonly performed?

IVF is no longer experimental. Use of IVF has increased dramatically since its inception nearly 25 years ago; 60,000 IVF cycles are performed in the United States annually. IVF is now a standard form of infertility therapy. Almost 25% of couples undergoing infertility treatment will require IVF.

4. Are children conceived through IVF normal?

There is a 3% risk of major congenital malformations among children conceived spontaneously or through IVF. There may be a minimally increased risk of chromosomal abnormalities and birth defects among children conceived with intracytoplasmic sperm injection (ICSI), where a single sperm is directly inserted into an egg's cytoplasm.

5. What are the indications for IVF?

With the advent of ICSI, male-factor infertility has been an increasingly common indication for performing IVF. See Fig. 2 for other common indications.

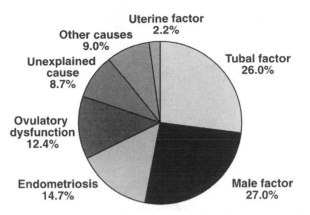

Figure 2. Primary diagnoses among couples undergoing assisted reproductive technology cycles. (From CDC, et al: 1998 Assisted Reproductive Technology Success Rates. Washington DC, U.S. DHHS, 2000.)

6. Does the success rate of IVF vary depending on the reason a couple requires it?

The indication for IVF does not generally confer a better or worse prognosis for establishing a pregnancy (Fig. 3).

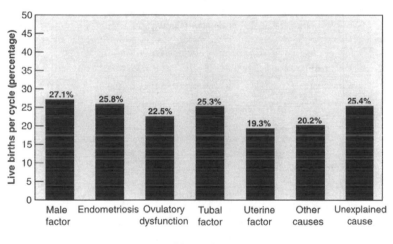

Diagnosis

Figure 3. Live birth rates among women undergoing assisted reproductive technology cycles by primary diagnosis. (From CDC, et al: 1998 Assisted Reproductive Technology Success Rates. Washington DC, U.S. DHHS, 2000.)

7. Is the IVF success rate dependent on maternal age?

Yes. IVF pregnancy rates decline with advancing maternal age (see Fig. 4, top of next page).

8. What screening studies are performed prior to IVF?

- A **semen analysis** evaluates the volume of the ejaculate, the concentration of sperm (normal > 20 million/ml), the percentage of motile sperm (normal > 50%), and morphology (normal appearance).
- **Evaluation of ovarian reserve** is performed in all women undergoing IVF. Serum levels of follicle-stimulating hormone (FSH) are measured on the third day of a menstrual cycle. Women over the age of 30 and those with only one ovary, prior ovarian surgery, or prior

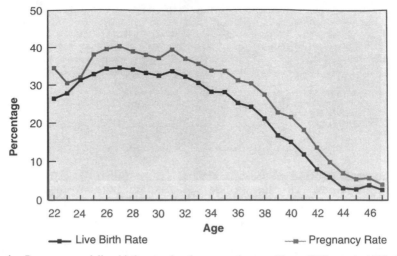

Figure. 4. Pregnancy and live birth rates by the woman's age. (From CDC, et al: 1998 Assisted Reproductive Technology Success Rates. Washington DC, U.S. DHHS, 2000.)

poor response to ovulation induction medication should undergo a clomiphene citrate challenge test. Clomiphene citrate 100 mg is taken daily from the fifth through the ninth day of a menstrual cycle. FSH levels are drawn on days 3 and 10. Women with even a single elevated FSH level have a 1% success rate per cycle with IVF.
• A **hysterosalpingogram, hysteroscopy, or sono-hysterography** assesses the uterine cavity.

9. What options are available to women with advanced maternal age or diminished ovarian reserve?

These couples can expect a 50% pregnancy rate using donor eggs. Eggs can be obtained from known donors (typically sisters and nieces) or anonymous donors. The eggs are fertilized with the husband's sperm and returned to the wife's uterus.

10. What medications are needed to create mature eggs in an IVF cycle?

Most women are made transiently menopausal with a gonadotropin-releasing hormone (GnRH) agonist such as leuprolide (Lupron), started 1 week after ovulation. A second medication with FSH as its active ingredient is then added for approximately 10 days. Medications like Pergonal and Repronex contain FSH derived from the urine of post-menopausal women. Follistim and Gonal-F consist of purified recombinant FSH. These medications are injected by the subcutaneous or intramuscular route. (*See last page for manufacturers.)

11. How are women monitored during an IVF cycle to optimize egg quality and number?

Serial transvaginal ultrasounds of dominant follicles, as well as serum measurements of estradiol and progesterone concentrations, are critical for a successful IVF stimulation. Alterations in dose and duration of medication can be tailored to the individual response of each patient. When the lead follicles reach approximately 18 mm in diameter, with an appropriate estradiol level, human chorionic gonadotropin (hCG) is administered to trigger the resumption of meiosis. Oocyte retrieval is performed approximately 37 hours after the hCG injection.

12. How is the egg retrieval performed?

Ultrasound-guided needle aspiration through the vagina is now routine. Intravenous sedation is used. Risks include blood loss and injury to bowel and bladder. These events are rare.

13. What is intracytoplasmic sperm injection (ICSI)? What are its indications?
Eggs can be fertilized conventionally by incubation with tens of thousands of motile sperm. However, many men have severe abnormalities in sperm count, motility, and morphology. In those cases, ICSI is indicated. A single sperm is injected into a single egg with a microscopic needle. Couples with poor fertilization in previous IVF cycles also benefit from ICSI.

14. Can men with no sperm in their ejaculate father children with ICSI?
Approximately 50% of men with congenital absence of the vas deferens are carriers of the cystic fibrosis gene. In these patients, a testicle can be biopsied and isolated sperm used successfully for ICSI. Similarly, men with no sperm in their ejaculate and patent vas deferens occasionally have a small number of useable sperm in their seminiferous tubules—amenable to testicular biopsy.

15. In a typical IVF cycle, what percentage of eggs are fertilized?
Approximately 70% of eggs fertilize. Only mature eggs, which have matured to meiosis II with formation of a polar body, can undergo ICSI.

16. Do all fertilized eggs develop into quality embryos?
Approximately 30–70% of embryos are chromosomally abnormal, and often do not develop into normal embryos. For that reason, it is common practice to observe many fertilized embryos, picking out only the best-looking ones for uterine transfer.

17. Which embryos benefit from assisted hatching?
The cleaved embryo needs to hatch out of its protective covering, called a zona pellucida, prior to implantation. Some couples benefit from thinning the zona with an acid solution prior to uterine transfer. Thinning is typically beneficial for:
• Reproductively older women
• Women with elevated day 3 FSH levels
• Couples with prior failed IVF cycles
• Subjectively thick zonas.

18. How many embryos are returned to the uterine cavity?
Most programs transfer three or four embryos into the uterus each cycle. In general, more embryos are transferred if they are of lesser quality (Fig. 5).

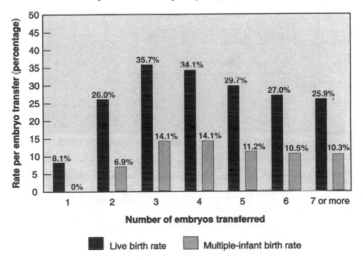

Figure 5. Live-birth and multiple-infant-birth rates for assisted reproductive technology cycles. (From CDC, et al: 1998 Assisted Reproductive Technology Success Rates. Washington DC, U.S. DHHS, 2000.)

19. Are multiple births common with IVF?

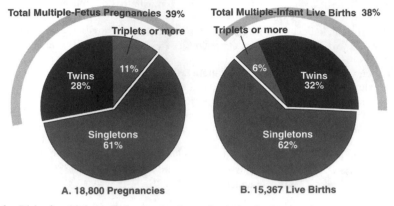

Figure 6. Risk of multiple births from assisted reproductive technology cycles. Many triplets reduce to twin pregnancies spontaneously or via intervention. (From CDC, et al: 1998 Assisted Reproductive Technology Success Rates. Washington DC, U.S. DHHS, 2000.)

20. Can extra embryos be safely frozen?

Ideally, embryos are frozen 1 day after oocyte retrieval at the two-pronuclear stage, or several days later at the blastocyst stage. Embryos must be dehydrated prior to freezing, then rehydrated after thawing. The process can be destructive, and it is not surprising that transfer of frozen embryos is half as successful as using their fresh counterparts. Successful pregnancies have been reported with embryos frozen up to 10 years. Children conceived through frozen embryo transfers do not have any increased risk for congenital anomalies or mental retardation.

21. How can uterine receptivity be optimized in an IVF cycle?

We currently lack a complete understanding of what makes the uterus sticky for an embryo to implant. Because GnRH agonists and oocyte aspiration impair the ovary's ability to produce endogenous progesterone, supplemental progesterone started after oocyte retrieval is standard in all IVF programs. Many patients also receive glucocorticoids, antibiotics, and supplemental injections of hCG in an effort to boost uterine receptivity.

22. What is ovarian hyperstimulation syndrome (OHSS)?

OHSS is an infrequent but potentially severe complication of IVF. It is most commonly seen in young women with very high estradiol concentrations and many intermediate-sized follicles. OHSS usually presents 1 week after oocyte retrieval. It is characterized by ascites, weight gain, and intravascular volume depletion. In severe cases, prerenal azotemia, hemoconcentration, and a hypercoaguable state can be present. Treatment with aggressive hydration is indicated, even if it worsens the ascites. Paracentesis early in the course of OHSS, and repeated as needed, is often indicated.

23. What are the reasons some couples fail to conceive through IVF?

- Less than optimal ovarian stimulation, due to diminished ovarian reserve/advanced maternal age or inappropriate stimulation medication dosing/regimen.
- Poor fertilization
- Poor embryo quality (often noted among women with diminished ovarian reserve and advanced maternal age)
- Poor technique for transferring the embryos into the uterus.

24. What is the maximum number of IVF cycles that a couple should attempt?

In general, IVF success rates do not fall significantly for couples who have failed one or two prior cycles. Significant differences exist between IVF laboratories; therefore, even several prior

IVF failures may not be indicative of a low pregnancy rate with future attempts in a different program. Most couples do not attempt more than three IVF cycles.

CONTROVERSIES

25. Why would you prefer a GnRH agonist or antagonist in an IVF cycle?

GnRH antagonists have the potential to shorten the IVF stimulation protocol, requiring fewer injections and less FSH-containing medication. Women who make few eggs or have high FSH levels may produce more eggs with a GnRH antagonist. Pregnancy rates with GnRH antagonists are similar to the more traditional cycles using GnRH agonists.

26. Should blocked fallopian tubes (hydrosalpinges) be removed prior to IVF?

Despite the fact that IVF bypasses the blocked tubes, their presence often leads to implantation failure. Meta-analyses have suggested that hydrosalpinges lower pregnancy rates by 50%. While many women with blocked tubes conceive through IVF, most practitioners recommend prophylactic salpingectomies prior to IVF.

27. At what stage of development are embryos transferred to the uterus?

Embryos are most often transferred 3 days after oocyte retrieval when they are cleaved into four to eight cells. If embryos are kept in culture until 5–6 days after ooctye retrieval, fewer of these blastocyst-stage embryos are usually transferred. Many IVF programs have had lower pregnancy rates with blastocyst transfers. Successful blastocyst programs may have fewer triplet gestations

28. How can uterine receptivity be evaluated?

Over the past decade, extensive studies evaluating cell adhesion molecules, such as integrins, have been conducted. The endometrial glandular integrin $\alpha v \beta 3$ appears to be closely tied to normal uterine receptivity. It initially appears coincident with the establishment of normal uterine receptivity. $\alpha v \beta 3$ expression is diminished in women suffering from endometriosis, hydrosalpinges, primary unexplained infertility, recurrent pregnancy loss, and polycystic ovarian disease. Note that strategies to optimize uterine receptivity allow for transfer of fewer embryos.

*Question 10: Personal and Gonal-F are made by Serono; Repronex is made by Ferring; Follistim is made by Organon.

BIBLIOGRAPHY

1. Castelbaum AJ, Lessey BA: Infertility and implantation defects. Infertil Reprod Med Clin North Am 12:427–446, 2001.
2. Fluker M, Grifo J, Leader A, et al: Efficacy and safety of ganirelix acetate versus leuprolide acetate in women undergoing controlled ovarian hyperstimulation. Fertil Steril 75:38–45, 2001.
3. Karande VC, Morris R, Chapman C, et al: Impact of the "physician factor" on pregnancy rates in a large assisted reproductive technology program: Do too many cooks spoil the broth? Fertil Steril 71:998–1000, 1999.
4. Langley MT, Marek DM, Gardner DK, et al: Extended embryo culture in human assisted reproduction treatments. Hum Reprod 16:902–8, 2001.
5. Nackley AC, Muasher SJ: The significance of hydrosalpinx in in vitro fertilization. Fertil Steril 70:787–788, 1998.
6. Scott RT Jr, Hofmann GE: Prognostic assessment of ovarian reserve. Fertil Steril 63:1–11, 1995.
7. U.S. Department of Health and Human Services: 1998 Assisted Reproductive Technology Success Rates. National summary and fertility clinic reports. Washington DC, DHHS, Centers for Disease Control and Prevention. December 2000.

16. PELVIC ORGAN PROLAPSE

Catherine S. Bradley, M.D., and Lily A. Arya, M.D., M.S.

1. Describe pelvic organ prolapse.

Pelvic organ prolapse (also called pelvic relaxation) is the prolapse or protrusion of pelvic structures into the vaginal canal. It results from weakening or damage to pelvic support structures, which can occur generally throughout the vagina or at specific sites. Common clinical terms for prolapse include cystocele, uterine prolapse, vault prolapse, enterocele, and rectocele.

2. What is a cystocele?

A cystocele is the protrusion of the bladder into the vagina and beyond. It appears as a protrusion of the anterior vaginal wall (Fig. 1).

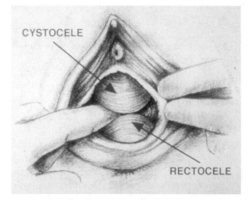

Figure 1. Cystocele and rectocele. Courtesy of Milex Products, Inc. Chicago, Illinois

3. What is uterine prolapse? What is procidentia?

Uterine prolapse is descent of the uterus into the vagina and beyond. Procidentia is a more advanced form of uterine prolapse, when the entire uterus has prolapsed outside the introitus.

4. What is vaginal vault prolapse?

Vaginal vault prolapse is the prolapse of the vaginal apex in a patient who has had a hysterectomy. It appears as a protrusion of the top of the vagina into the vagina or beyond.

5. What is an enterocele?

An enterocele is prolapse of the small bowel into the vagina. It appears as a protrusion of the upper or posterior vagina into the lower vagina or beyond.

6. What is a rectocele?

A rectocele is prolapse of the rectum behind the posterior vaginal wall. It appears as a protrusion of the posterior vaginal wall into the vagina and beyond (see Fig. 1).

7. List the causes of pelvic organ prolapse. When does it occur?

Many factors can lead to a loss of pelvic support and the development of prolapse. The most important risk factor for prolapse is a history of vaginal childbirth. Vaginal delivery of an infant stretches the birth canal and may damage or weaken pelvic support structures. Genetic factors also predispose to the development of prolapse. Pelvic organ prolapse is more common in Caucasian women than in black or Asian women, although the reasons for this association are still unknown. Chronic and repetitive increases in intra-abdominal pressure related to chronic constipation, chronic coughing, obesity, ascites, and strenuous physical activity increase the risk.

Although prolapse can occur at almost any age, it is more common in women older than 40. This is likely due to a generalized weakening of supporting tissues with age, as well as a loss of hormonal support after menopause.

8. How common is pelvic organ prolapse?

Pelvic organ prolapse is very common, but accurate prevalence rates are unknown. It has been estimated that up to 50% of all parous women lose some pelvic support, and 10–20% of them seek care for prolapse. Prolapse is one of the most common indications for gynecologic surgery. One study has shown that women have an 11% risk of undergoing surgery to repair pelvic organ prolapse or urinary incontinence in their lifetime.

9. Which structures provide normal pelvic support?

Pelvic support structures include both muscles and fascia of the pelvic floor, which close the pelvic outlet and surround the external vaginal opening, the urethra, and the anal canal.

10. What is the pelvic floor?

The levator ani (including the puborectalis, pubococcygeus and iliococcygeus muscles) and the coccygeus muscles form the pelvic floor. These muscles create a hammock-like sling between the pubis and coccyx, and are attached laterally along the pelvic sidewalls. The levator ani muscle is tonically contracted, providing a firm shelf posteriorly to support the pelvic contents and aiding with urinary and fecal continence.

11. Define endopelvic fascia.

Endopelvic fascia is a loose network of connective tissue, containing small vessels, lymphatics, and nerves, that surrounds the pelvic organs and the vagina. Historically, thicker areas of the endopelvic fascia in the pelvis have been described as ligaments, such as the cardinal and uterosacral ligaments, which help to support the uterus and cervix. The supportive endopelvic fascia that separates the vagina from the bladder and from the rectum is called *pubovesical* and *rectovaginal* fascia, respectively. Many experts believe that discreet breaks in the endopelvic fascia that lines the vagina lead directly to prolapse in those areas.

12. What are the symptoms associated with pelvic organ prolapse?

Mild forms of prolapse are usually asymptomatic and identified only on physical exam. The most common symptom of prolapse is a bulge of tissue protruding from the vaginal opening; it may interfere with sitting or walking. Some women with pelvic organ prolapse report pelvic pressure, especially after prolonged standing. Prolapse may interfere with sexual intercourse. Longstanding prolapse that protrudes beyond the introitus may result in ulceration and bleeding from the prolapsed vaginal skin. Advanced forms of prolapse may also cause difficulty with urination or defecation, and urinary or fecal incontinence are often associated with the disorder.

13. How is pelvic organ prolapse evaluated?

Pelvic organ prolapse is evaluated by pelvic examination in both the lithotomy and standing positions. The patient is asked to strain or to perform a Valsalva maneuver during the examination, which often demonstrates a higher grade of prolapse than seen at rest.

14. How is prolapse graded?

One common prolapse grading system classifies prolapse by the underlying pelvic organ and its location in relation to the hymen (Table 1). The POP-Q (pelvic organ prolapse quantification) exam is a more standardized classification system that identifies several points within the vagina and measures the distance of each point from the vaginal hymen. Measurements of the perineal body and genital hiatus are also included.

Table 1. *A Classification System for Pelvic Organ Prolapse*

Grade 0	No prolapse
Grade 1	Descent halfway to the hymen
Grade 2	Descent to the hymen
Grade 3	Descent halfway past the hymen
Grade 4	Maximum possible descent for each site

15. What nonsurgical treatments are available for pelvic organ prolapse?

The finding of asymptomatic pelvic organ prolapse on exam does not require treatment. However, if the patient is symptomatic, conservative treatments are usually recommended for milder grades of prolapse. These may include pelvic floor muscle exercises (Kegel exercises), which contract the pubococcygeus muscles isometrically to achieve increased strength and bulk. Estrogen replacement therapy may improve minor degrees of pelvic relaxation or slow the progression of mild prolapse. A pessary can be placed to support the prolapsed vagina. Finally, patients should avoid exacerbating factors by losing weight, limiting heavy lifting, and treating constipation or conditions that lead to a chronic cough.

16. What are pessaries?

Pessaries are supportive vaginal devices, usually made from inert materials such as silicone, that are designed to be placed into the vagina to return and hold pelvic structures in their normal position. Pessaries are used when surgery is not elected or contraindicated. They can also be used as temporary treatment in a patient awaiting a surgical procedure. Pessaries are very effective in relieving symptoms of pelvic organ prolapse.

A wide variety of pessary shapes and sizes is available (Figs. 2 and 3). Commonly used devices are the ring, donut, and Gellhorn pessaries. A careful fitting by an experienced healthcare provider is important to avoid complications related to poor sizing, such as urethral obstruction or vaginal erosion. The pessary must be removed and cleaned regularly, either by the patient or by her healthcare provider, every 2–3 months. Side effects include urinary tract or vaginal infections and vaginal odor, discharge, or bleeding. Some women with severe laxity of the pelvic floor may not be able to retain a pessary successfully.

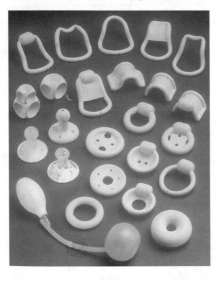

Figure 2. Vaginal pessaries. Courtesy of Milex Products, Inc. Chicago, Illinois

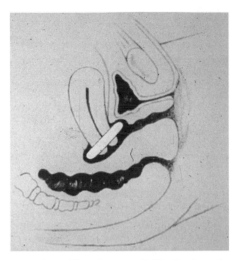

Figure 3. Ring pessary in position. Courtesy of Milex Products, Inc. Chicago, Illinois

17. What types of surgery are performed for pelvic organ prolapse?

Many different surgeries are used to repair prolapse and pelvic support defects (Table 2). Most procedures are performed from a vaginal approach, although they may also be performed through an abdominal incision or laparoscopically. Typically, several procedures are combined, since prolapse tends to occur at more than one site in most patients. For instance, a vaginal hysterectomy and paravaginal repair may be performed for a patient with both uterine prolapse and a cystocele. Patients with genuine stress incontinence may need a concomitant anti-incontinence procedure as well. In patients with severe or recurrent prolapse, a graft (either natural or synthetic) may be placed under the vaginal wall to increase longevity of the surgical repair.

Table 2. *Common Surgical Procedures for the Treatment of Pelvic Organ Prolapse*

DEFECT LOCATION	CLINICAL CONDITION	PROCEDURES
Anterior	Cystocele	Anterior colporrhapy Paravaginal repair
Superior	Uterine prolapse	Hysterectomy Colpocleisis
	Enterocele	Vaginal enterocele repair McCall culdeplasty Abdominal enterocele repair (Halban or Moschcowitz procedures)
	Vault prolapse	Uterosacral ligament suspension Sacrospinous ligament suspension Abdominal sacral colpopexy
Posterior	Rectocele	Posterior colporrhaphy Rectovaginal fascia defect repair
Perineal body	Perineal body defect	Perineoplasty

18. What is colpocliesis? When is it indicated?

Colpocleisis is the surgical obliteration of the vagina. It is indicated for the treatment of severe uterine or vaginal vault prolapse in the elderly woman who no longer desires to retain sexual function. Colpocleisis can be performed under local anesthesia and is a relatively short procedure, so it is also indicated in women with prolapse who have medical contraindications to general or regional anesthesia.

BIBLIOGRAPHY

1. American College of Obstetricians and Gynecologists: Pelvic Organ Prolapse. ACOG Tech Bull Number 214, 1995.
2. Baden WF, Walker TR: Fundamentals, symptoms, and classification. In Baden WF, Walker TR (eds): Surgical Repair of Vaginal Defects. Philadelphia, JB Lippincott Co., 1992.
3. Bump RC, Mattiasson A, Bo K, et al: The standardization of terminology of female pelvic organ prolapse and pelvic floor dysfunction. Am J Obstet Gynecol 175:10, 1996.
4. DeLancey JOL: Anatomy and biomechanics of genital prolapse. Clin Obstet Gynecol 36: 897, 1993.
5. Olsen AL, Smith VJ, Bergstrom JO, et al: Epidemiology of surgically managed pelvic organ prolapse and urinary incontinence. Obstet Gynecol 89:501, 1997.
6. Wall LL: Incontinence, prolapse, and disorders of the pelvic floor. In Berek JS, Adashi EY, Hillard PA (eds): Novak's Gynecology, 12th ed. Baltimore, William & Wilkins, 1996, pp 619–676.

17. URINARY INCONTINENCE

Lily A. Arya, M.D., M.S., and Catherine S. Bradley, M.D., MSCE

1. Define urinary incontinence.

Incontinence is defined as involuntary urine loss that is a social or hygienic problem. Urinary incontinence is two to three times more common in women than in men, and the prevalence increases with age. Its presence has a significant effect on the quality of life of women, and it is a leading cause of admission of elderly women to nursing homes.

A myriad of etiologies can be responsible for incontinence. Two common causes that gynecologists are asked to diagnose and treat are stress (50–70% cases) and detrusor instability or mixed causes (20–40%). Less common causes are bladder overdistension and genitourinary fistulas.

2. What is genuine stress incontinence (GSI)?

Stress incontinence (also called genuine stress incontinence) is loss of urine due to **increased intra-abdominal pressure**. Urethral hypermobility following childbirth is the most common cause of GSI. Normally, the vagina is attached bilaterally to the pelvic diaphragm, providing a stable base on which the bladder neck and proximal urethra rest. This positioning allows increases in intra-abdominal pressure to be transmitted equally to the bladder and urethra, maintaining urethral closure and continence. In women with urethral hypermobility, there is descent of the proximal urethra and bladder neck such that these structures are no longer compressed against the vagina during increased intra-abdominal pressure, and leakage of urine occurs.

In a subset of patients with severe GSI, there is **weakness of the internal urethral sphincter**, resulting in intrinsic sphincter deficiency. In these women, stress incontinence occurs with minimal exertion or even at rest. Common causes are advanced age, prior bladder neck surgery, and radiation treatment.

3. What is detrusor instability (DI)?

Detrusor instability, also called overactive bladder, is a condition in which the bladder contracts involuntarily in response to filling. It was called detrusor dyssynergia in the past. It commonly presents as **urge incontinence**—leakage of urine associated with a strong desire to void. No cause is identified in more than 90% of these patients. Advancing age is an important risk factor. Detrusor instability caused by neurologic diseases such as cerebrovascular disease, multiple sclerosis, or spinal cord injury is called *detrusor hyperreflexia*. Irritation of the bladder by inflammation (such as urinary tract infection) or prior pelvic surgery can also cause detrusor instability.

4. What is overflow incontinence?

Overflow incontinence is involuntary loss of urine following **overdistension of the bladder**. Overflow incontinence, usually short-term, can occur after vaginal delivery—especially if epidural anesthesia was used. Other causes include diabetes, neurological diseases, severe genital prolapse, and postsurgical obstruction.

5. What is continuous incontinence?

This is continuous leakage of urine such as that caused by genitourinary fistulas. These fistulas may be congenital, or may follow pelvic surgery or radiation.

6. Which aspects of the patient's history are important in differentiating GSI and DI?

With GSI, the patient often complains of loss of urine with *physical activity*, such as coughing, sneezing, climbing stairs, laughing, bouncing, and intercourse. Urine loss is instantaneous. In DI, women typically complain of *urgency* followed by a large loss of urine.

Voiding logs can be helpful in the history. The patient keeps track of the number of times per day that she urinates, oral intake, urine output, and timing of any involuntary urine loss. In taking a history, carefully review systems to identify the causes of incontinence listed in Questions 2–5.

7. List the significant physical findings.

The physical exam is performed to rule out other causes of incontinence. In patients with GSI, a pelvic exam typically reveals evidence of pelvic relaxation, such as cystocele, rectocele, or uterine prolapse. A cystocele is often associated with GSI; however, it does not cause incontinence. A pelvic mass also may contribute to GSI. It is frequently possible to demonstrate GSI when the patient coughs with a full bladder. In postmenopausal women, pay attention to the estrogen status of the vagina and bladder, because estrogen deficiency can contribute to incontinence. Remember, too, that a neurologic examination is essential in evaluating urinary stress incontinence.

8. What laboratory tests are helpful in evaluating incontinence?

Postvoid residual is an easy initial test to obtain. After the patient voids, in general, there should be less than 50 ml of urine in the bladder. Postvoid residual is measured by ultrasound or catheterizing the patient in the office. A patient with an elevated postvoid residual (repeat measurements greater than 100–200 ml) may have an underlying neurologic disorder. The presence of an elevated postvoid residual is a relative contraindication to surgical treatment of GSI and to anticholinergic medications for DI. Catheterization also provides a good opportunity to obtain urine for analysis and culture.

Urinalysis and urine culture help to diagnose urinary tract infection. Blood work is required only if compromised renal function, diabetes, syphilis, or other systemic diseases are suspected.

9. Which tests are *most* helpful in differentiating between GSI and DI?

A **cystometrogram** involves filling the bladder to measure volume-pressure relationships. As the bladder is filled to its normal capacity of 300–500 ml, the pressure inside the bladder should remain low. The patient usually experiences the first urge to void at 150–200 ml. Patients with DI often have reduced bladder capacity (< 300 ml) and demonstrate urinary incontinence that is associated with involuntary bladder contractions (pressure increase above baseline). In patients with GSI, incontinence is demonstrated when the patients coughs or strains (e.g., Valsalva maneuver). The intravesical pressure at which leakage is noted (leak point pressure) is generally < 60 cm of water pressure if intrinsic sphincter deficiency is present.

Cystoscopy should be performed especially in patients with irritative bladder symptoms such as urgency, frequency, and hematuria to rule out inflammation, tumors, or anatomic deformities.

10. Which tests are *less* helpful in differentiating between GSI and DI?

The **Q-tip test** checks urethral motility. A sterile Q-tip swab is placed in the urethra to a depth of 3 cm to evaluate the angle between the urethra and bladder. In women with a positive test, the angle of the Q-tip changes by > 35° on Valsalva maneuver. This is considered to be evidence of poor bladder neck support, but it is not a reliable test; all patients with GSI do not have a positive test (see table). Even women without incontinence can have a positive test.

The **Marshall test** assesses pelvic support. The tips of a Kelly clamp are placed on each side of the urethra to restore the urethra to its normal anatomic position. If incontinence is corrected, the test is believed to be positive for GSI, and the patient is judged a good candidate for surgical correction. Current studies show that the Marshall test causes obstruction of the urethra and is not helpful in differentiating between GSI and DI.

11. What are indications for more extensive testing with multichannel urodynamics?

These urological tests can simultaneously record urethral, vesical, and intra-abdominal pressures as well as electromyographic activity of the pelvic musculature. They can be used to confirm the type of incontinence in a patient with mixed incontinence symptoms or for whom prior continence procedures have failed. Multichannel urodynamics should be done for patients with stress incontinence prior to surgical correction and in patients with urge incontinence not responsive to medical therapy.

The presence of DI in a woman with a suggestive history but negative simple cystometry should be further evaluated. Intrinsic sphincter dysfunction can be diagnosed or the voiding mechanism can be determined to attempt to predict which patients may experience postoperative urinary retention.

Differential Diagnosis and Treatment of Urinary Incontinence

	DETRUSOR INSTABILITY	GSI WITH URETHRAL HYPERMOBILITY	INTRINSIC SPHINCTER DEFICIENCY
Basic pathology	Irritable detrusor muscle	Loss of support to UVJ	Weakness of urethral sphincter
Symptoms	Urge incontinence, frequency, urgency, nocturia	Stress incontinence	Stress incontinence with minimal exertion, large volume leaks
Q tip test	No characteristic finding	Hypermobility of UVJ (Q tip > 35)	Hypermobility of UVJ, fixed scarred urethra if due to prior surgery
Findings on cystometrogram	Involuntary detrusor contractions	Leak point pressure (> 60 cm of water pressure)	Leak point pressure (< 60 cm of water pressure)
Treatment	Bladder training, pelvic muscle rehabilitation, medications (anti-cholinergics).	Pelvic muscle rehabilitation, surgery	Pelvic muscle rehabilitation, bladder training, medications, surgery

GSI = genuine stress incontinence, UVJ = urethrovesical junction

12. Describe medical treatments that are available for genuine stress incontinence.

No good medical treatment exists for GSI with urethral hypermobility. Oral or vaginal estrogen may have some limited benefit in postmenopausal women with stress or mixed incontinence. Phenylpropanolamine (an alpha-adrenergic agonist) is useful for mild GSI caused by sphincteric deficiency. Pelvic muscle rehabilitation (Kegel exercises with or without biofeedback and/or electrical stimulation) is helpful in controlling symptoms. Behavioral modification (fluid intake regulation, improving accessibility to toilet for patients with limited mobility, and change of medications such as diuretics) is also useful.

13. What medical treatments are available for detrusor instability?

Bladder contractions are caused by stimulation of the parasympathetic nervous system, which is mainly accomplished through the release of acetylcholine. Therefore, anticholinergics are often successful in controlling DI. Examples include oxybutynin, tolterodine, propantheline, and imipramine. Imipramine is advantageous in treating mixed stress incontinence and DI because of its combined alpha-adrenergic and anticholinergic properties.

Estrogen replacement in postmenopausal women may improve urgency, but has not been conclusively shown to reduce urge incontinence. Bladder training (to suppress urgency and prolong the interval between voids) and behavioral modification are also useful.

14. Which surgical repairs are best for GSI?

Surgical management of genuine stress incontinence can be divided into: (1) procedures that restore the anatomic support of the proximal urethra and the urethrovesical junction in women with hypermobility and normal intrinsic urethral sphincter, and (2) procedures designed to compensate for a poorly functioning urethral sphincter (intrinsic sphincter deficiency). Over the past century, a large number of different surgical repairs have been used to correct GSI. No one method has proved to be best.

Abdominal and vaginal procedures use different techniques to resuspend the urethrovesical angle in its normal anatomic position. Abdominal approaches include the Burch procedure (attaches vagina to the Cooper's or the pectineal ligament) and the Marshall-Marchetti-Krantz procedure. The Burch procedure may be performed laparoscopically. Older vaginal approaches include the Pereyra, Raz, and Stamey procedures; newer vaginal approaches have been developed using the Cooper's ligament.

For intrinsic sphincter deficiency, a sling is placed under the urethra to support it. Periurethral collagen injections under local anesthesia are used to treat intrinsic sphincter deficiency in women unwilling or unable to tolerate surgery. Experimental techniques include artificial sphincters and Teflon injections.

15. What are the surgical outcomes?

The traditional vaginal approach to stress incontinence has been the Kelly plication, but recent studies have suggested that it does not provide adequate long-term support of the urethrovesical junction. The cure rate for stress incontinence following anterior colporrhaphy (for cystocele) is only 40%.

Treatment of stress urinary incontinence resulting from urethral hypermobility is best performed with the Marshall-Marchetti-Krantz or Burch procedure, both of which have an overall success rate of 85%. Surgical failures often result from inadequate preoperative evaluation of the cause of incontinence.

The success rate of the suburethral sling procedure to treat intrinsic urethral sphincter dysfunction is 80–90%. Periurethral bulking injections with GAX-collagen have a lower success rate of 45–65%.

BIBLIOGRAPHY

1. Agency of Health Care Policy and Research: Urinary Incontinence in Adults: Acute and Chronic Management. Clinical Practice Guideline No. 2. AHCPR Publication no. 96-0682. Rockville, MD, U.S. Department of Health and Human Services, 1996, pp 5–73.
2. American Urogynecologic Society: Diagnosis of the Incompetent Urethral Sphincteric Mechanism. Quarterly report. Vol XVIV No. 2, Summer 2000.
3. Nichols DH, Randal CL: Choice of operation for urinary stress incontinence. In Nichols DH, Randal CT (eds): Vaginal Surgery, 4th ed. Baltimore, Williams & Wilkins, 1996.
4. Walters MD, Newton ER: Pathophysiology and obstetric issues of genuine stress incontinence and pelvic floor dysfunction. In Walters MD, Karram MM (eds): Urogynecology and Reconstructive Pelvic Surgery, 2nd ed. St. Louis, MO, Mosby, 1999, pp 135–143.

18. SPONTANEOUS ABORTIONS

Yu-Hsin Wu, M.D.

1. What is the incidence and differential diagnosis of vaginal bleeding in the first trimester?

Approximately 30% of women bleed during the first trimester of pregnancy. The differential diagnosis includes threatened abortion, ectopic pregnancy, abnormal pregnancy, vaginal lesions, increased friability of the cervix, and infections.

2. What is the risk of miscarriage for patients who have first-trimester bleeding?

About 50% of women who experience first-trimester bleeding will spontaneously abort. Those who do not miscarry may have a slightly increased incidence of fetal anomalies, preterm birth, and fetal growth restriction.

3. What percentage of pregnancies end in a miscarriage?

Of all *clinically* recognized pregnancies, 15–20% end in a miscarriage. However, the incidence of total human embryonic loss is much greater. Up to 40% of all human embryos fail to implant or are aborted before the time of expected menses, resulting in spontaneous miscarriage of a *subclinical* pregnancy. When considering clinical and subclinical pregnancies, approximately 50% of all pregnancies end in miscarriage.

4. What is the definition of an abortion?

An abortion can either be spontaneous or induced. It is defined as:
- A termination of pregnancy before 20 weeks gestation as calculated from the date of onset of last menses, or
- Delivery of a fetus weighing < 500 grams.

5. When do most clinical spontaneous abortions occur?

Approximately 80% of spontaneous abortions, or miscarriages, occur in the first trimester. The incidence of miscarriage decreases with increasing gestational age. Once embryonic cardiac activity is seen sonographically at 6 weeks' gestation, the subsequent abortion rate is 6–8%. Once fetal viability is confirmed at 8 weeks' gestation, the abortion rate is only 2–3%.

6. What causes spontaneous abortions?

The causes for spontaneous abortions can be divided into two categories: genetic and environmental (see table). Overall, genetic abnormalities account for 50–70% of spontaneous abortions, with decreasing incidence as gestation progresses. Fetal chromosomal abnormalities cause 70% of first-trimester miscarriages and 30% of second-trimester miscarriages, but only 3% of stillbirths. Also note that the incidence of a chromosomally abnormal abortus markedly increases after a maternal age of 35 years.

Causes of Spontaneous Abortion

Genetic Causes	
Trisomy, polyploidy/aneuploidy, translocations	
Environmental Causes	
Uterine	Congenital uterine anomalies
	Leiomyoma
	Intrauterine adhesions or synechiae

(*Table continued on next page.*)

Causes of Spontaneous Abortion (cont.)

Environmental Causes (cont.)	
Cervical	Incompetent cervix
Endocrine	Progesterone deficiency (inadequate luteal phase) Thyroid disease (uncontrolled) Diabetes mellitus (uncontrolled) Hypersecretion of LH
Immunologic	Autoimmunity: antiphospholipid syndrome, SLE Alloimmunity
Infections	*Toxoplasma gondii, Listeria monocytogenes, Chlamydia trachomatis, Ureaplasma urealyticum, Mycoplasma hominis,* herpes simplex, *Treponema pallidum, Borrelia burgdorferi, Neisseria gonorrhoea, Streptococcus agalactiae*
Toxins	Alcohol, caffeine, smoking Anesthetic gases High doses of radiation Medications (methotrexate, misoprostol, tretinoin)

LH = luteinizing hormone, SLE = systemic lupus erythematosus

7. What is the most common type of chromosomal anomaly found in spontaneously aborted fetuses?

Autosomal trisomies are the most common type of chromosomal abnormality found in aborted fetuses. They result from nondisjunction during meiosis and account for about half of the abnormal karyotypes found in fetal wastage. **Trisomy 16** is the most common trisomy found (accounts for about one-third of trisomies).

8. What is the single most common karyotype seen in spontaneously aborted fetuses?

Monosomy X or 45, XO is the single most common karyotype seen in fetal wastage. It is found in 10–20% of aborted fetuses that have a chromosomal anomaly.

9. Describe the different types of abortions. How is each initially managed?

TYPE	DEFINITION	MANAGEMENT
Complete Abortion	Spontaneous expulsion of all fetal and placental tissue from uterus prior to 20 weeks' gestation. Cervix closed on examination.	No further intervention necessary; ultrasound to confirm an empty uterus may sometimes be helpful.
Incomplete Abortion	Passage of some fetal or placental tissue, but not all, from uterus prior to 20 weeks' gestation. Cervix dilated on examination.	IV hydration, type and screen/cross, immediate suction curettage
Threatened Abortion	Uterine bleeding prior to 20 weeks' gestation, without any cervical dilation or effacement.	Ultrasound to document fetal viability; modified activity and pelvic rest until bleeding stops
Inevitable Abortion	Uterine bleeding prior to 20 weeks' gestation, accompanied by cervical dilation, but no expulsion of fetal or placental tissue through cervical os.	Expectant management or evacuation of pregnancy (surgical or medical termination)

(Table continued on next page.)

TYPE	DEFINITION	MANAGEMENT
Missed Abortion	Fetal death before 20 weeks' gestation without explusion of any fetal or maternal tissue for at least 8 weeks thereafter.	Suction curettage or medical termination of pregnancy
Septic Abortion	Any of the abortions above, accompanied by uterine infection.	IV antibiotics followed by suction curettage

10. How do I clinically differentiate between the different types of abortions when a woman presents with vaginal bleeding?

History: Last menstrual period? How much bleeding and for how long? Cramping? Passage of fetal tissue? Fever, chills, abdominal tenderness?

Exam: Temperature and vital signs? Abdominal tenderness? Rebound and/or guarding?
  • Speculum exam: tissue at os? Purulent discharge?
  • Bimanual exam: Cervix—closed or dilated? cervical motion tenderness? Uterus—size? tenderness? Adnexa—masses? tenderness?

Labs: CBC—hemoglobin, white cell count, platelets. Type and screen—Rh status (Rh-negative patients need Rho[D] immunoglobulin [e.g., RhoGAM]); blood typed if transfusion necessary. βhCG—serial levels can help make the diagnosis.

Ultrasound: An intrauterine pregnancy with βhCG > 1500 mIU/mL should be visualized by transvaginal ultrasound; with a βhCG > 6000 mIU/mL, by transabdominal ultrasound.

Diagnostic flowchart (US = ultrasound):

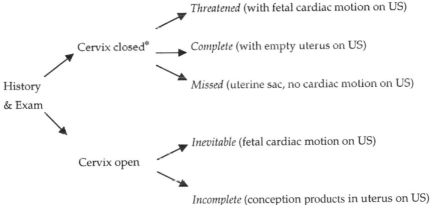

Threatened (with fetal cardiac motion on US)

Cervix closed* ———→ *Complete* (with empty uterus on US)

History & Exam

Missed (uterine sac, no cardiac motion on US)

Cervix open

Inevitable (fetal cardiac motion on US)

Incomplete (conception products in uterus on US)

*Don't forget that ectopic pregnancy must be ruled out!

11. What is the utility of quantitative hCG measurement in a patient with a threatened miscarriage?

In a normal viable pregnancy, the βhCG level should double every 48 hours. In patients with abnormal gestation or ectopic pregnancy, the βhCG level would be slowly rising, plateauing, or dropping.

12. Which patients with miscarriage should receive RhoGAM?

All patients who are Rh negative and experience vaginal bleeding due to miscarriage or ectopic pregnancy should receive Rhogam. If the patient is at < 12 weeks' gestation, she should receive MICRhoGAM (50 mcg). After 12 weeks' gestation, a full dose of RhoGAM (300 mcg) should be administered IM.

13. What is the definition of recurrent pregnancy loss?
Recurrent pregnancy loss (RPL) is classically defined as three or more *consecutive* spontaneous abortions.

14. When should evaluation of recurrent pregnancy loss begin?
Generally, evaluation is begun after three consecutive losses. However, it sometimes is begun after two consecutive losses, depending on the patient's age and level of concern.

15. How often is an identifiable cause for recurrent pregnancy loss found?
An identifiable cause is found in 50–60% of cases.

16. What is the differential diagnosis for RPL?
Genetic factors
Anatomic abnormalities of the uterus
Endocrine disorders: uncontrolled diabetes or thyroid dysfunction, luteal phase deficiency
Autoimmune disorders: antiphospholipid syndrome, lupus anticoagulant
Alloimmune disorders
Environmental causes: alcohol, tobacco, anesthetic agents
Infectious causes: *Ureaplasma urealyticum, Mycoplasma hominis*
Thrombophilias

17. What does the initial work-up for RPL include?
• Karyotype of both parents and/or products of conception to rule out genetic factors
• Labs to rule out endocrine factors: TSH, serum glucose, prolactin, luteal phase assessment
  (progesterone levels and endometrial biopsy)
• Ultrasound or hysterosalphingogram to rule out uterine abnormalities

18. What is a luteal phase defect?
A luteal phase defect is attributed to deficient secretion of progesterone by the corpus luteum early in pregnancy, resulting in inadequate stimulation of the endometrium. Many attempts have been made to link low levels of progesterone to RPL, and subsequently use exogenous progesterone supplementation to decrease rates of RPL. However, these attempts have been unsuccessful and many specialists doubt the existence of this "syndrome" as a cause.

19. How is a luteal phase defect (LPD) diagnosed and treated?
The diagnosis is made with two endometrial biopsies done 7 days after ovulation which show a lag in histological development of more than 2 days. In addition, two other diagnostic methods can suggest LPD: (1) A basal body temperature chart showing a luteal phase of less than 11 days, and (2) a serum progesterone level < 10 ng/ml 1 week after ovulation.

Treatment is by progesterone replacement. No well-controlled studies provide convincing evidence that exogenous replacement works, but there is likewise no evidence that harm may be incurred.

20. What is the chance of a live birth after two consecutive miscarriages? After three consecutive miscarriages?
After two consecutive miscarriages, the chance of a live birth is about 70–75%. After three consecutive losses with a previous live birth, the chance of a subsequent live birth is 70%. After three consecutive losses without a previous live birth, the chance of a live birth is 50–65%.

21. Describe the proposed mechanism of antiphospholipid antibody and lupus anticoagulant in RPL.
These antibodies block prostocyclin formation (a vasodilatior and inhibitor of platelet aggregation), resulting in thromboxane excess. Thromboxane is a potent vasoconstrictor that promotes platelet aggregation, and its excess can lead to increased risk of thrombosis and therefore RPL.

22. How are patients with antiphospholipid syndrome and lupus anticoagulant treated during pregnancy?

Generally these patients are placed on a low-dose aspirin (75–80 mg). Depending on the situation, subcutaneous heparin is sometimes added. Studies show that adding corticosteriods to aspirin or heparin does not produce additional benefit.

BIBLIOGRAPHY

1. American College of Obstetricians and Gynecologists, Committee on Technical Bulletins: Early Pregnancy Loss. ACOG Technical Bulletin No. 212. Washington, DC, ACOG, 1995.
2. Mishell DR, Stenchever MA, Droegemueller W, Herbst AL: Comprehensive Gynecology, 8th ed. St. Louis, Mosby-Year Book, Inc., 1997, pp 403–430.
3. Scroggins KM, Smucker WD, Krishen AE: Spontaneous pregnancy loss: Evaluation, management, and follow-up counseling. Prim Care 27(1):153–167, 2000.
4. Speroff L, Glass RH, Kase NG: Clinical Gynecologic Endocrinology and Infertility, 6th ed. Baltimore, Lippincott Williams & Wilkins, 1999, pp 1043–1056.

19. INDUCED ABORTION

Abike James, M.D.

1. What are the major methods used to terminate a pregnancy?
  • Surgical evacuation, using either dilation and suction curettage, or dilation and extraction
  • Medical abortion
  • Labor induction

2. What are the advantages and disadvantages of medical versus surgical abortion?

MEDICAL ABORTION	SURGICAL ABORTION
Usually avoids invasive procedure	Involves invasive procedure
Usually avoids anesthesia	Allows use of sedation if desired
Requires two or more visits	Usually requires only one visit
May take days to weeks to complete	Is completed in a predictable period
Use is confined to early pregnancy (may be available sooner in pregnancy than surgical abortion)	May be used in early pregnancy but also available for later gestations
High success rate (~95%)	High success rate (~99%)
Requires follow-up to ensure complete abortion	Does not require follow-up in all cases
Generally is a multi-step process	Tends to be a single-step process

Adapted from American College of Obstetricians and Gynecologists: Practice Bulletin—Clinical management guidelines for obstetrician-gynecologists. Number 26, April 2001.

3. How does the method of surgical evacuation vary according to the weeks of gestation?
  < 6 weeks: Use suction curettage with a smaller cannula (6 mm) and *manual* vacuum aspiration. Post procedure, make an effort to identify villi (they have a characteristic powder-puff pattern when floated in water). If none are identified, follow serial B-hCGs to rule out ectopic pregnancy and to confirm pregnancy termination.
  6–13 weeks: Perform vacuum aspiration, generally with an electric vacuum pump. Use suction cannulas sized according to gestational age. Inspect tissue for villi, sac, and fetal parts (over 10 weeks).
  > 13 weeks (second-trimester abortions): Cervical softening and dilation is achieved using lamicel and/or laminaria several hours before the procedure. Uterine evacuation is performed using special instruments, and is followed by suction and/or sharp curettage. Fetal parts are identified post procedure to ensure completeness.

4. What are the medications currently used to perform medical abortions? How effective are they? What are their mechanisms of action?
  Mifepristone (RU-486): Acts as a progesterone receptor antagonist. Usually is used in combination with a prostaglandin analogue (misoprostol). Efficacy when used with misoprostol is usually ~96% for pregnancies up to 49 days of gestation.
  Methotrexate: Blocks dihydrofolate reductase, an enzyme involved in producing thymidine during DNA synthesis. It therefore inhibits the syncytialization of the cytotrophoblast, ultimately preventing implantation. Also used in combination with misoprostol with an efficacy rate of 92–96% for pregnancies up to 49 days of gestation. Of note, although the efficacy rate is similar

to that of mifepristone/misoprostol, 15–20% of patients will have to wait up to 4 weeks for the abortion to occur.

5. What are the side effects from the various methods of medical abortion?
Bleeding and pain, nausea (12–47%), vomiting (9–45%), diarrhea (7–67%), warmth or chills (14–89%), headache (12–27%), dizziness (14–37%), and fatigue.

6. What are the major complications of medical abortion?
Hemorrhage requiring emergency dilatation and curettage (< 1%), post abortal endometritis (0.09–0.5%), incomplete abortion (~5%).

7. What are the major complications of surgical abortions?
Uterine perforation (< 1%), hemorrhage (< 1%), post abortal endometritis (0.4–4.7%), incomplete abortion (~1%).

8. When is labor induction performed? What are the methods currently employed?
Labor induction techniques are available for early and mid second-trimester gestations. They allow abortion of the fetus without dismemberment. These techniques are usually performed when the patient wants to see the fetus intact. Methods include intra-amniotic instillation of hypertonic saline, urea, or prostaglandin F2α, extra-amniotic administration of prostaglandin E2 via the vaginal route, and high-dose oxytocin IV.

9. What serious complications may occur with instillation of hypertonic saline?
Hyperosmolar coma, hypernatremia, and/or disseminated intravascular coagulation.

10. What is the preferred method of second-trimester termination?
Intra-amniotic infusions have been replaced with dilation and extraction (D&E) or vaginal prostaglandins because of the high incidence of complications with intra-amniotic instillation. Up to 20 weeks' gestation, D&E is safer than vaginal prostaglandins in experienced hands. After 20 weeks, the optimal technique is debatable.

11. Did the 1973 U.S. Supreme Court decision in Roe v. Wade result in any change in maternal mortality?
Yes. The maternal mortality rate from induced abortions was 39% in 1972, and 6% in 1974. Today, the overall risk of death from legal abortion is less than 1 per 100,000 procedures.

12. How does the number of terminations performed today compare with the number performed before legalization?
There is no way to know how many illegal pregnancy terminations were performed, but the incidence of patients hospitalized for incomplete and septic pregnancy terminations has decreased markedly. About 1.3 million legal abortions are performed in the U.S. annually. Each year, 2–3% of all women of reproductive age have an abortion.

BIBLIOGRAPHY

1. ACOG Practice Bulletin. Clinical management guidelines for obstetrician-gynecologists. Medical management of abortion. Obstet Gynecol 97(4 Suppl):S1–13, 2001.
2. Castadot RG: Pregnancy termination: Techniques, risks and complications and their management. Fertil Steril 45:5, 1986.
3. Creinin MD, Edwards J: Early abortion: Surgical and medical options. Curr Probl Obstet Gynecol Infertil 20(1):1–32, 1997.
4. Creinin MD: Medical termination of pregnancy. In Sciarra JJ (ed): Gynecology and Obstetrics, revised ed. Philadelphia, Lippincott Williams and Wilkins, 1999, pp 1–27.
5. Grimes DA: Medical abortions: Public health and private lives. Am J Obstet Gynecol 183(2 Suppl):S1–2, 2000.

6. Hern WM, et al: Outpatient abortion for fetal anomaly and fetal death from 15–34 menstrual weeks' gestation: Techniques and clinical management. Obstet Gynecol 81:301, 1993.
7. Kruse B, Poppema S, Creinin MD, Paul M: Management of side effects and complications in medical abortion. Am J Obstet Gynecol 183 (2 Suppl):S65–75, 2000.
8. Stubblefield PG: Surgical techniques of uterine evacuation in first- and second-trimester abortion. Clin Obstet Gynaecol 13:53, 1986.

20. ECTOPIC PREGNANCY

Ty B. Erickson, M.D.

1. What is an ectopic pregnancy?

An ectopic pregnancy is one that develops at any site other than the endometrium.

2. What is the incidence of ectopic pregnancy?

The true incidence is difficult to determine because of the varied populations studied, but it ranges from 1 of 64 to 1 of 241 pregnancies, with an average of approximately 20 per 1000 pregnancies. There has been a fourfold increase over the past 20 years. Ectopic pregnancy continues to be the most common cause of maternal death in the first half of pregnancy, and the second most common overall, accounting for 10–15% of all maternal deaths.

3. Why has the incidence increased over the past 20 years?

The increase is due to a combination of increasing salpingitis and better antibiotics, which allow tubal patency following infection. The resultant tube is patent, but has luminal damage.

4. What is the cause of ectopic pregnancy?

The major cause of ectopic pregnancy is **salpingitis**. The incidence of histologic evidence of prior salpingitis is 40%. Any mechanism that causes abnormal tubal motility, so that the blastocyst remains in the tube at the time of implantation, will also cause an ectopic gestation. Examples include infection (particularly Chlamydia), exposure to diethylstilbestrol (DES), prior tubal surgery, and smoking at the time of conception. Failure of tubal sterilization methods has been reported to account for 3% of ectopic pregnancies. Chromosomal and structural anomalies of the conceptus may predispose to ectopic pregnancy.

5. Where do the majority of ectopic pregnancies occur?

Of ectopic pregnancies, 97.7% occur in the fallopian tube, 1.4% are abdominal, and < 1% are ovarian or cervical. The majority of tubal pregnancies occur in the ampulla, 12% in the isthmus, and 5% in the fimbriated end.

6. What are Spiegelberg's criteria for identification of an ovarian pregnancy?

- The tube, including fimbria ovarica, must be intact.
- The gestational sac must occupy normal ovarian position.
- The sac must be connected to the uterus by the utero-ovarian ligament.
- Ovarian tissue must be identified histologically in the wall of the gestational sac.

7. What is the incidence of an intrauterine pregnancy with an ectopic pregnancy (heterotopic pregnancy)?

The classic estimate is 1 of 30,000, but a more likely estimate is 1 of 4000–15,000. Newer ovulation induction methods and in vitro techniques have increased the risk to as high as 3% of successful transfer cycles. These are difficult to diagnose, and 50% are identified after rupture.

8. Does the risk of ectopic pregnancy vary according to contraceptive methods?

Yes.

Contraceptive Method	Risk of Ectopic Pregnancy
None	1%
Oral contraceptives	1%
Diaphragm	1%
Intrauterine device (IUD)	5%
Progestasert IUD	15%

9. What is the likelihood that a woman with one ectopic pregnancy will have a subsequent ectopic pregnancy?

Recurrence risk varies from 7% to 15%.

10. List the risk factors for an ectopic pregnancy.
• Tubal surgery (reconstructive or tubal ligation, particularly if done by coagulation)
• History of pelvic inflammatory disease
• Previous ectopic pregnancy
• IUD use
• Progestin-only oral contraceptives
• DES exposure
• Endometriosis
• Cigarette smoking

11. What is the differential diagnosis of an ectopic pregnancy?

Threatened or incomplete abortion	Dysfunctional uterine bleeding
Gestational trophoblastic disease	Adnexal torsion
Ruptured corpus luteal cyst	Degenerating uterine leiomyomata
Salpingitis	Endometriosis
Appendicitis	

Up to one-third of patients with ectopic pregnancy will be seen once before the diagnosis is confirmed; delayed diagnosis increases morbidity substantially.

12. What are the most common symptoms of an ectopic pregnancy?

Over 90% of patients have abdominal pain; however, only 35% report totally missing a period, although careful history reveals some abnormality with the preceding cycle. Abnormal bleeding at the time of presentation is not uncommon.

13. Why do some patients have shoulder pain?

Shoulder pain is referred from diaphragmatic irritation due to hemoperitoneum and occurs in up to 25% of patients.

14. What are the most common signs?

Patients are usually afebrile, and orthostasis is not commonly seen unless massive hemoperitoneum is present. Abdominal tenderness is seen in over 90% of patients. A palpable pelvic mass is not helpful, because it is present in only 50% of patients, 20% of whom have the ectopic pregnancy on the side contralateral to the mass. Uterine size is normal in 70% of patients.

15. What is the role of human chorionic gonadotropin (HCG) titers in the diagnosis and management of ectopic pregnancy?

HCG, a glycoprotein produced by trophoblastic tissue, can be measured in the serum within 8–12 days after fertilization. Two reference standards are used by various labs to report the titers. The first is the International Reference Preparation (IRP), which is identical to the third international standard of the World Health Organization. The second is the Second International Standard (SIS), which approximates one-half the value of the IRP. The IRP is most commonly used.

During the first 6–7 weeks, the serum HCG values approximately double every 48 hours in 90% of intrauterine pregnancies. A subnormal rise < 66% is seen in 85% of nonviable pregnancies, and a rise of < 20% is 100% predictive of a nonviable pregnancy. Seventeen percent of ectopic pregnancies meet criteria for normal doubling times. Doubling times are not valid after 7 weeks of gestation. Following titers in the stable patient is helpful in early gestations to rule out ectopic pregnancies.

16. When is ultrasound helpful in the diagnosis of ectopic pregnancy?

Ultrasound is definitive if cardiac activity is identified either in the tube or uterus. In conjunction with HCG titers, it is also helpful in confirming intrauterine pregnancy. Endovaginal probes allow earlier detection of pregnancy location at least 1 week before transabdominal scans. A *discriminatory zone*, using HCG titers with ultrasound, has been identified at a level of 6500 mIU/ml (IRP), at which transabdominal ultrasound should identify an intrauterine gestational sac, or 2000 mIU/ml (IRP) if endovaginal ultrasound is available. Specific findings using endovaginal probes for ectopic pregnancy include a **tubal ring** (1- to 3-cm mass with a 2- to 4-mm concentric echogenic rim surrounding a hypoechoic center) in 68% of tubal pregnancies. The probe also allows better evaluation of the pseudosac, fluid in the cul-de-sac, and character of pelvic masses.

Each medical center should establish criteria for evaluating possible ectopic pregnancies with combined modalities of ultrasound and HCG values, including which reference standards are to be used. The criteria must take into consideration the quality of ultrasound equipment and personnel.

17. Describe the role of culdocentesis in the diagnosis of ectopic pregnancy.

With the advent of accurate serum HCG values and endovaginal probe ultrasound, culdocentesis is less frequently needed. It still has a role for the patient with a positive pregnancy test and fluid in the cul-de-sac in whom a definitive intrauterine sac is not identified, or when titers or ultrasound are not available.

18. Why is the blood obtained by culdocentesis nonclotting?

The nonclotting blood results from lysis of blood that has clotted previously. The hematocrit of the nonclotting blood should exceed 15% to be significant.

19. What is the role of progesterone levels in the diagnosis of ectopic pregnancies?

Serum progesterone levels are not dependent on gestational age; therefore, a single value gives a snapshot view of pregnancy viability. In 98% of viable pregnancies, values exceed 10 ng/ml, and in 98% of ectopic pregnancies not associated with ovulation induction, values are less than 20 ng/ml. A single level < 15 ng/ml is highly suggestive of a nonviable pregnancy, but does not distinguish between pending miscarriage and ectopic pregnancy. Unfortunately, because of differences in populations, assay kits, and overlap in the 10–20 ng/ml range, the clinical use of serum progesterone levels is limited.

20. Describe the role of laparoscopy in the diagnosis of tubal pregnancy.

If a patient has a subnormal rise in HCG titers or an abnormal ultrasound, frozen-section dilatation and curettage may be performed; if the result is negative, the laparoscope will allow visualization of the tube. However, false-negative rates approach 4% and may be higher if surgery is performed early in the pregnancy.

21. What about expectant management of ectopic pregnancies?

If patients are hospitalized for observation, with surgery only for hemorrhage, 57% of ectopic pregnancies spontaneously resolve. However, 60% of patients are in hospital for more than 4 weeks, which is not practical.

22. What surgical options are available?

Traditionally a laparotomy with partial salpingectomy of the ipsilateral side has been performed. The trend currently focuses on *tubal preservation*. Fimbrial evacuation by digital expression is not advocated because of the high failure rate with persistent trophoblast (> 25%). **Linear salpingostomy**, either by laparotomy or, more recently, laparoscopy, is the method of choice, even with tubes dilated as much as 4 cm. There is, however, a 10% risk of persistent trophoblast, and titers should be followed weekly until they reach nondetectable levels. The recurrent ectopic rate is not increased by this technique, and subsequent fertility is equal and possibly slightly better than with salpingectomy.

23. Describe the role of methotrexate (MTX) in treating ectopic pregnancy.

Economics and patient morbidity have driven the nonsurgical management of ectopic pregnancy. Clinical studies have demonstrated success with varying treatment regimens in ectopic pregnancy: multidose MTX with citrovorum rescue or single-dose protocols have been advocated. MTX also has been reported to be successful in treating interstitial, abdominal, and cervical pregnancies, which have substantial surgical risk. Perhaps the most commonly used technique is to give a single intramuscular dose based on body surface area, 50 mg/m^2, without citrovorum. Median success rates are 85% (range 65–95%), with the remainder requiring either a second dose or surgical intervention. Tubal patency after treatment approaches 80%.

24. How does MTX work?

MTX acts as a folic acid antagonist and interferes with DNA synthesis and cellular multiplication. It has been used in treating gestational trophoblastic disease for years with excellent results.

25. What risks are associated with MTX treatment?

The traditional complications of stomatitis, dermatitis, pleuritis, and altered liver function have been reported. Additionally, 60% of patients experience increased pelvic pain during the first few days after treatment.

26. What are the contraindications to MTX therapy for ectopic pregnancy?

Known sensitivity to MTX	Chronic liver or lung disease
Breast-feeding	Blood dyscrasias
Immunodeficiency	Embryonic ectopic cardiac activity

Some advocate as a relative contraindication an HCG titer > 10,000 or a sac size > 35mm.

27. What is the most common protocol for nonsurgical management of ectopic pregnancy?

Once an ectopic pregnancy has been confirmed, 50 mg/m^2 is administered intramuscularly. Weekly HCG titers are followed until the absence of HCG is detected. This may take 4 weeks, and initially there may be a continued rise in the first week. If a 15% reduction is not achieved during the first week, or in subsequent weeks a plateau occurs, then an additional injection of MTX is given or surgical exploration is advocated.

28. Are other pharmacologic treatments available?

Actinomycin-D, a more potent chemotherapeutic agent than MTX, has been used successfully in treating a limited number of ectopic pregnancies, especially in advanced gestations (HCG levels > 10,000 mIU/ml), in which MTX has a higher failure rate. Potassium chloride (KCl) injected into the fetal heart in advanced ectopic pregnancy has been reported to induce asystole, and may have a role in treating heterotopic pregnancy.

29. What is the role of mifepristone (RU486)?

Mifepristone is an antiprogestin used for pregnancy terminations. Therapy has not been successful in treating ectopic pregnancy as a single agent. However, recent data suggest in combination with MTX (600 mg of mefepristone) the success rates are significantly improved, approaching 97%. Although controversial, this combination may prove to be most efficacious in the future nonsurgical management of ectopic pregnancy.

30. What about subsequent fertility after an ectopic pregnancy?

The intrauterine pregnancy rate for patients with previous full-term pregnancies approaches 80%. The rate is about 40% if the patient is nulliparous. Patients with ruptured ectopic pregnancies have improved rates compared with unruptured ectopic pregnancies (65% vs. 82%, respectively).

BIBLIOGRAPHY

1. ACOG Practice Bulletin: Medical management of tubal pregnancy. No. 3. Washington DC, American College of Obstetricians and Gynecologists, 1998.
2. Balasch J, Barri P: Treatment of ectopic pregnancy: The new gynaecological dilemma. Hum Reprod 9:547, 1994.
3. Buster JE, Heard MJ: Current issues in medical management of ectopic pregnancy. Curr Opin Obstet Gynecol 12(6):525–527, 2000.
4. Fleischer A, Pennell R, McKee M, et al: Ectopic pregnancy: Features at transvaginal sonography. Radiology 174:377, 1990.
5. Kadar N, Caldwell B, Romero R: A method of screening for ectopic pregnancy and its indications. Obstet Gynecol 58:162, 1981.
6. Perdu M, et al: Treating ectopic pregnancy with the combination of mifepristone and methotrexate: A phase 11 nonrandomized study. Am J Obstet Gynecol 179(3):640–643, 1998.
7. Sau AK, Sau M: Diagnosing suspected ectopic pregnancy. Can we offer completely non-surgical management for ectopic pregnancy? BMJ 322(7289):793–794, 2001.
8. Shalev E, Ben-Shlomo I: Treatment of ectopic pregnancy. New Engl J Med 344(5):384–385, 2001.
9. Stabile I, Grudzinskas J: Ectopic pregnancy: A review of incidence, etiology and diagnostic aspects. Obstet Gynecol Surv 45:335, 1990.
10. Stovall TG, Ling FW: Single-dose methotrexate: An expanded clinical trial. Am J Obstet Gynecol 168:1759, 1993.
11. Vermesh M, Silva P, et al: Management of unruptured ectopic gestation by linear salpingostomy: A prospective randomized clinical trial of laparoscopy versus laparotomy. Obstet Gynecol 73(Pt 1): 400, 1989.

21. CONTRACEPTION

Molina Dayal, M.D., *and Steven Sondheimer*, M.D.

1. **What methods of contraception are currently available to women in the United States?**
   - Abstinence, withdrawal, and fertility awareness
   - Permanent sterilization
   - Hormonal
     (a) Oral contraceptives (OCPs; combination and progestin-only)
     (b) Injectables:
        Depot medroxyprogesterone acetate (Depo-Provera)
        Lunelle (estradiol cypionate and medroxyprogesterone acetate)
     (c) Implant:
        Norplant (6 rods of levonorgestrel)
     (d) Vaginal ring (NuvaRing: ethinyl estradiol and etonorgestrel)
     (e) Transdermal patch (Evra: ethinyl estradiol and norgestimate)
   - Intrauterine device (IUD)
     (a) Levonorgestrel (Mirena)
     (b) Copper (Paragard)
   - Barrier methods
     (a) Diaphragm
     (b) Cervical cap
     (c) Condoms (male and female)
   - Spermicides
   - Emergency contraception (hormonal and copper IUD)

2. **With typical use (as opposed to perfect use) of a given method of contraception, what percentage of women will have an unintended pregnancy within the first year of use?**

No method	85
Spermicides	26
Fertility awareness	25
Female condoms	21
Diaphragm/cervical cap	20
Withdrawal	17
Male condoms	14
Progestin-only OCPs	7
Combination OCPs	5
Vaginal ring*	1.2
IUD	0.8
Transdermal patch*	0.7
Tubal ligation	0.55
Depo-Provera	0.3
Vasectomy	0.15
Norplant	0.05

   * Limited data on "typical use" for these methods

3. **What is the mechanism of action of OCPs?**

   Estrogenic effects: inhibition of ovulation in part by the suppression of follicle-stimulating hormone (FSH) and luteinizing hormone (LH)

Progestational effects: inhibition of ovulation by suppressing LH; thickening of cervical mucus, thus hampering sperm transport; possible inhibition of sperm capacitation; production of a decidualized endometrium with exhausted and atrophic glands; altered motility of the uterus and fallopian tubes

4. What is the association of OCPs with myocardial infarction?

Recent evidence shows that the association between current combined OCP use (containing 35 micrograms of ethinyl estradiol) and myocardial infarction (MI) is weak, with a relative risk ranging from 0.9 to 2.5. There is no evidence to support an increased or decreased risk of MI due to past OCP use compared to no use. Smoking has been identified as an independent risk factor for MI; the combination of smoking and OCP use can be synergistic for increasing the risk of an MI.

5. What is the association of OCPs with stroke?

The link between *high-dose* OCP pills and ischemic stroke has historically been reported. Subsequent studies showed a decrease in the odds ratio and relative risk with a decrease in the estrogen dose. There is no significant increase in risk of ischemic stroke in women younger than 45 years old who use OCPs. In addition, there is no consistent, strong evidence linking OCP use to hemorrhagic stroke. Since smoking, hypertension, and migraine headaches all are independent risk factors for stroke, women with other independent risk factors (e.g., smoking, diabetes) may have a slightly increased risk of stroke while taking an OCP.

6. What is the relationship between second- and third-generation OCPs and the risk of deep vein thrombosis?

Deep vein thrombosis (DVT) and pulmonary embolism are the most common, serious side effects of estrogen-containing hormonal contraception. Risk increases approximately **three-fold** with *modern OCPs* (35 mcg of ethinyl estradiol)—less than the increase associated with pregnancy. There is no biological evidence that specific progestins have different effects on clotting factors.

In the mid 1990s, however, epidemiological studies reported that women using *third-generation OCPs* (containing the progestins gestodene and desogestrel) had a higher risk of venous thromboembolism compared to women using *second-generation OCPs* (containing norethindrone and levonorgestrel). Studies performed since then have shown a weak association between OCP use and venous thromboembolism (strength of association ranging from 0.7 to 2.3). After reanalysis of the data, the U.S. Food and Drug Administration issued a statement that the risk of DVT with the third-generation progestins "is not great enough to justify switching to other products."

Factor V Leiden mutation occurs in 3–5% of Caucasians and is responsible for the majority of cases of venous thrombosis in which there is an identifiable risk factor. This mutation may independently increase the risk of DVT.

7. What are some of the therapeutic uses of OCPs?

Hyperandrogenism: Combination OCPs suppress ovarian, adrenal, and peripheral androgen metabolism. The estrogen component of OCPs also increases sex hormone-binding globulin levels and inhibits 5 alpha-reductase in the skin, resulting in lower levels of dihydrotestosterone. OCPs, alone or with other agents, can successfully treat both acne and hirsuitism. No randomized controlled trial has found one formulation to be better than another in the treatment of acne. From a clinical standpoint, over 60% of women with hirsuitism respond to OCPs. Current low-dose progestin-only pills do not stimulate an androgenic response.

Menstrual disorders: Primary dysmenorrhea in most women can be successfully treated with OCPs. Oral contraceptives should be used after an attempt of the first-line treatment of nonsteroidal anti-inflammatory medications is unsuccessful. OCPs can be used to treat heavy and inter-menstrual bleeding by restoring synchrony to the endometrium. For acute episodes of menorrhagia (seen commonly with anovulation) with associated anemia, high-doses (three or four pills a day) of combination formulations can effectively suppress bleeding. Once the bleeding has stopped, the high-dose regimen can be tapered and then stopped to allow withdrawal bleeding. For episodes of heavy bleeding without anemia, one or two pills of a high-dose formulation can be effective until bleeding abates, followed by a withdrawal bleed.

Endometriosis: Clinicians often use OCPs to reduce pelvic pain associated with endometriosis and for long-term suppression after initial medical or surgical therapy. A recent Cochrane Collaboration review supported the use of OCPs as a "long-term alternative treatment for the painful symptoms of endometriosis."

Hypoestrogenic states: OCPs have been used in women with hypothalamic amenorrhea as a method of hormone replacement therapy. The majority of these patients are adolescents with eating disorders or exercise-induced amenorrhea. OCP use in the perimenopausal period has several distinct advantages: it prevents pregnancy, regulates uterine bleeding in a predictable fashion, and treats vaso-motor and vaginal dryness symptoms at the same time. Estrogen replacement in the form of OCPs can also benefit patients who are amenorrheic after radiation, chemotherapy, or bilateral oophorectomy.

Ovarian cysts: Even though OCPs are sometimes prescribed to induce regression of ovarian cysts, little evidence exists to support this treatment.

Other menstrual-related disorders: OCPs may be useful in managing premenstrual related mood disturbances (premenstrual dysphoric disorder). Some randomized controlled studies have shown benefits of OCPs for this purpose, while others have not. Menstrual migraines occur immediately prior to the onset of menses and not at any other time during the cycle. These headaches may be triggered by changes in estrogen levels immediately prior to menstrual flow and can be treated with OCPs that deliver a continuous dose of estrogen, thereby minimizing hormone fluctuation.

8. What are the non-contraceptive benefits of OCPs?
Reduction of ovarian and endometrial cancer risk
Decreased risk of benign breast disease (fibroadenomas, fibrocystic change)
Decreased risk of symptomatic pelvic inflammatory disease
Decreased risk of ectopic pregnancy
Increase in bone mineral density
Possible reduction in colorectal cancer risk
Possible improvement in symptoms of rheumatoid arthritis
Decrease in menstrual flow
Decreased incidence of anemia
Decrease in primary dysmenorrhea
Improvement in hirsutism and acne

9. What is the association of OCPs with cancer?
Ovarian cancer: Users of OCPs are less likely to develop ovarian cancer than never-users. The risk of developing epithelial ovarian cancer decreases by 40% with as little as 3–6 months of OCP use. Further declines in risk are seen with longer periods of use. The protective effect persists for at least 15 years after OCP discontinuation. OCPs may provide primary prevention for women at risk for hereditary ovarian cancer as well.

Endometrial cancer: Pill users have a 50% reduction in endometrial cancer risk compared to never-users. Risk is reduced by 20% with 1 year of use, 40% with 2 years of use, and 60% with 4 or more years of use. This reduction in risk persists for at least 15 years after discontinuation. Protection is seen with all monophasic preparations, including pills with less than 50 mcg of ethinyl estradiol, but there is no data thus far with multiphasic or progestin-only preparations.

Breast cancer: Evidence suggest that there is a slight increase in the relative risk of localized breast cancer associated with current (relative risk 1.24) or recent (relative risk 1.16 for use within 1–4 years) use of OCPs compared to never use. However, breast cancers diagnosed in OCP users were significantly less advanced than those in never-users. Family history of breast cancer does not influence the association between current or recent OCP use and breast cancer risk. Also, duration of use, dosage, and formulation do not influence the risk of breast cancer. Young women have a very low baseline risk of breast cancer. This risk is slightly increased by the use of OCPs, but does not persist beyond 4 years after cessation of use.

10. List the contraindications for OCP use.

Women with the following conditions should not use oral contraceptives:
- Known presence or history of deep venous thrombosis or pulmonary embolism
- History of cerebral vascular accident, coronary artery or ischemic heart disease
- Diabetes with microvascular complications (neuropathy, retinopathy), or duration greater than 20 years
- History of estrogen-dependent cancer including known or history of breast cancer
- Current pregnancy
- Migraines with focal neurologic symptoms
- Age > 35 years in the setting of smoking more than 20 cigarettes a day
- Hypertension (blood pressure > 160/100 mmHg) or with vascular disease
- Active liver disease (benign hepatic adenoma, liver cancer, active viral hepatitis, or severe cirrhosis)
- Major surgery with prolonged immobilization or any surgery of the legs
- Presence or family history of hypercoagulable disorder

11. Describe some other methods of hormonal contraception, aside from oral contraceptives.

Depo-Provera: intramuscular injection every 12 weeks of medroxyprogesterone acetate

Lunelle: monthly injection of estradiol cypionate and medroxyprogesterone acetate

Norplant : levonorgestrel; progestin-only implant lasting for 5 years

NuvaRing: a vaginal ring combination of ethinyl estradiol and etonorgestrel placed every 3 weeks

Evra: a transdermal combination patch of norgestimate and ethinyl estradiol placed every week

12. What potential problems and side effects are attributed to long-acting hormonal contraception?

Menstrual side effects are the most common side effects of hormonal contraception, particularly the progestin only methods. Almost all women using Depo-Provera, Norplant, and progestin-only OCPs experience irregular bleeding and spotting initially. With Depo-Provera, amenorrhea is common after 1 year of use (50%). Headaches are the most common non-menstrual side effect. Both of these complaints often lead to method discontinuation. With the exception of Depo-Provera, return of fertility tends to be rapid for hormonal methods of contraception (approximately 1 month for most methods; 8.5 months for Depo-Provera).

The clinical significance of decreased bone mineral density (BMD) in Depo-Provera users is still under investigation. Studies have shown that small decreases in BMD do occur shortly after initiation of Depo-Provera use, but reverse after discontinuation—a trend that is similar to that seen during lactation.

13. What is the effect of hormonal contraception on pregnancy?

The use of any hormonal method of contraception early in pregnancy does not increase the risk of congenital anomalies or early pregnancy loss.

14. What methods of emergency contraception are currently available?

The emergency contraception formulations available in the United States include combined OCP tablets, progestin-only contraceptive tablets, and the copper-T IUD.
- Combination methods: With the **Yuzpe method**, 200 mcg of ethinyl estradiol and 1 mg of levonorgestrel in two divided doses 12 hours apart is given. The risk of pregnancy is reduced by 74%. **Preven** is a prepackaged kit containing instructions for emergency contraceptive pill use, appropriately dosed estrogen and progestin pills, and a pregnancy test.

• Progestin (levonorgestrel)-only methods: **Plan B** is a prepackaged form of progestin-only pills for emergency contraceptive use. It has similar or better effectiveness as the combination Yuzpe method and fewer side effects (nausea, vomiting).

All oral emergency contraception is best used within 72 hours of unprotected intercourse; use sooner, however, may be more effective.

• Copper IUD: The IUD is a less frequently used method of emergency that can be inserted up to 7 days after ovulation to prevent pregnancy. The failure rate is very low, 0.1%. Also, this method has the additional advantage of providing long-term contraception.

15. What is the mechanism of action of emergency contraceptives?

Emergency contraception likely inhibits or delays ovulation and may also impair endometrial receptivity. Other possible mechanisms include interference with corpus luteum function, thickening of cervical mucus, and alterations in tubal transport of sperm, egg, or embryo. Emergency contraceptives do *not* interrupt an already established pregnancy.

16. What is the mechanism of action of an IUD?

An IUD causes a foreign-body reaction within the uterine cavity, thus altering sperm motility/integrity. It alters tubal fluids, thereby interfering with ova and sperm transport and interaction. Finally, an IUD alters the uterine lining so that it becomes unfavorable for implantation.

17. List the absolute contraindications for an IUD insertion.
• Confirmed or suspected pregnancy
• Known or suspected pelvic malignancy
• Undiagnosed vaginal bleeding
• Acute or chronic pelvic infection
• High-risk behavior for sexually transmitted diseases (i.e., multiple sexual partners, having partners at risk for sexually transmitted infections)
• Hyperbilirubinemia secondary to Wilson's disease (for copper-containing devices only)

18. What are the major risks associated with IUD use?
• Displaced string
• Uterine perforation and difficult removal
• Pelvic infection: the IUD itself does not cause pelvic infection; in general, with IUDs there is an increased risk for pelvic inflammatory disease with exposure to sexually transmitted infections. The modern progestin-only IUDs may actually decrease the risk of pelvic infection by thickening cervical mucus.

19. What is the appropriate time for IUD insertion?

The levonorgestrel IUD should be inserted within 7 days of onset of menstruation or immediately after early pregnancy loss; it can then be replaced by a new system at any time of the menstrual cycle. The Copper IUD can be inserted at any point in the cycle as long as the patient is not pregnant. This IUD can be inserted immediately postpartum, postabortion, or as an "interval" insertion. An 'interval' insertion is defined as insertion in women who are neither postpartum nor postabortion, or an insertion in women 6 weeks after delivery.

20. Describe the mechanism of action of barrier methods of contraception.

Both the male and female condoms provide a physical barrier that prevents sperm and egg interaction. Diaphragms, caps, and sponges use two different mechanisms, a physical barrier as well as a spermicidal chemical.

21. What are some of the advantages and disadvantages of barrier methods of contraception?

Vaginal barriers have many *advantages*, including protection against sexually transmitted infections, provision of immediate protection without much prior planning, easy access, and no systemic side effects. *Disadvantages* include the need for a high degree of motivation for use, discomfort with placement/use, possible latex allergy (condoms), and increased incidence of urinary tract infections (diaphragm).

22. What is the role of permanent sterilization as a contraceptive method?

Sterilization (female tubal sterilization and vasectomy) has become one of the most widely used methods of family planning worldwide. In fact, sterilization is the most common method of contraception used by couples over the age of 30 in the U.S. today. Both types are meant to be permanent and are comparable in effectiveness. Less than 1% of women will become pregnant after tubal sterilization in the first year. The risk of failure, however, persists for years after the procedure and varies by method of tubal occlusion and age of the patient.

BIBLIOGRAPHY

1. American College of Obstetricians and Gynecologists: Sterilization. ACOG Tech Bull 222, 1996.
2. American College of Obstetricians and Gynecologists: Emergency Contraception. ACOG Tech Bull 25, 2001.
3. Barnhart KB, Dayal M: Contraception. In Rakel RE, Bope ET (eds): Conn's Current Therapy 2002. Philadelphia, W.B. Saunders, 2002, pp 1103–1111.
4. Dayal MB, Barnhart KB: Noncontraceptive benefits and therapeutic uses of the oral contraceptive pill. Semin Reprod Med 19(4):295–303, 2001.
5. Grimes DA: Intrauterine device and upper genital tract infection. Lancet 356:1013–1019, 2000.
6. Iyer V, Farquahr C, Jepson R: Oral contraceptive pills for heavy menstrual bleeding (Cochrane Review). In The Cochrane Library, Issue 2, 1999. Oxford: Update Software.
7. Schlesselman JJ: Net effect of oral contraceptive use on the risk of cancer in women in the United States. Obstet Gynecol 85:793–801, 1995.
8. Schwingl PJ, Ory HW, Visness CW: Estimates of the risk of cardiovascular death attributable to low-dose oral contraceptives in the United States. Am J Obstet Gynecol 180:242–249, 1999.
9. Speroff L: Oral contraceptives and breast cancer risk: Summary and application of data. Int J Fertil 45(suppl 2):113–120, 2000.
10. Vandenbroucke JP, Rosing J, Bloemenkamp KWM, et al: Oral contraceptives and the risk of venous thrombosis. N Engl J Med 344(20):1527–1535, 2001.

22. FEMALE SEXUAL DYSFUNCTION

Saifuddin T. Mama, M.D., M.P.H.

1. What aspects of sexuality should a gynecologist be familiar with?

The physiology underlying the sexual response and the phases of the sexual response cycle. These are influenced by all aspects (e.g., societal, cultural, physiological, and emotional) of a woman's life. Chronological events and others—such as menarche, age of first sexual activity, contraception, sexual abuse, rape, surgery, childbearing, changes in marital status, menopause, and death of a partner—are all events that affect sexuality.

The perception that physicians are not comfortable discussing sexuality still hinders patients from relating their concerns. The physician should discuss with the patient events in her life that impact on her self-image and sexual health. Assessment of sexual dysfunction, as well as treatment and referral, are necessary components of the gynecologic doctor-patient relationship.

2. List the normal physiologic changes seen in the sexual response.
- Vasocongestion and increased muscle tone in the genitalia, breasts, and skin
- Generalized elevations in pulse, blood pressure, and respiration

3. What are the phases of the sexual response cycle?

Masters and Johnson described the phases in 1966; they are excitement, plateau, orgasm, and resolution. These phases can occur simultaneously or overlap, with wide variability in the same individual at different times. Kaplan modified this cycle to desire, arousal, and orgasm.

4. Describe the physiologic changes during desire and arousal.

The initial response in women is vaginal lubrication with transudate from the vaginal walls due to vasocongestion. The upper two-thirds of the vagina expand, the cervix and uterus elevate, and the clitoris and labia increase in size. Concomitantly, an increase in breast size and nipple erection occurs. The "orgasmic platform" develops upon vasocongestion of the lower third of the vagina, a slowing of vaginal lubrication, and retraction of the shaft and glands of the clitoris. A sex flush along the chest wall and back develops in 50–75% of women.

5. What characterizes orgasm?

In women, simultaneous rhythmic contractions of the orgasmic platform, uterus, and rectal sphincter occur at 0.8-second intervals, which then diminish in intensity, duration, and regularity. There is generalized myotonia, tachycardia, and tachypnea, and an elevation in blood pressure. This response is also seen in women who have previously undergone hysterectomy and infundibulectomy. Note that women can be multi-orgasmic. The resolution of vasocongestion results in a return to normal anatomy and physiology.

6. What is sexual dysfunction?

This is a broad diagnosis incorporating many types of sexual disorders. An impaired physiologic response, along with and impacted by multifactorial psychosocial issues, constitutes sexual dysfunction.

7. What is the prevalence of sexual dysfunction?

Studies show a range of 10% to 63%; the average is 41%.

8. Which epidemiologic factors suggest an increased risk for sexual dysfunction?

Women with low incomes, lower educational levels, unmarried status, or a prior history of emotional or psychological stressors are more likely to report sexual dysfunction.

9. What are the types of disorders seen in female sexual dysfunction?

Types of disorders in females include sexual desire disorders, sexual arousal disorder, orgasmic disorder, and sexual pain disorders. They are subtyped by life-long versus acquired, generalized versus situational, and specific etiology.

10. Describe sexual desire disorders.

Hypoactive sexual desire disorder is characterized by a deficiency of sexual thoughts and/or desire for or receptivity to sexual activity. This can have an organic etiology and/or a psychosocial component. *Sexual aversion* disorder is a phobia with avoidance of sexual contact and severe anxiety associated with contemplation of sexual activity. These patients have a normal physiologic sexual response.

11. What is sexual arousal disorder?

The inability to generate or maintain sufficient sexual excitement, both anatomically and physiologically, with decreased vasocongestion, lack of lubrication, and (subjectively) diminution of excitement. Patients with pelvic floor dysfunction and incontinence are an example.

12. Define orgasmic disorder.

An absence of, or difficulty in attaining, orgasm despite sufficient sexual stimulation and arousal. This can be primary or situational; in the latter case, orgasm can be attained only under certain circumstances.

13. What are the sexual pain disorders?

Dyspareunia, which is genital pain associated with intercourse, and vaginismus, which involves involuntary spasm of the muscles of the outer third of the vagina, preventing vaginal penetration. Dyspareunia is often associated with specific conditions such as vaginal atrophy, dryness, pelvic adhesions, endometriosis, myomas, vaginitis, vulvitis, and vestibulitis, but it is also impacted by factors such as insufficient time for or lack of stimulation, prior abuse, and cultural perceptions regarding sexuality.

Patients with **vaginismus** have a normal physiologic sexual response cycle, including arousal, vaginal lubrication, and even pleasurable non-coital sexual activity, but are unable psychologically to engage in sexual activity involving penetration. The muscles of the lower third of the vagina and the introitus constrict, in response to actual or perceived penetration. It may be related to a history of sexual trauma or abuse.

14. What is the etiology of sexual dysfunction?

The etiology is multifactorial, generally a combination of organic and pyschosocial factors. Changes in **vascularity**, such as insufficiency of the pudendal artery, with atherosclerosis caused by hypertension, elevated cholesterol, smoking, and diabetes could affect vaginal vasocongestion. **Neurogenic causes** involving spinal cord dysfunction or injuries and hormonal conditions such as premature ovarian failure and menopause can play a part. Underlying **depression** or **anxiety disorders** affect sexuality.

Medications that decrease desire include some antidepressants (e.g., selective serotonin reuptake inhibitors, tricyclic antidepressants), H_2 blockers, some antipsychotics, and some antihypertensives (e.g., beta blockers, thiazide diuretics, and spironolactone). Antidepressants that increase sexual desire include trazodone.

Psychosocial factors run the gamut from religious and cultural expectations, prior history of abuse or trauma, fear of rejection, and fear of intimacy, to body image issues, among others.

15. How is sexual dysfunction evaluated?

Since most patients do not spontaneously report a sexual problem, a routine sexual history should be taken only after rapport has been established between the physician and the patient. Ask about sexual orientation, type and frequency of sexual activity, information on partners past and present, and sexual satisfaction. The patient must feel that complete confidentiality will be observed at all times.

16. What medications are used to treat female sexual dysfunction?

In postmenopausal women, both oral and intravaginal estrogen replacement therapy is used to alleviate vaginal atrophy, dryness, and dyspareunia. A decrease in libido is often treated with estrogen and methyltestosterone—side effects of this treatment include elevated cholesterol, acne, voice changes, and hirsuitism. Sildenafil (Viagra) in female patients with intact peripheral neural stimulus for nitric oxide release can increase genital blood flow and increase clitoral and vaginal smooth muscle relaxation. This may be helpful for patients with sexual arousal disorder. Its use presently is not FDA-approved.

17. What devices are used for female sexual dysfunction?

A clitoral vacuum device, battery powered for home use, applies a gentle vacuum over the clitoris to enhance blood flow. This has been used in sexual arousal disorder.

18. What other treatments are available for female sexual dysfunction?

Treatment may involve correcting the underlying condition associated with the dysfunction. For example, in dyspareunia, treating the immobility from adhesions or endometriosis with laparoscopic lysis of adhesions can help. In inflammation stemming from vaginitis or vulvitis, symptom alleviation with antifungals and, if needed, steroid creams will resolve the dyspareunia. A referral to a therapist experienced in sexual dysfunction is needed in most situations. The patient's partner is usually included in the therapy process.

BIBLIOGRAPHY

1. Basson R, Berman J, Burnett A, et al. Report of the International Consensus Development Conference on Female Sexual Dysfunction: Definitions and classifications. J Urol 2000;163:888–893.
2. Basson R, McInnes R, Smith MD, et al. Efficacy and safety of sildenafil in estrogenized women with sexual dysfunction associated with female sexual arousal disorder. Obstet Gynecol 2000;95:S54.
3. Berman JR, Goldstein I. Female sexual dysfunction. Urol Clin North Am 2001;28(2):405–416.
4. Kaplan HS. Disorders of sexual desire and other new concepts and techniques in sex therapy. New York, Brunner/Mazel, Inc., 1979.
5. Laumann EO, Paik AMA, Rosen RC. Sexual dysfunction in the United States: Prevalence and predictors. JAMA 1999;281:537–554.
6. Masters WH, Johnson VE. Human sexual response. Boston, Little, Brown and Company, 1966.

23. MENOPAUSE

Stephen W. Sawin, M.D.

1. What are the differences between menopause, peri-menopause and the climacteric?

The North American Menopause Society defines *menopause* as "the permanent cessation of menstruation resulting from the loss of ovarian follicular activity." Natural menopause is defined as 12 months of amenorrhea without another pathologic cause. The average age at which this occurs is 51.4 years. Menopause before age 40 is called premature ovarian failure.

Peri-menopause is "the period immediately prior to menopause and the first year after menopause." The average age that peri-menopause starts is 47.5 years and it lasts on average 4 years.

The *climacteric* is "the phase during the aging of women marking the transition from the reproductive to the non-reproductive state." This time period includes events such as decreased fertility that precedes peri-menopause and extend beyond menopause.

2. What causes menopause to occur? What endocrine changes are seen?

Menopause is due to a gradual depletion of functioning ovarian follicles. Declining inhibin levels from the granulosa cells lead to increased follicle-stimulating hormone (FSH) production from the pituitary that accelerates the follicular phase of the menstrual cycle. High basal estradiol levels during menses can be seen, often in association with follicular cysts. As the granulosa cells gradually lose their ability to produce estradiol, FSH levels rise (as do luteinizing hormone [LH] levels, to a lesser extent). After menopause, androgen levels decline by 50%, but the greater decline of estradiol favors a higher androgen-to-estrogen ratio, leading to signs of hirsutism and alopecia in some women. Estrogen production after menopause is principally estrone produced by aromatazation of androstenedione in adipose tissues.

3. What are the major symptoms of menopause?

One major symptom of menopause is the irregularity of the menstrual cycles, initially seen as a shortening of the cycle, due to both shorter follicular and luteal phases. Anovulation then occurs and leads to skipped menstrual periods, oligomenorrhea, and eventually amenorrhea. Another predominate symptom is the hot flash, which occurs in approximately 70% of women. Sleep and mood disturbances also have been described. Symptoms of urogenital atrophy such as dyspareunia, vulvar pruritus, and incontinence can also occur.

4. Describe available treatments for menstrual irregularities at menopause.

Irregular menstrual cycles can be treated with low-dose oral contraceptive pills (20 µg of ethinyl estradiol) in many women in the perimenopause—as long as they don't smoke or have hypertension or vascular disease. Monthly withdrawal with progestins is another effective way to control irregular bleeding while reducing the risk of endometrial hyperplasia. Also with this approach, when the patient does not withdraw after progestin, hypoestrogenism is diagnosed and estrogen replacement therapy can be considered. Continuous progestins can be given, but can lead to breakthrough bleeding. Estrogen and progestin combination therapy can also be given.

5. What is a hot flash?

A hot flash is a sudden sensation of warmth, often accompanied by a flushed sensation of the upper body and face, typically lasting 1–5 minutes. It is due to alterations in the hypothalamic thermoregulatory center due to fluctuations in steroid and peptide hormone levels. Increases in serum LH are associated with the hot flash, but do not appear to be the cause. The exact cause is unknown. Hot flashes can least 5–7 years after menopause.

8. Define osteopenia and osteoporosis. How are they assessed?

The World Health Organization (WHO) defines osteopenia as a bone mineral density (BMD) that is > 1.0 to < 2.5 standard deviations (SD) below the young adult mean (called a "T" score). Osteoporosis is ≥ 2.5 SD below the young adult mean. A "Z" score is the BMD of the patient compared to her own age. A "Z" score > 1 SD below the mean is abnormal.

BMD is best assessed by a dual energy x-ray absorptiometry (DEXA) study. Biochemical markers of bone remodeling include serum markers of bone formation (osteocalcin, bone-specific alkaline phosphatase, and precollagen extension peptides) and urinary markers of bone resorption (pyridinoline cross-link peptides, N telopeptides, hydroxyproline, and hydroxylysine). In general, bone markers increase with increasing bone turnover.

9. How common is osteoporosis? Why is it such a health concern?

Osteoporosis affects 25 million Americans and results in 1.5 million fractures annually in the U.S. at an estimated cost of 10 billion dollars. Approximately 15% of women over age 50 have osteoporosis, and up to 50% of osteopenia. Fifty percent of women over age 65 years will have a fracture. Up to 25% of fractures (particularly hip fractures) lead to death within 1 year, and another 25% of patients remain bedridden. Fractures commonly occur in the vertebrae (spinal compression fractures) leading to loss of height, pain, and the "dowager's hump." Other sites are the hip (femur) and distal radius (Colles fractures).

10. What are the types and causes of osteoporosis?

Primary osteoporosis (type 1) is due to estrogen deprivation, advancing age, excessive smoking and alcohol consumption, poor nutrition (particularly lack of calcium, vitamin D, and protein), inadequate weight-bearing exercise, and hereditary factors such as race (Asians and Caucasians are at higher risk) and a slender body build. **Secondary osteoporosis (type 2)** can be due to: endocrine abnormalities such as parathyroid, thyroid, and cortisol excess, diabetes, and hypogonadism; gastrointestinal abnormalities such as malabsorption and anorexia; medications such as anticonvulsants, cyclosporine, glucocorticoids, GnRH agonists, heparin, isoniazid, lithium, methotrexate, and thyroid hormone.

11. Describe the treatments available for osteoporosis.

The treatments available for the prevention and treatment of osteoporosis include weight-bearing exercise, smoking and alcohol cessation, calcium supplementation (500 mg/day if on estrogen and 1000 mg/day if not on estrogen), vitamin D supplementation (especially patients in nursing homes who get limited sunlight exposure), estrogen and/or progestin replacement therapy, bisphosphonates (etidronate, alendronate, risedronate), calcitonin, selective estrogen receptor modulators (tamoxifen, raloxifene), tibolone, and parathyroid hormone. Sodium fluoride (NaF) increases bone density but may increase fracture risk. A new slow-release formulation of NaF shows more promising results. Parathyroid hormone is also under study for increasing BMD. (Please see table, next page.)

12. Why is hormone replacement therapy (HRT) often recommended in menopause?

HRT with estrogen (and a progestin if a uterus is still present) is given in menopause to replace deficient hormones. Some view the hypogonadism that defines menopause as an endocrinopathy similar to failure of other glands, therefore requiring treatment. Studies have shown a 70–80% improvement in vasomotor symptoms and urogenital atrophy, and a 2–5% increase in BMD with a 25–50% decrease risk of vertebral and hip fractures. Other studies have suggested a 20% decrease in risk of colorectal cancer, possible decreased risk of Alzheimer's and Parkinson's diseases, a 25% reduction in risk of tooth loss, and a possible decreased risk of age-related macular degeneration. While observational studies have pointed to a cardio-protective benefit of HRT, randomized controlled trials have not substantiated this effect.

Major Studies Demonstrating Efficacy of Treatment Modalities for Osteoporosis

TREATMENT	STUDY	DOSE	STUDY TYPE	BMD		FRACTURE		
				VERTEBRAL	FEMUR	VERTEBRAL	FEMUR	NONVERTEBRAL
HRT	PEPI (1996)	0.525 mg	RCT (3 yrs)	Inc 5.0%	Inc 1.7%			
	Torgerson (2001)		Meta-analysis					Dec 27%
Bisphosphonates								
Alendronate	FIT (1996)	10 mg/d	RCT (3 yrs)			Dec 55%	Dec 51%	Dec 47%
	FOSIT (1999)	10 mg/d	RCT (1 yr)	Inc 4.9%	Inc 3%			
Risedronate	VERT (1999)	5 mg/d	RCT (3 yrs)	Inc 5.4%	Inc 1.6%	Dec 41%		Dec 39%
SERMs								
Tamoxifene	NSABP PI (1998)	20 mg/d	RCT (5 yrs)			Dec 26%	Dec 45%	
Raloxifene	MORE (1999)	60 mg/d	RCT (3 yrs)	Inc 2.6%	Inc 2.1%	Dec 30%	No Change	No Change
Calcitonin	PROOF (2000)	200 IU/d	RCT (5 yrs)	Inc 1.5%		Dec 33%		
Flouride	Pak (1995)	25 mg bid	RCT (4 yrs)	Inc 4%		Dec 68%		
Vitamin D	Chapuy (1994)	800 IU/d	RCT (3 yrs)				Dec 27%	Dec 28%

Inc = increase, Dec = decrease

FIT = Fracture Intervention Trial, FOSIT = Fosamax Intervention Trial, MORE = Multiple Outcomes of Raloxifene Evaluation, NSABP = National Surgical Adjuvant Breast and Bowel Project, PEPI = Postmenopausal Estrogen/Progestin Interventions Trial, PROOF = Prevent Recurrence of Osteoporotic Fractures Study, RCT = randomized controlled trial, VERT = Vertebral Efficacy with Risedronate Therapy

13. What estrogen preparations are available for hormone replacement therapy?

Currently Available Preparations for Hormone Replacement Therapy

17 β Estradiol	**Conjugated Equine**
Oral	Premarin (po, iv, vaginal)
Activella (with norethindrone acetate)	PremPhase (with Provera, 5 mg × 14 d)
Estrace	PremPro (with 2.5 mg Provera QD)
Gynodiol	**Synthetic Conjugated**
OrthoPrefest (with norgestrel)	Cenestin
Vaginal	**Estropipate**
Estrace cream	Ogen (po and vaginal)
Estring (ring)	Ortho-Est
Vagifem (tablets)	**Esterified**
Transdermal	Estratab
Alora	Estratest (with 2.5 mg methyl-testosterone)
Climara	Menest
CombiPatch (with norethindrone acetate)	**Other**
Esclim (stretchable)	Biest (estradiol and estriol)
Estraderm	Triest (estrone, estradiol, and estriol)
FemPatch	Delestrogen (estradiol valerate-IM)
Vivelle ("Dot" is smallest patch available)	Estrocare (black cohosh extract)
Ethinyl Estradiol	
Estinyl (20 and 50 μg EE tablets)	
FemHrt (5 μg EE/1 mg norethindrone acetate)	

EE = ethinyl estradiol

14. What progestins are available, when are they used, and what are their side effects?

Currently available progestins used for HRT include medroxyprogesterone acetate (MPA), norethindrone, and micronized progesterone. A progestin-containing intrauterine device can also be used. MPA has been associated with mood disturbance (mainly depression) in some women, while micronized progesterone can lead to sedation. The role of progestins in HRT is to reduce the risk of endometrial hyperplasia that occurs with estrogen-only therapy in women who have not had a hysterectomy (a four- to eight-fold increased risk without progestin). Recent studies have shown that progestins can reverse some of the beneficial effects of estrogens on lipids, and one study suggested women on estrogen plus progestin had a higher risk of breast cancer than patients on estrogen alone.

15. What are the contraindications to estrogen replacement therapy?

Estrogen replacement therapy is contraindicated in pregnancy, and in patients with active thromboembolic disease, chronic liver impairment, undiagnosed genital bleeding, or estrogen-dependent neoplasms. Estrogen therapy has been associated with an increased risk of cholelithiasis and deep venous thrombosis as well as an increased risk of endometrial cancer if a concomitant progestin is not used. The effect, if any, on the occurrence of breast cancer is controversial.

16. What are selective estrogen receptor modulators (SERMs)? What are their advantages and disadvantages?

The ideal HRT would have positive estrogen-like effects in the urogenital system, hypothalamic thermoregulatory center, cardiovascular system, and bone as well as anti-estrogenic properties in the breast and endometrium (to prevent estrogen-dependent neoplasms). SERMs are a class of drugs that have differential estrogen agonistic and antagonistic properties in various tissues, and have been called "designer estrogens." Raloxifene is currently approved for the treatment of osteoporosis and is being studied for potential cardioprotective effects. It appears not to promote endometrial hyperplasia and may reduce the risk of breast neoplasms. Unfortunately it does not improve hot flashes or urogenital atrophy.

CONTROVERSIES

17. What is the effect of HRT on cardiovascular disease?

The effect of estrogen on cardiovascular disease is unclear. Estrogen has been shown to decrease LDL and total cholesterol while raising HDL and triglycerides. It also decreases Lp(a) lipoprotein, fibrinogen, and plasminogen-activator inhibitor type 1; inhibits oxidation of low-density lipoprotein; and improves vascular endothelial cell function. Many observational studies have shown a 30–50% decrease in coronary heart disease in estrogen users. A recent randomized controlled trial (Heart and Estrogen/Progestin Replacement Study II) found no benefit of HRT over the 6.8 years of the study, and a slight increased risk of myocardial infarction in the first year of use. The relative hazard of a cardiac event did decrease from 1.52 in the first year to 0.60 by year four, but the trend toward fewer cardiac events over time did not reach statistical significance after 6–8 years of follow-up. The Women's Health Initiative Study, recently completed, shows a relative hazard for coronary heart disease of 1.29 after 5.2 years of follow-up.

18. Does HRT increase the risk of breast cancer?

More than 50 epidemiological studies and over a half-dozen meta-analyses have tried to answer this question. With few exceptions, these studies have been observational and subject to bias. In addition, the types of hormones used, their respective doses, and their duration of administration vary from study to study, as do the criteria for the diagnosis of breast cancer. The majority of meta-analyses did *not* find compelling evidence for an association between HRT and breast cancer.

A re-analysis of the world's literature was performed by a collaborative group of epidemiologists who collected the original data from all previous studies. This re-analysis found that "ever-users" of HRT had a relative risk of breast cancer of 1.14 and "current-users" for 5 or more years had a relative risk of 1.35. It also found that HRT users had significantly less mortality from breast cancer than "never-users." The improved survival rates may be due to less aggressive tumor types in HRT users.

Recently, the Women's Health Initiative Study was halted prematurely due to an increased relative hazard for breast cancer of 1.26 after 6 years of follow-up.

BIBLIOGRAPHY

1. The North American Menopause Society: A decision tree for the use of estrogen replacement therapy or hormone replacement therapy in postmenopausal women: Consensus opinion. Menopause 7:76–86, 2000.
2. Bush TL, Whiteman M, Flaws JA: Hormone replacement therapy and breast cancer: A qualitative review. Obstet Gynecol 98:498–508, 2001.
3. Collaborative Group on Hormonal Factors in Breast Cancer: Breast cancer and hormone replacement therapy: Collaborative reanalysis of data from 51 epidemiological studies of 52,705 women with breast cancer and 108,411 women without breast cancer. Lancet 350:1047–1059, 1997.
4. Chestnut CH, et al: A randomized trial of nasal spray salmon calcitonin in postmenopausal women with established osteoporosis: The Prevent Recurrence of Osteoporotic Fractures Study (PROOF). Am J Med 109:267–276, 2000.
5. Effects of hormone therapy on bone mineral density: Results from the Postmenopausal Estrogen/Progestin Interventions (PEPI) Trial. JAMA 276:1389–1396, 1996.
6. Ettinger B, et al: Reduction of vertebral fracture risk in postmenopausal women with osteoporosis treated with raloxifene: Results from a 3-year randomized clinical trial (MORE). JAMA 282:637–645, 1999.
7. Fisher B, et al: Tamoxifen for prevention of breast cancer: Report of the National Surgical Adjuvant Breast and Bowel Project P-1 Study (NSABP P-1). J Natl Cancer Inst 90:1371–1388, 1998.
7a. Grady D, Herrington D, Bittner V, et al: Cardiovascular disease outcomes during 6.8 years of hormone therapy. Heart and Estrogen/Progeston Replacement Study Follow-up (HERS II). JAMA 288:49–57, 2002.

8. Harris ST, et al: Effects of risedronate treatment on vertebral and nonvertebral fractures in women with postmenopausal osteoporosis: A randomized controlled trial (VERT). JAMA 282:1344–1352, 1999.
9. Manson JE, Martin KA: Postmenopausal hormone replacement therapy. N Engl J Med 345:34–40, 2001.
10. Meunier PJ: Evidence-based medicine and osteoporosis: A comparison of fracture risk reduction data from osteoporosis randomise clinical trials. Int J Clin Pract 53:122–129, 1999.
11. Pak CY, Sakhaee K, Adams-Huet B, et al: Treatment of postmenopausal osteoporosis with slow-release sodium fluoride. Final report of a randomized controlled trial. Ann Intern Med 123:401–408, 1995.
12. Pols HAP, et al: Multinational, placebo-controlled, randomized trial of the effects of alendronate on bone density and fracture risk in postmenopausal women with low bone mass: Results of the FOSIT Study. Osteoporos Int 9:461–468, 1999.
13. Physicians' Desk Reference, 55th ed. Montvale, NJ, Medical Economics, 2001.
14. Speroff L, Glass RH, Kase NG (eds): Clinical Gynecologic Endocrinology and Infertility, 6th ed. Baltimore, MD, Lippincott Williams & Wilkins, 1999.
15. Torgerson DJ, Bell-Syer SEM: Hormone replacement therapy and prevention of nonvertebral fractures: A meta-analysis of randomized trials. JAMA 285:2891–2897, 2001.
16. World Health Organization: Assessment of fracture risk and its application to screening for postmenopausal osteoporosis: Report of a WHO Study Group. (Technical report series 843). Geneva, Switzerland, World Health Organization, 1994.
17. Writing Group for the Women's Health Initiative Investigators: Risks and benefits of estrogen plus progestin in healthy postmenopausal women. Principle results from the Women's Health Initiative randomized controlled trial. JAMA 288:321–333, 2002.

24. BREAST DISEASE

Alfredo Gil, M.D.

1. How is the breast exam performed?

In general, be methodical and consistent. Examine the patient in the sitting and supine positions. Have the patient flex the pectoralis muscle and open the axilla. This is easily accomplished by asking the patient to place the ipsilateral hand behind her head.

2. If a mass is discovered, how is it best described?

Size, contour, consistency, and mobility are noted, along with attachment to skin or underlying fascia. Careful examination of the axillary and supraclavicular nodes should be part of the exam. Note nipple discharge or rashes. A simple diagram of the breasts with findings drawn facilitates subsequent exams.

3. Why is a newly discovered breast mass important?

In the United States, approximately 180,000 women will be diagnosed with breast cancer in the next year. Most will present with a palpable breast mass.

4. In regard to the mass, what aspects of the history are important to highlight?

Most newly discovered breast masses are found by the patient herself. It is important to ask when it was first found, how it has changed, whether it changes with the menstrual cycle, and whether it is painful.

5. What characteristics of a breast mass suggest malignancy?

Palpable breast cancers usually have irregular or indistinct borders and may be attached to the skin, to its dermal attachments, or to the underlying fascia. However, these characteristics are not invariable. No physical characteristics allow one to distinguish reliably between benign and malignant lesions. Any breast mass should be biopsied.

6. What is the breast cancer gene? Why is it important?

The breast and ovarian cancer genes (BRCA 1 and 2) are found on two separate chromosomes. Mutations in these genes carry a greatly increased risk of breast and ovarian cancers (as well as colon, prostate, and pancreatic cancers in males). The lifetime risk of breast cancer in women with these mutations may be as high as 87%. These gene mutations are present in less than 1% of the population. So, most breast cancers are *not* due to these mutations.

Women with a strong family history may choose to be screened for the gene. Depending on the outcome of this test, the woman's age, family history, and pregnancy plans, consideration may be given to an increased cancer surveillance program or even to prophylactic mastectomy or oophorectomy.

7. What are the risk factors for breast cancer?

Age, family history of breast cancer, history of breast cancer in the opposite breast, hormone replacement therapy for longer than 10 years, early menarche and/or late menopause, nulliparity, and a history of colon or uterine cancer.

The Gail model is a computer model that analyzes a woman's various risk factors to give her an "accurate," individualized risk assessment. This model includes some of the above identified risk factors. It does not include whether or not a woman has been tested for the BRCA gene. It also does not consider the use of hormone replacement therapy.

8. Does the use of hormone replacement therapy (HRT) increase a woman's risk of breast cancer?

The bulk of epidemiologic data appears to support a slight increase in the risk of breast cancer with the use of HRT. Duration of use appears to correlate with risk.

Women should include consideration of their baseline risk of breast cancer in their assessment of the risks and benefits of HRT. A family history of breast cancer does not in itself preclude the use of HRT.

9. Is there anything a woman can do to reduce her risk of breast cancer?

Unfortunately, there is not a great deal that a woman can do to reduce her risk. Most of the risk factors (e.g., family history, age at menarche) are not under her control. It would be difficult to further complicate family planning decisions with consideration of breast cancer risk.

A woman should consider her baseline risk when deciding whether or not HRT is appropriate for her. For women at very high risk, prophylactic therapy with tamoxifen has been shown to be beneficial, with a reduction in new breast cancers. However, this therapy has not yet been shown to reduce the incidence of cancer deaths or death overall. Also, tamoxifen has side effects and effects on the uterus, which limit its use.

10. What initial diagnostic step can be taken to evaluate a newly discovered mass?

Needle aspiration of the palpable breast mass is easily and safely performed in an office or clinic setting. It distinguishes cystic from solid masses and provides cells for subsequent cytologic evaluation. Mammogram and ultrasound can aid in describing the characteristics of the mass, but alone neither study should be used to reassure the physician or the patient that the mass is benign. Magnetic resonance imaging may be helpful in the management of a palpable mass or an abnormal finding on ultrasound or mammography. It is not a screening tool.

11. If a breast cyst is aspirated, should the fluid be sent for microscopic exam?

Only if it is bloody. A clear or yellow fluid does not need to be sent for cytologic analysis.

12. What characteristics of an aspirated cyst require further work-up?

As noted, aspiration of bloody fluid is suspicious. Also, if there is a residual mass after aspiration or if the cyst recurs, the likelihood of cancer increases, and further diagnostic studies should be performed.

13. If attempted aspiration of a palpable breast mass reveals a solid lesion, what further diagnostic studies can be performed?

The aspirated sample can be prepared on a slide and sent for cytologic analysis. The technique requires some experience and the availability of a cytopathologist.

14. List the advantages of fine-needle aspiration of a solid breast mass over open biopsy.

Fine-needle aspiration is cheaper and more comfortable, has a better cosmetic result, and, in experienced hands, is very accurate.

15. What are the disadvantages of fine-needle aspiration of a solid breast mass over open biopsy?

A considerable amount of skill is required to obtain a satisfactory sample. An experienced cytopathologist is required to interpret the sample. There is a small but measurable number of false-negative and false-positive results compared with open biopsy.

16. Describe the role of mammography in the evaluation of palpable breast masses.

The purpose of mammograms is to detect non-palpable, suspicious areas in either breast. Mammography along with ultrasound can also serve as an adjunct in the evaluation of a palpable mass.

17. Does a normal-appearing mammogram in a woman with a palpable mass exclude the possibility of cancer?

No. In general, the false-negative rate for mammograms is reported to be as high as 16%. Even in the presence of clinically evident cancer, mammograms can be interpreted as normal.

18. In what settings are mammograms particularly difficult to interpret?

Dense breasts are difficult for radiologists to evaluate. Overall, this problem is found in 25% of women and is particularly common in younger women.

19. Describe the role of ultrasound in the evaluation of solid breast masses.

Ultrasound is useful for differentiating solid from cystic masses. The study can be used in women with large breasts who have deep, inaccessible lesions or who cannot undergo needle aspiration.

20. What is the approach to a woman whose mammogram shows a non-palpable lesion that is read as "probably benign" by the radiologists?

There are two choices: biopsy or repeat mammography within 6 months. Recent studies indicate that the second approach is probably safe, but much depends on the comfort of the physician with the mammographic appearance and availability of the patient for follow-up.

21. If a lesion is regarded as suspicious on mammogram, but is not palpable, how is it approached?

Mammographic localization techniques (including wires and dyes) are used to guide the surgeon for an open, excision biopsy.

22. Are techniques other than open biopsy available to sample suspicious, non-palpable breast lesions?

Recently, radiologists have developed techniques of stereotactic core biopsies of non-palpable breast lesions. The technique is well tolerated and accurate, but its role in the approach to patients with suspicious, non-palpable breast lesions is currently being defined.

23. What pathologic findings on breast biopsy put patients at a higher risk for subsequent development of breast cancer?

Most breast biopsies return as benign with some variation of fibrocystic disease. Of these lesions, approximately 30% show a proliferative pattern that is associated with an increased risk for the subsequent development of cancer. In this 30%, atypical hyperplasia shows the highest relative risk.

24. Discuss the significance of nipple discharge in a woman who is not breastfeeding.

The character of the discharge is important. Milky discharge is termed galactorrhea and is usually benign. Bloody discharge may be a symptom of a breast neoplasm, specifically an intraductal papilloma. Yellow or green discharge also may be associated with breast disease.

Galactorrhea can be caused by medications (e.g., phenothiazines, oral contraceptives), hypothyroidism, pituitary tumors, and a variety of other less common causes. Evaluation should begin with a review of current medications and assessment of the prolactin level and thyroid function.

25. What is the differential diagnosis of a breast mass?

Breast cancer, fibrocystic disease, fibroadenoma, trauma (fat necrosis). The frequency varies with age. Fibrocystic change of the breast is the most common cause of a breast mass.

26. What is fibrocystic change of the breast?

Fibrocystic change or fibrocystic disease is a benign change in breast tissue characterized by fibrosis of breast stroma and the formation of cysts within the breast. It typically affects women between ages 20 and 50 and is unusual after menopause. Some women can palpate changes in the breast, but most women with fibrocystic change are only aware of breast pain that varies with their menstrual cycle; the symptoms are worse prior to menses. Women with fibrocystic disease are *not* at increased risk for breast cancer.

27. What causes mastalgia? How can it be treated?

Breast pain, termed mastalgia, has a variety of nonspecific causes. Fibrocystic change is associated with mastalgia. Hormones—either oral contraceptives or HRT—can cause mastalgia. Various treatments have been used, including analgesics, low-dose diuretics, danazol, and reduction in caffeine intake. Women with mastalgia are *not* at increased risk for breast cancer.

28. Describe the major types of breast cancer.

Most breast cancers involve the ductal tissue. Ductal carcinoma is divided into **infiltrating ductal carcinoma** and **ductal carcinoma in situ** (DCIS). Approximately 10% of breast cancers are lobular. Again, this category is subdivided into *infiltrating lobular carcinoma* and *lobular carcinoma in situ*.

Ductal carcinoma in situ identifies a woman at increased risk of invasive breast cancer. Most women with DCIS develop an infiltrating carcinoma, and a small percentage have an invasive tumor present in the breast at the time of diagnosis of DCIS. Lobular carcinoma in situ is also associated with an increased risk of invasive breast cancer, but the development of breast cancer is somewhat less likely than with DCIS, and the time to diagnosis of invasive disease is longer.

BIBLIOGRAPHY

1. Donegan W: Evaluation of a palpable breast mass. N Engl J Med 327:937–942, 1992.
2. Dupont WD, Page DL: Risk factors for breast cancer in women with a proliferative breast disease. N Engl J Med 312:146–151, 1985.
3. Fisher B, Costantino JP, Wicherham DL, and other National Surgical Adjuvant Breast and Bowel Project Investigators: Tamoxifen for prevention of breast cancer: Report of the National Surgical Adjuvant Breast and Bowel Project P-1 Study. J Natl Cancer Inst 90:1371, 1998.
4. Grant CS, Goellner JR, Welch JS, Martin JK: Fine needle aspiration of the breast. Mayo Clinical Proc 61:377–381, 1986.
5. Layfield LJ, Chrischilles EA, Cohen MB, Bottles K: The palpable breast nodule: A cost-effective analysis of alternate diagnostic approaches. Cancer 72:1642–1651, 1993.
6. Parker SH, Lovin JD, Jobe WE, et al: Sterotactic breast biopsy with a biopsy gun. Radiology 176:741–747, 1990.
7. Sickles EA: Periodic mammographic follow-up of probably benign lesions: Results in 3184 consecutive cases. Radiology 179:463–468, 1991.
8. Speroff L, Glass RH, Kase NG: Clinical gynecologic endocrinology and infertility, 6th ed. Philadelphia, Lippincott Williams & Wilkins, 1999.
9. Stenchever MA, Droegemueller W, Herbst AL, Mishell DR: Comprehensive gynecology, 4th ed. St. Louis, Mosby, 2001.

II. Gynecologic Oncology

25. VULVAR AND VAGINAL CANCERS

Peter Argenta, M.D.

1. How is vulvar cancer different than vulvar dysplasia?

Dysplasia refers to abnormally differentiated cells contained entirely within the epithelium—above the basal membrane. Violation of the basement membrane indicates invasion and therefore cancer.

2. What is the incidence of vulvar cancer?

It is estimated that 3600 new cases of vulvar cancer were diagnosed during 2001, accounting for 5–8% of all genital tract cancers detected in women. The incidence appears to have increased during the last century; however, this may reflect the longer average life-span of women compared with earlier decades.

The most common cancers of the vulva are epidermoid squamous cell (85%), melanoma (5%), undifferentiated (4%), and sarcoma (2%). Adenocarcinomas and Bartholin's gland cancer are rare, comprising about 1% of vulvar cancers each. Except where specified, this chapter focuses on squamous cell cancers.

3. What are the causative agents and risk factors?

There is no confirmed causative agent, but multiple risk factors have been identified. They include: advanced age (the highest incidence occurs between ages 65 and 75), history of vulvar dysplasias, low socioeconomic status, and smoking. Obesity, hypertension, and diabetes are more common in these patients, probably reflecting comorbid disease of the elderly rather than causation. Human papilloma virus (HPV) is found in up to 60% of vulvar cancers, though it is epidemiologically linked more strongly to cervical cancer.

4. List the symptoms of vulvar cancer.

The most common presenting complaint is itch (45%) or palpable mass (45%). Pain, bleeding, ulceration, or dysuria are present in at least 10% of cases. In most patients, symptoms are mild and persist for months (sometimes more than a year) before medical attention is sought. Failure of apparently routine infection (Candida) to respond to standard therapy tips the clinician to the possible presence of cancer.

5. How is the diagnosis made?

The diagnosis is made by vulvar biopsy. Unfortunately, most reports indicate that diagnosis is often delayed by weeks or months while topical medical treatments are applied in the absence of a tissue diagnosis.

6. Describe the pattern of spread.

Most vulvar cancers behave similarly, with relatively indolent growth followed by metastasis through lymphatic tissue. Lymphatic flow in the vulva runs anteriorly from the labia toward the mons, and then laterally to the ipsilateral groin. The most common site of initial metastasis is to the superficial inguinal nodes. From there spread is usually through the fossa ovalis to the deep femoral nodes, then proximally to the iliac chains. Lymph channels do cross the midline; therefore, centrally occurring lesions have an increased incidence of contralateral groin involvement.

There are lymphatics in the anterior introitus and clitoris which drain under the symphysis, directly into the pelvic lymph channels, but they are of little clinical significance as pelvic metastasis without inguinal pathology is exceedingly rare.

7. How is vulva cancer staged?

Staging for Carcinoma of the Vulva

Stage 0 Tis	Carcinoma in situ: intraepithelial carcinoma
Stage I T1N0 M0	Tumor confined to the vulva and/or perineum; ≤ 2 cm in greatest dimension; nodes not palpable
Stage II T2N0 M0	Tumor confined to vulva and/or perineum—> 2 cm in greatest dimension; notes are not palpable
Stage III T3N0 M0 T3N1 M0 T1N1 M0 T2N1 M0	Tumor of any size with (1) adjacent spread to lower urethra and/or vagina or anus and/or (2) unilateral regional lymph node metastasis
Stage IVA T1N2 M0 T2N2 M0 T3N2 M0 T4 any N M0	Tumor invades any of the following: Upper urethra, bladder mucosa, rectal mucosa, pelvic bone, and/or bilateral regional node metastasis
Stage IVB Any T Any N, M1	Any distant metastasis, including pelvic lymph nodes

TNM Classification of Carcinoma of the Vulva

T	**Primary tumor**	**N**	**Regional lymph nodes**
Tis	Preinvasive carcinoma (carcinoma in situ)	N0	No lymph node metastasis
T1	Tumor confined to vulva and/or perineum; ≤ 2 cm in greatest dimension	N1	Unilateral regional lymph node metastasis
T2	Tumor confined to vulva and/or perineum; > 2 cm in greatest dimension	N2	Bilateral regional lymph node metastasis
T3	Tumor of any size with adjacent spread to urethra and/or vagina and/or to anus	**M**	**Distant metastasis**
		M0	No clinical metastasis
T4	Tumor of any size infiltrating bladder mucosa and/or rectal mucosa, including upper part of urethral mucosa and/or fixed to bone	M1	Distant metastasis (including pelvic lymph node metastasis)

From International Federation of Gynecology and Obstetrics: Annual report on the results of treatment in gynecological cancer. Int J Gynecol Obstet 28:189–190, 1989.

8. How is vulvar cancer treated?

Surgery is the primary therapy for vulvar cancer. Traditionally, radical vulvar excision with bilateral inguinal and pelvic lymph node dissection was the standard of practice for all invasive lesions. This procedure provided excellent survival rates, but carried considerable morbidity and was profoundly disfiguring. Recently, more conservative approaches such as wide and radical local excisions have been demonstrated to provide similar efficacy with substantially reduced morbidity.

Lesions demonstrating poor prognostic features can be treated even more aggressively with combination therapies using surgery, radiation, and/or chemotherapy.

9. When is a groin dissection necessary?

Ipsilateral groin dissection is required for lesions that are unilateral (> 1 cm from midline) and that invade > 1 mm *or* are > 2 cm in width. If these nodes are negative, the risk for isolated contralateral metastasis is less than 3% overall. If any of the ipsilateral nodes are positive, however, the contralateral groin must be surgically evaluated. Some doctors advocate pelvic node dissection when groin nodes are positive, but adequate data from prospective, randomized trials indicates that postoperative radiation to the groin and hemipelvis is superior to pelvic lymph node dissection in maintaining local control.

Lesions that are < 1 cm from the midline require bilateral groin evaluation if dissection is required, because the propensity for contralateral spread is much higher as the midline is approached.

10. Is there a role for radiation or chemotherapy?

Radiation is used predominantly for locally advanced disease. Due to the geometry of this body region, attaining homogeneous dosing is difficult at best, and impossible in some cases. When bulky disease exists, interstitial radiation can be applied (some reported success).

Chemotherapy is useful for disease that has metastasized out of the pelvis. In this setting, neither surgery nor radiation can address all of the lesions. Response rates to chemotherapy alone are up to 30%, but the duration of response is generally short. Using chemotherapy as a radiation-sensitizing agent, as has been successful for cervical cancer, is under investigation now.

11. What precautions are taken when the lesion is near the urethra?

Effort should be made to leave the urethra intact. When dictated by the proximity of the tumor, the distal 1–2 cm of the urethra can be excised without impairing continence. *Note*: When excision margins are close to, or include, the urethra, it it important to confirm that the repair is tension free, because stricture with healing may result in urethral dysfunction at a later date.

12. What is the prognosis for vulvar cancer?

Five-year survival rates are as follows:

Stage I	91%
Stage II	81%
Stage III	48%
Stage IV	15%

The presence of even one lymph node metastasis decreases survival rates in all stages by 50% or more in most series. Deep (pelvic) nodal metastases are even more ominous, with fewer than one in five patients surviving 5 years.

13. What is vulvar Paget's disease?

Paget's disease of the vulva is an intraepithelial lesion characterized by a superficial, velvety thickening with areas of intermixed redness and leukoplakia (the so-called "cake-icing effect"). Underlying adenocarcinomas were once reported in up to 20% of Paget's cases, prompting recommendations for radical excision. Recent studies, however, suggest a much lower incidence, with most lesions curable by simple local excision and sampling of the underlying tissue to exclude occult cancer.

14. What is the incidence of vaginal cancer?

Fewer than 2000 women are diagnosed with new vaginal cancers each year, approximately 1–3% of all female genital malignancies. Interestingly, **secondary cancers of the vagina** (from cervix, endometrium, vulva, bladder, urethra, and other locations) are more common than primary vaginal malignancies.

15. What are the predisposing factors to vaginal cancer?

As with vulvar cancer, there is no causative agent identified for squamous lesions, which compose the vast majority of cases. Bacterial infection, trauma (as with pessary or prolapse), and HPV exposure have all been postulated as predisposing factors, but scientific evidence of causation is lacking. Exposure to the synthetic estrogen diethylstilbestrol (DES) *in utero* is associated with increased incidence of adenocarcinomas of the vagina, specifically of the clear cell subtype.

16. Who gets vaginal cancer?

Though vaginal cancer has been reported in every decade of life, it is predominantly a disease of older women, with about 70% of patients diagnosed after the age of 70. Two notable exceptions to this rule are sarcoma botryoides and vaginal endodermal sinus tumor. These rare tumors demonstrate a predilection for infants and children.

17. How does vaginal cancer present?

The most common complaint is vaginal discharge, with or without bleeding. Difficulty with voiding and/or intercourse are also reported owing to the tendency of this cancer to restrict the normal pliability of the vagina. Often the diagnosis is delayed because of the subtlety of the symptoms, especially in sexually inactive women.

18. Does the pattern of spread in vaginal cancer follow that of cervical cancer or vulvar cancer?

It depends on the location of the lesion. Like both cervix and vulvar cancer, the route of metastasis is primarily via lymph channels; however, there are extensive anastomoses of lymphatic channels in the vagina, and any pelvic or inguinal node chain may be affected primarily. In general, though, the distal third of the vagina drains to the femoral and external iliac nodes; the middle third drains to the internal iliac chain; and the proximal third to the common iliacs and pre-sacral areas.

19. How is vaginal cancer staged?

Staging for vaginal cancer is based on clinical exam:

Stage 0	Carcinoma in situ
Stage I	Tumor limited to vaginal wall
Stage II	Tumor involves subvaginal tissue but does not extend to pelvic sidewall
Stage III	Tumor extends to the sidewall
Stage IV	Tumor extends beyond the true pelvis or has invaded bladder or rectal mucosa
IVa	Direct extension into adjacent organs, or beyond true pelvis
IVb	Distant metastases

Note: When cancer in the vagina is contiguous with an adjacent superficial structure (e.g., cervix, urethra, vulva), the cancer is most often secondarily involving the vagina.

20. What are the management options for vaginal cancer?

Both stage I and *in situ* lesions can be managed with surgical excision. In some patients, radical hysterectomy is performed to obtain adequate margins. When deep invasion is present, external beam radiation to the whole pelvis is given initially to reduce the primary tumor volume and sterilize the regional lymphatics. External beam therapy is followed by intracavitary or intrastitial treatment, which allows cytotoxic doses to be delivered directly to the tumor while minimizing collateral damage to surrounding normal tissue.

Persistent or recurrent disease can be treated with exenterative procedures if the disease has not spread distantly. The success rate for these procedures has been reported as high as 40%.

21. What is the prognosis for patients after treatment of vaginal cancer?

Five-year survival rates are as follows:

Stage I	70%
Stage II	40%
Stage III	30%
Stage IV	15–20%

BIBLIOGRAPHY

1. Chyle V, Zagars GK, Wheeler JA: Definitive radiotherapy for carcinoma of the vagina: Outcome and prognostic factors. Int J Radiat Oncol Biol Phys 891–905, 1996.
2. Homesley HD, Bundy BN, Sedlis A, et al: Assessment of current International Federation of Gynecology and Obstetrics staging of vulvar carcinoma relative to prognostic factors for survival (a Gynecologic Oncology Group Study). Am J Obstet Gynecol 156:1159–1164, 1987.
3. Kucera H, Vavra N: Primary carcinoma of the vagina: Clinical and histopathological variables associated with survival. Gynecol Oncol 40:12, 1991.
4. Levenback C, Burke TW, Morris M: Potential applications of intraoperative lymphatic mapping in vulvar cancer. Gynecol Oncol 59:216–220, 1995.
5. Manetta A, Gutrecht EL, Berman Ml DiSaia: Primary invasive carcinoma of the vagina. Obstet Gynecol 76:639–642, 1990.
6. Morrow CP, Curtin JP: Synopsis of Gynecologic Oncology. Philadelphia, Churchill-Livingstone, 1998.
7. Podratz KC, Symmonds RE, Taylor WF, Williams TJ: Carcinoma of the vulva: Analysis of treatment and survival. Obstet Gynecol 61:63–74, 1983.
8. Robboy SJ, Noller NL, O'Brien P, et al: Incidence of cervical and vaginal dysplasia in 3980 diethylstilbestrol-exposed young women. Experience of the National Collaborative DES Adenosis Project. JAMA 252:2979–2983, 1984.

26. PRECANCEROUS DISEASE OF THE LOWER GENITAL TRACT

Bruce Drummond, M.D.

1. Why is the Papanicolaou (Pap) smear a good screening test for cervical cancer?

The Pap smear is a noninvasive and inexpensive screening test for cervical precancerous disease that is easily performed in the office setting. For the past 40 years, the Pap smear has been instrumental in reducing the mortality from cervical cancer by 70%.

2. How frequently should Pap smears be performed?

The American College of Obstetricians and Gynecologists recommends an annual cervical smear and pelvic exam for all women who are 18 years or older, or who have been sexually active. If three consecutive, satisfactory, and normal smears are obtained, then less frequent Pap smears may be performed at the discretion of the physician.

3. What is the most effective tool used for the Pap test?

The extended tip spatula in combination with a cytobrush is the most effective tool for obtaining cervical cells.

4. What is the advantage of a ThinPrep Pap test over the conventional Pap smear test?

The ThinPrep test uses a liquid vial for transport of the specimen and the ThinPrep 2000 machine for slide preparation, which results in minimal obscuring elements on the slide. Compared to conventional smears, the ThinPrep Pap test increases the detection rate of low-grade squamous intraepithelial neoplasia (LSIL) by 72% and high-grade squamous intraepithelial neoplasia (HSIL) by 103%. The atypical squamous cells of undetermined significance (ASCUS) rates are reduced by 39%. In addition to a higher sensitive and specificity, the ThinPrep improves the adequacy of the specimens. The Food and Drug Administration therefore has permitted the claim "significantly more effective" for marketing the liquid-based Pap test.

5. What is the Bethesda System?

In 1988, the National Cancer Institute sponsored a consensus panel that developed the Bethesda system. The two-tiered system classified cytological abnormalities as either low- or high-grade squamous intraepithelial abnormalities. It was revised in 1991 to address the need for terminology to correlate well with histological findings. A third consensus panel, Bethesda 2001, was convened in an attempt to simplify the classification system. New recommendations reflect advances in technology and are intended to minimize equivocal diagnoses. These recommendations should also produce reports that are more adaptable to the clinical setting.

6. What are some of the recommendations of Bethesda 2001 that pathologists may adopt into their Pap smear reporting system?

The terms "within normal limits" and "benign cellular changes" have been eliminated in the current recommendations. The general categorization section reports abnormalities as "negative for intraepithelial lesion or malignancy," or "epithelial cell abnormality" and "other." Epithelial abnormalities are divided into squamous or glandular subcategories. The "other" category may document findings such as endometrial cells found on the smear in a patient over 40 years old. The term "bacterial vaginosis" is now used, as well.

The term "satisfactory but limited by" has been eliminated. Specimen adequacy is reported as either "satisfactory for evaluation" or "unsatisfactory for evaluation." Physicians should pay attention to reports that note a lack of endocervical cells. Depending on clinical suspicion and judgment, physicians may repeat the Pap smear at accelerated intervals. Rescreening should not exceed 1 year if endocervical cells are absent on the specimen. Pap smears obscured by inflammation or blood should be considered for repeat screening.

Bethesda 2001 attempted to reduce confusion in the atypical cell category. Atypical cells undergoing repair and inflammation are reported as normal. Atypical squamous cells (ASC) that share features of high-grade precancerous cells can be reported as ASC-H. Clinicians will then be more likely to follow-up with colposcopy. ASC of undetermined significance are termed ASC-US.

7. Why is the human papillomaviruses (HPV) clinically important?

The human papillomavirus is associated with genital precancerous lesions such as cervical intraepithelial neoplasia (CIN), vulvar intraepithelial neoplasia, and vaginal intraepithelial neoplasia. The virus is predominately transmitted by sexual contact. There is strong evidence demonstrating that HPV infection can lead to the development of invasive cervical cancer.

8. What are the cellular changes seen with HPV infection?

Based on strict criteria, the cellular changes seen in HPV-infected squamous cells are cytoplasmic vacuolization and nuclear enlargement, irregularity, and hyperchromasia.

9. What is the natural history of HPV infections and CIN lesions?

Over time, 70% of cervical HPV lesions spontaneously regress, 14% progress, and the remainder persist. Interestingly, the natural history of HPV and CIN lesions is almost identical (see table).

For CIN I lesions with HPV (HPV-CIN I), 65% regress, 14% progress to CIS, and the remainder persist. For HPV-CIN III lesions, 11% regress, 79% progress, and the remainder persist.

Comparison of the Natural History of CIN and Genital HPV

LESION	REGRESSION (%)	PERSISTENCE (%)	PROGRESSION TO CIS (%)	PROGRESSION TO INVASIVE CANCER (%)
CIN 1	57.0	32.0	11.0	1.0
CIN 2	43.0	35.0	22.0	5.0
CIN 3	32.0	< 56.0	—	> 12.0
HPV-NCIN	79.9	14.6	5.2	0.0
HPV-CIN 1	65.1	20.8	14.2	0.0
HPV-CIN 2	58.6	18.6	21.4	0.0
HPV-CIN 3	11.6	9.3	79.1*	0.5†

Table compiled from the data reviewed by Östör (1993), and from the figures of Kuopio Prospective Follow up Study (1981–98) (Syrjänen et al., 1996a,b).
• Progression based on colposcopy (lesion severity and extent) and histology (progress from severe dysplasia to CIS in two subsequent biopsies). HPV-NCIN: HPV lesion without CIN.
† One lesion progressed to invasion in less than 3 years.

10. Why are CIN I and HPV cellular changes included in the same category of low-grade squamous intraepithelial neoplasia in the Bethesda system?

The Bethesda system includes HPV cellular changes and CIN I in the same category of low-grade squamous intraepithelial neoplasia because they cannot be consistently distinguished on the basis of morphology, molecular biology, or clinical behavior.

11. Why are CIN II and CIN III included in the same category of high-grade squamous intraepithelial neoplasia?

The Bethesda system lumps CIN II and CIN III together because reproducibility in distinguishing them is low, the natural history is similar, and the treatment recommendations are the same. (See figures.)

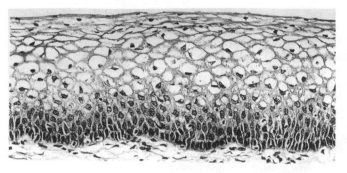

Normal cervical epithelium, uniform in pattern and cytology. The cells mature progressively as they move toward the surface, the nuclei become pyknotic, and glycogenation occurs.

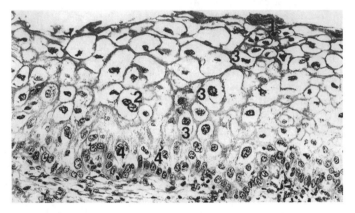

HPV infection "alone" (low-grade intraepithelial neoplasia), with mild, full-thickness cellular enlargement, and hyperchromasia with superficial dyskeratosis accompanied by (1) karyopyknosis, (2) binucleation, and (3) koilocytosis. In the bottom three cell layers are variable nuclear and cell size; irregular, variable, condensed chromatin aggregation; degenerative nucleoplasmic clearing; nucleolar increase; and (4) some visible early koilocytes.

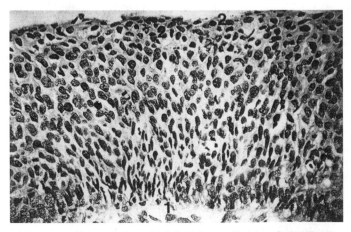

CIN III (high-grade intraepithelial neoplasia), with full-thickness effacement by small-cell suprabasal cells exhibiting characteristic neoplastic "coarse-pepper" chromatin without conspicuous macronucleation. (1) Flat basal margin. (2) Mitoses close to the surface.

12. What is an effective triage strategy for the presence of atypical squamous cells of undetermined significance (ASCUS) on cytology?

Testing for cancer-associated HPV subtypes may be an effective triage strategy. This strategy uses the presence or absence of high-risk HPV subtypes to determine the need to proceed to the next diagnostic step—colposcopy and cervical biopsy. Under this strategy, the liquid-based cytology media is saved during cytologic evaluation. When ASCUS is found, the saved sample is tested with the Hybrid Capture 2 HPV DNA test. If the test is positive for high-risk viruses, colposcopy is done, and when it is negative, a repeat Pap test is done at 6 to 12 months.

13. What is the ASCUS/LSIL triage study?

The ASCUS/LSIL Triage Study (ALTS) is a multi-center, randomized trial that compares the sensitivity and specificity of different triage methods for women found to have ASCUS or low-grade intraepithelial neoplasia on Pap smear. Thus far, the authors have concluded that all low-grade squamous intraepithelial lesions on cytology should be evaluated by colposcopy. That is, the use of HPV testing was not found to be helpful in determining the need for colposcopy.

However, for women with ASCUS on Pap, HPV typing was helpful. Testing for high-risk HPV subtypes using the Hybrid Capture 2 (HC2) viral assay was 96% sensitive for the diagnosis of CIN 3 or cervical cancer. Repeat Pap smear was only 85% sensitive. Moreover, the addition of the HPV assay allowed approximately half the women with ASCUS on Pap to forgo colposcopy.

So a strategy including HPV testing eliminates the need for repeat Pap smears and unnecessary colposcopic exams for patients with ASCUS not associated with high-risk HPV subtypes. The negative predictive value of the HC2 test is 99%. Further outcomes from the ongoing ALTS and the cost of HPV testing will determine the future clinical application of this triage method.

14. What criteria make a colposcopic exam satisfactory?

A satisfactory colposcopy is one where the squamocolumnar junction and the full extent of abnormal epithelium are visible. An exam is unsatisfactory when the extent of lesion is not seen. This occurs when the lesion extends into the endocervix or is obscured by inflammation or atrophy.

15. How do abnormal epithelial tissues look on a colposcopic examination?

Abnormal epithelium, with its higher cellular count and increased nuclear content, reflects light, giving it an opaque appearance after application of dilute acetic acid. Patterns of the abnormal ectocervical epithelium containing CIN are described as acetowhite, mosaic, and punctated (see table). Leukoplakia and atypical blood vessels are more likely to be seen in an endocervical lesion. Foci of invasive carcinoma may be detected by atypical blood vessel patterns. Early invasion may have the above stated abnormalities in a larger lesion with ulceration, increased vascularity, or the presence of other epithelial types.

International Colposcopic Terminology

Normal Colposcopic Findings
   Original Squamous epithelium
   Columnar epithelium
   Normal transformation zone

Abnormal Colposcopic Findings (within the transformation zone)
   Acetowhite epithelium*
      Flat
      Micropapillary or microconvoluted
   Punctation*
   Mosaic*
   Leukoplakia*
   Iodine negative
   Atypical vessels

(*Table continued on next page.*)

International Colposcopic Terminology (cont.)

Colposcopically Suspect invasive carcinoma

Unsatisfactory Colposcopy
  Squamocolumnar junction not visible
  Severe inflammation or severe atrophy
  Cervix not visible

Miscellaneous Findings
  Non-acetowhite micropapillary surface
  Exophytic condyloma
  Inflammation
  Atrophy
  Ulcer
  Other

---

* Indicates minor or major changes. Minor changes: acetowhite epithelium, fine mosaic, fine punctation, thin leukoplakia. Major changes; dense acetowhite epithelium, coarse mosaic, coarse punctation, thick leukoplakia, atypical vessels, erosion. (Ratified by the International Federation of Cervical Pathology and Colposcopy, at Rome, Italy, May 1990.)

16. What colposcopic features suggest the presence of adenocarcinoma in-situ?
Although the precursor glandular lesions of invasive disease are linked to HPV, they are not as well defined as squamous lesions. Intense acetowhite changes, non-uniform or fused papillae, large crypt openings with excessive mucus production, and abnormal blood vessels suggest the presence of adenocarcinoma in-situ.

17. What considerations are given to a pregnant patient with abnormal cytology?
The diagnostic management of abnormal cytology in pregnancy is the same as in the non-pregnant state. An experienced colposcopist can determine the precancerous nature and extent of the lesion with careful inspection and, if necessary, selective punch biopsy. If there is a suggestion of *invasive cancer*, punch, wedge, or cone biopsy should be done, with consideration for the increased vascularity of the pregnant cervix. For *precancerous lesions*, vaginal delivery and delay of treatment until after delivery is recommended. The evaluation during pregnancy includes counseling to addresses the pregnant women's fears and concern for the well-being of the unborn child.

18. What is the importance of human immunodeficiency virus (HIV) status in precancerous disease?
There is a high prevalence of abnormal Pap smears, condyloma, and precancerous disease corresponding directly to the severity of the immunodeficiency. The lower genital tract, including the cervix, vagina, vulva, perineum, and anus is more likely to be involved in women with HIV. Finally, there are higher rates of persistence, recurrence, and progression of precancerous disease in women infected with HIV. Therefore, it is necessary to screen more frequently—at 6-month intervals—and to have a low threshold for colposcopy. With ASCUS on a Pap smear from an HIV-positive woman, the likelihood of precancerous disease may be as high as 38%.

19. What are the indications for a conization of the cervix?
After a colposcopy is performed, a cold knife cone, loop electrosurgical excision procedure (LEEP), or carbon dioxide laser may be employed in the following conditions:
  • The colposcopy is unsatisfactory because the extent of the lesion cannot be seen and biopsied.
  • The cytology suggests a more serious lesion or invasion, and there is no colposcopic evidence confirming this finding.
  • There is suggestion of invasive disease on cytology, colposcopy, or biopsy.
  • An abnormal glandular lesion is present.
  • The endocervical curettage is positive for a precancerous or cancerous lesion.

20. Do LEEP specimens with dysplasia found at the margins indicate inadequate treatment?

The LEEP specimen with dysplasia noted at the margins does not indicate inadequate treatment. On close follow-up, in most cases, there will be no residual disease.

21. When is a hysterectomy indicated for treatment of precancerous disease of the cervix?

Hysterectomy is rarely indicated for the routine treatment of CIN. If a conization specimen has CIS present at the margins, the patient's age, desire for fertility, anxiety, and ability to adhere to a very close follow-up schedule are important factors in the decision for hysterectomy.

If a hysterectomy is planned for coexisting benign gynecologic conditions, an adequate evaluation of the cervix is necessary for precancerous lesions.

22. After conization of the cervix, how can recurrence of precancerous disease be detected?

Cytology alone can be used for completely resected lesions. This should take place at 4- to 6-month intervals for 2 years. For specimens with residual lesion at the endocervical margins, endocervical brush cytology or endocervical curettage is performed. For positive ectocervical margins, colposcopy may be used to detect residual disease. HPV-DNA typing can be considered for partially resected lesions.

23. How is future pregnancy affected by conization of the cervix?

Removal of greater than 10 mm depth of cervical tissue is an independent risk factor for preterm labor and low birth weight. Cervical stenosis may require dilation for evaluation of recurrence and facilitating progressive labor. Loss of fertility has not been proven following excisional biopsy.

24. What are the risk factors for vaginal intraepithelial neoplasia (VAIN)?

VAIN is found in women who have had cervical or vulvar intraepithelial neoplasia, have received previous radiation for cervical cancer, or are in an immunosuppressed state from transplant or HIV infections. HPV has been implicated as the cause of vaginal neoplasia.

25. How can VAIN be diagnosed and treated?

Most lesions are detected by colposcopy in the upper one-third of the vagina as acetowhite changes or abnormal vasculature. Lugol's solution may stain the lesions yellow. Local anesthesia aids biopsy. Vaginal precancer may be found in association with cervical or vulvar precancerous disease. For lesions VAIN II or greater, treatment consists of excisional or ablative therapy.

26. What are the hallmarks of vulvar intraepithelial neoplasia (VIN)?

VIN is classified as VIN I, II, III, and carcinoma-in-situ with increasing degrees of atypia in the epithelium. Precancerous vulvar disease is associated with sexually transmitted infections, HIV, smoking, and other lower genital tract neoplasia. HPV is often found in VIN lesions. Unlike the natural history of cervical precancerous disease, the progression of VIN III to cancer is unusual.

27. What is the presentation of vulvar precancer?

Patients usually complain of chronic itching. The lesions found on the vulva may be red, pigmented, or white. There may be single lesions or multiple lesions that can be flat or raised. The anal region should also be evaluated during the colposcopic exam.

28. What is the management of vulvar precancer?

After the diagnosis is established with punch biopsy, wide local excision, laser ablation, or application of 5 fluorouracil cream may be used for treatment. Recurrence of vulvar precancer is common, warranting reevaluation at 4- to 6-month intervals.

BIBLIOGRAPHY

1. American College of Obstetricians and Gynecologists: Cervical Cytology: Evaluation and Management of Abnormalities. ACOG Tech Bull 183, 1993.
2. Cover Story/Symposium, Bethesda 2001: How the new Pap terminology will impact clinical practice. Contemp OB/GYN, Oct 2001.
3. Diaz-Rosario LA, Kabawat SA: Performance of a fluid based, thin-layer Papinicolaou smear method in the clinical setting of an independent laboratory and an outpatient screening population in New England. Arch Path Lab Med 123:817–821, 1998.
4. Singer A, Monaghan J: Lower Genital Tract Precancer—Colposcopy, Pathology, and Treatment, 2nd ed. Oxford, Blackwell Science Ltd., 2000.
5. Solomon D, Schiffman M, Tarone R: ALTS Study Group. Comparison of three management strategies for patients with atypical squamous cells of undetermined significance: Baseline results from a randomized trial. J Natl Cancer Inst 193:293–299, 2001.

27. CERVICAL CANCER

Peter Argenta, M.D.

1. Differentiate cervical dysplasia, carcinoma *in situ*, and cervical cancer.

Cervical dysplasia refers to a neoplastic process that has not violated the basement membrane. For this reason it is also called cervical intraepithelial neoplasia. Carcinoma *in situ* refers to high-grade dysplasia involving the full thickness of the epithelium, usually with marked nuclear atypia. The term "cancer" implies that there has been invasion through the basement membrane. Untreated carcinoma *in situ* progresses to cancer in about 15–33% of patients if follow-up is extended to 10 years.

2. What causes cervical cancer?

The cause of cervical cancer is unknown. However, extensive evidence indicates that infection with certain subtypes of human papilloma virus is an important risk factor. Increased incidence of cervical cancer is seen with: lower socioeconomic status, early age of first coitus, higher numbers of sexual partners or spouses with high numbers of sexual partners, and cigarette smoking. Most recently cervical cancer has been associated with autoimmune deficiency, with increased incidence seen in patients after organ transplant, and in those with HIV/AIDS disease. In fact, cervical cancer has become an "AIDS-defining" condition.

3. How many people get cervical cancer?

In the United States, it is estimated that 12,900 women got cervical cancer during 2001, making it the 10th most common cancer diagnosed. Worldwide incidence approaches 500,000 cases/year, and half of these patients will die of their disease, making it among the leading causes of cancer death for women in many developing nations.

4. Is the incidence of cervical cancer increasing or decreasing? Why?

Decreasing. There is solid evidence that the incidence of cervical cancer has decreased steadily in areas where screening programs are employed. These programs, in general, improve detection of preinvasive disease and allow for therapeutic intervention. The risk may be reduced in an individual by 90% when regular screening is employed. Additionally, patients who are screened regularly are much more likely to present with an early-stage lesion if cancer is detected.

5. Can cervical cancer be diagnosed by Pap smear?

No. The diagnosis of cervical cancer depends on tissue biopsy. Cytologic changes that are highly suggestive of cancer can be detected on Pap smear, but biopsy is required to demonstrate: (1) violation of the basement membrane, and (2) the origin of the cells. Occasionally, primary cancers of the endometrium, fallopian tube, vagina, ovary, and peritoneum can present with abnormal cells on Pap smear as a result of exfoliated cells.

6. True or false: There is only one type of cervical cancer.

False; there are many types. Carcinomas (cancers derived from epithelial tissues) are the vast majority, with squamous cell carcinoma comprising 85–90% of all cases. Adenocarcinomas make up most of the remainder (10–15%). Sarcomas, neuroendocrine tumors, melanoma, and primary cervical lymphoma also occur, but rarely.

7. How is stage of disease assigned?

Staging for cervical cancer is based on clinical exam, preferably under anesthesia. It usually includes a cystoscopy and proctoscopy as well as a bimanual examination. Once assigned, the stage does not change based on progression or intraoperative findings.

Here is the Federation of Gynecology and Obstetrics' 1995 staging system:

Stage I: The carcinoma is strictly confined to the cervix (extension to the corpus should be disregarded).

• Stage IA: Invasive cancer identified only microscopically. All gross lesions, even with superficial invasion, are stage IB cancers. Invasion is limited to measured stromal invasion with maximal depth of 5.0 mm and maximal width of 7.0 mm.

• Stage IA1: Measured invasion of stroma no deeper than 3.0 mm and no wider than 7.0 mm.

• Stage IA2: Measured invasion of stroma deeper than 3.0 mm but no deeper than 5.0 mm and no wider than 7.0 mm.

• Stage IB: Clinical lesions confined to the cervix or preclinical lesions larger than stage IA.

• Stage IB1: Clinical lesions no larger than 4.0 cm.

• Stage IB2: Clinical lesions larger than 4.0 cm.

Stage II: The carcinoma extends beyond the cervix but has not extended to the pelvic wall. The carcinoma involves the vagina but not as far as the lower third.

• Stage IIA: No obvious parametrial involvement.

• Stage IIB: Obvious parametrial involvement.

Stage III: The carcinoma has extended to the pelvic wall. Rectal examination reveals no cancer-free space between the tumor and pelvic wall. The tumor involves the lower third of the vagina. All cases with hydronephrosis or nonfunctioning kidney are included unless kidney disease is known to be due to other causes.

• Stage IIIA: No extension to the pelvic wall.

• Stage IIIB: Extension to the pelvic wall and/or hydronephrosis or nonfunctioning kidney.

Stage IV: The carcinoma has extended beyond the true pelvis or has clinically involved the mucosa of the bladder or rectum. Bullous edema does not assign a case to stage IV.

• Stage IVA: Spread of carcinoma to adjacent organs.

• Stage IVB: Spread to distant organs.

8. What is the 5-year survival rate?

Prognosis, as with other gynecologic malignancies, correlates with stage. Overall 5-year survival rates by stage are:

I	85–92%
IIA	75–83%
IIB	58–67%
III	25–35%
IV	8–14%

9. When is surgery appropriate in the treatment of cervical cancer?

Surgery is appropriate only when the tumor can be entirely removed. In general, this applies to disease that is stage IIA or lower. Survival for surgery is essentially equivalent to that of radiation with chemotherapy. Advantages of surgery in the treatment of cervical cancer include: ovarian preservation, better sexual function, and decreased incidence of cystitis and enteritis. If intraoperative findings indicate that the disease cannot be resected with clear margins, most authors advocate aborting surgery in favor of radiation therapy.

Surgery may also be used in the treatment of centrally recurrent disease.

10. Does surgical therapy always involve a hysterectomy?

No. In stage IA (microscopic) disease there may be a role for conservative therapy (cone biopsy followed by strict observation) if the patient desires preservation of fertility. Conservative therapy should only be offered when the margins of the cone biopsy are negative (see below).

11. How is radical hysterectomy different from a simple hysterectomy?

A radical hysterectomy is designed to remove both the primary cancer *and* the proximal portion of the lymphatic drainage routes. To achieve this, the specimen must include the parametria on both sides, the upper vaginal cuff , the uterosacral and cardinal ligament complexes, and the local vascular supply. Additionally, lymph nodes are routinely removed from the pelvic chains (obturator, external iliac, hypogastric, and ureteral) at the time of radical hysterectomy. *Note*: Oophorectomy is not necessarily indicated when performing a radical hysterectomy.

12. What are the complications of radical hysterectomy?

The most common complication is transient bladder dysfunction, which results from interruption of the sensory and motor nerve supply to the detrusor muscles. The extent of dysfunction correlates with the extent of the dissection, but is usually self-limited. Lymphocyst formation, infection, pulmonary embolism, and hemorrhage are more common in radical than simple hysterectomy, probably reflecting both the increased technical difficulty and operative duration of radical surgery. Ureteral fistula, owing to devascularization during ureteral mobilization is an uncommon but dreaded complication.

13. What is a total pelvic exenteration? Who are candidates for this procedure?

A total pelvic exenteration involves removing the bladder and distal ureters, any remaining mullerian structures, the vagina, the rectum and sigmoid colon, and the muscles of the pelvic floor. The classic total pelvic exenteration has in many places been replaced by more conservative, less morbid approaches, such as an anterior (bladder and mullerian structures) or posterior (sigmoid/rectum and mullerian structures) exenteration, or a supralevator exenteration (spares the musculature of the pelvic floor).

Exenteration is reserved for patients with central recurrence after primary therapy, usually recurrent cervical cancer. Exenteration can also be used to palliate severe symptoms such as postradiation fistulas or hemorrhage from a tumor.

14. Success rate for exenteration?

The 5-year survival rate for patients after exenteration ranges from 20% to 60% in the literature. Survival rates have generally increased over the last 50 years both within and between studies, with many authors now reporting 5-year survival rates around 50%. Patients who experience recurrence after exenteration are candidates for chemotherapy only, and have a 1-year mortality rate in excess of 90%.

15. When is radiation appropriate in the treatment of cervical cancer?

Radiation is appropriate when the disease is confined to the pelvis, generally stages IB through stage III. Radiation is the only viable treatment for people with locally advanced disease, as defined by spread to the sidewall or lymph nodes. Radiation may be appropriate for early stage disease in patients who are unable to tolerate surgery, or in elderly patients for whom ovarian preservation is not an issue and/or for whom maintenance of sexual function is not important. Radiation can also be used for symptomatic control of metastasis or bleeding from a central tumor.

Multiple randomized prospective studies have demonstrated a significant survival advantage when platinum-based chemotherapy is given, as a sensitizing agent, with the radiation.

16. How is radiation given?

Radiation in the treatment of cervical cancer is typically given in two phases. During the first phase, the entire pelvis receives **external beam radiation**, to shrink the tumor volume and to sterilize the regional lymph nodes. Between 4500 cGy and 5000 cGy are usually administered in this fashion, but up to 6000 cGy can be directed to known lymph node deposits.

Brachytherapy is the second phase and involves the insertion of a catheter through the cervix into the uterine cavity. Radiation can be administered directly to the tumor by placing a source in the lumen of the catheter. Local doses of over 10,000 cGy can be given in this way.

The optimum dosing schedule for chemotherapy during radiation has not been entirely worked out, but most studies advocate weekly platinum for 2–6 weeks.

17. What are the complications of radiation therapy?

Radiation therapy has few acute side effects and is generally well tolerated. The most common complaints during treatment are watery diarrhea, radiation cystitis, and a sunburn-like skin reaction. Long-term side effects are also uncommon, but can include infertility as a result of toxicity to the ovaries, small bowel obstruction (especially if para-aortic lymph nodes are irradiated), large bowel stricture, and chronic intermittent enteritis or cystitis. Vaginal atrophy is virtually assured without regular use of a dilator.

18. When is chemotherapy the best treatment?

Chemotherapy is employed when the disease has spread beyond the pelvis. Because not all organs can tolerate radiation doses high enough to treat cancer, radiation is not an option. Likewise, surgery is not useful because not all metastases are detectable on clinical or radiologic exam. Chemotherapy is delivered intravenously and thus reaches the entire body. Unfortunately, cervical cancer, like most squamous cancers, is relatively chemoresistant, with response rates of 10–25% for most agents.

19. Is adenocarcinoma treated differently than squamous lesions?

Though stage for stage the survival and treatment regimens for patients with adenocarcinoma are the same as for those with squamous lesions, adenocarcinomas tend to present at a more advanced stage. Further, conservative treatment of stage IA lesions is not recommended because microinvasive adenocarcinoma is difficult to characterize pathologically, may be multifocal, and is not as reliably assessed by follow-up Pap smears.

BIBLIOGRAPHY

1. Brophy PF, Hoffman JP, Eisenberg BL: The role of palliative pelvic exenteration. Am J Surg 167:386–390, 1994.
2. Keys HM, Bundy BN, Stehman FB, et al: Cisplatin, radiation, and adjuvant hysterectomy compared with radiation and adjuvant hysterectomy for bulky stage IB cervical carcinoma. N Engl J Med 340:1154–1161, 1999.
3. Lahousen M, Haas J, Pickel H, et al: Chemotherapy versus radiotherapy versus observation for high risk cervical carcinoma after radical hysterectomy: A randomized, prospective, multicenter trial. Gynecol Oncol 73:196–201, 1999.
4. Morror CP: Is pelvic radiation beneficial in the postoperative management of stage IB squamous cell carcinoma of the cervix with pelvic lymph node metastasis treated by radical hysterectomy and pelvic lymphadenectomy? Gynecol Oncol 37:74, 1990.
5. Morrow CP, Curtin JP: Synopsis of Gynecologic Oncology. Philadelphia, Churchill-Livingstone, 1998.
6. Peters III WA, Liu PY, Barrett II RJ, et al: Concurrent chemotherapy and pelvic radiation therapy compared with pelvic radiation therapy alone as adjuvant therapy after radical surgery in high risk early stage cancer of the cervix. J Clin Onc 18:1606–1613, 2000.
7. Shingleton HM, Orr JW: Cancer of the Cervix. Philadelphia, JB Lippincott, 1995.
8. Whitney CW, Sause W, Bundy BN, et al: Randomized comparison of fluorouracil plus cisplatin versus hydroxyurea as an adjunct to radiation therapy in stage IIB-IVA carcinoma of the cervix with negative para-aortic lymph nodes: A Gynecologic Oncology Group and Southwest Oncology Group study. J Clin Once 17:1339–1348, 1999.

28. ENDOMETRIAL HYPERPLASIA AND UTERINE CANCER

Christina S. Chu, M.D.

1. What is the incidence of endometrial cancer?

Endometrial cancer is the most common gynecologic cancer, and the fourth most common cancer in women. In the United States, approximately 35,000 cases are diagnosed each year. About 6000 women die each year of endometrial cancer. The incidence of the disease has been increasing over the last few decades.

2. What are the risk factors associated with endometrial cancer?

Most endometrial cancers are thought to arise as a result of increased exposure to unopposed estrogen. Factors such as unopposed estrogen replacement therapy, obesity, anovulatory menstrual cycles, early menarche, late menopause, nulliparity, and tamoxifen use predispose patients to developing endometrial cancer. The risk is threefold for patients who are 21–50 pounds overweight, and tenfold for those more than 50 pounds overweight. A nulliparous patient is twice as likely to develop the disease as a woman with one child, and three times as likely as a woman with five or more children. Women who undergo menopause later than age 52 have more than twice the risk for developing endometrial cancer. Even when controlling for weight and age, diabetes mellitus is associated with an almost three times greater risk for the cancer.

3. Is age associated with endometrial cancer?

Endometrial cancer is predominantly a disease of postmenopausal women. The average age for developing endometrial cancer is about 60, with most sufferers diagnosed in their 50s. It is important to note, however, that 5% of women are diagnosed under the age of 40, and that almost a quarter of women with endometrial cancer present prior to menopause.

4. Is there a screening test for endometrial cancer?

There is currently no good screening tool for asymptomatic patients. Pap smears are unreliable for diagnosing endometrial cancer, given that only 50% of patients with cancer have abnormal cells detected on Pap. However, some women at increased risk for disease—such as postmenopausal women on unopposed estrogen, obese postmenopausal women, women with late menopause, premenopausal women with anovulatory cycles, and women on tamoxifen—may benefit from screening. Screening may be performed by office endometrial biospy, or with ultrasound to measure the thickness of the endometrial stripe complex (endometrial cancers have not been reported in women with stripes less than 4 mm in thickness).

5. How does endometrial cancer present?

Ninety percent of patients with endometrial cancer have abnormal uterine bleeding—most commonly, postmenopausal bleeding. Ten percent of patients may present with leukorrhea. Occasionally, patients with cervical stenosis will not present with bleeding, but may have a pyometra or hematometra.

6. What is the differential diagnosis for postmenopausal bleeding?

The most common cause of postmenopausal bleeding is endometrial and/or vaginal atrophy caused by the lack of endogenous estrogen. Exogenous hormone replacement therapy is also a frequent cause of postmenopausal bleeding. Endometrial or cervical polyps, and endometrial hyperplasia may also cause bleeding. Endometrial cancer is only responsible for about 15–20% of postmenopausal bleeding. Other factors such as cervical cancer, urethral caruncles, and trauma are also infrequent causes of bleeding.

7. List the important elements in the work-up of a patient with abnormal bleeding.

All patients with abnormal bleeding should undergo office endometrial biospy. If a patient with a negative biospy continues to have symptoms, a D&C (with or without hysteroscopy) should be performed because the false negative rate of an office biopsy is approximately 10%. Any patient with suspicious findings on office biopsy (such as necrosis or hyperplasia) should also undergo D&C. Ultrasound has also been used to evaluate the endometrium. Patients with endometrial stripes < 4 mm on ultrasound likely have atropy as a source of bleeding, rather than hyperplasia or carcinoma.

8. What is endometrial hyperplasia? What is its relationship to endometrial cancer?

Hyperplasia of the endometrium, which refers to abnormal proliferation of both glands and stroma, can only be diagnosed based on pathologic examination of a tissue specimen. Hyperplasia may be characterized as simple (with regular gland shapes) or complex (irregular glands with back-to-back crowding). Endometrial cells may also display cytologic atypia (enlarged nuclei, irregularity, hyperchromasia). Patients who have hyperplasia with atypia are at increased risk for progressing to endometrial cancer.

Risk for Progressing to Endometrial Cancer Based on Type of Hyperplasia

	ATYPIA ABSENT	ATYPIA PRESENT
Simple	1%	8%
Complex	3%	29%

9. How is endometrial hyperplasia treated?

Depending on age and desires for fertility, patients with hyperplasia may be treated with progestin therapy or hysterectomy. Young women with simple hyperplasia are often treated successfully with oral contraceptive pills, periodic progesterone withdrawal, or high-dose progestins. Hysterectomy is recommended for patients with atypical complex hyperplasia. Those who are still desirous of future childbearing, or those with serious medical problems making them poor surgical candidates may also be treated with high-dose progestins and followed closely with repeat endometrial biopsies every 3–6 months.

10. What is the histology of endometrial cancers?

Here is a summary of the classification scheme of the International Society of Gynecologic Pathologists:
Endometrioid adenocarcinoma
Mucinous carcinoma
Serous carcinoma
Clear cell carcinoma
Squamous carcinoma
Undifferentiated carcinoma
Mixed types
Miscellaneous carcinoma
Metastatic carcinoma
The vast majority of endometrial carcinomas are endometrioid in histology (75–80%). Papillary serous tumors comprise less than 10% of endometrial carcinomas, display early intraperitoneal spread, and are very aggressive cancers. Clear cell carcinomas are rare (only about 4%), but are also a more aggressive subtype. Common metastatic tumors to the endometrium include breast, ovary, stomach, colon, and pancreas. Not all tumors of the endometrium are carcinomas. Approximately 3% of endometrial cancers are sarcomas, such as malignant mixed mullerian tumors and endometrial stromal tumors.

11. How is endometrial cancer staged?

Since 1988, endometrial cancer has been surgically staged by the International Federation of Gynecologists and Obstetricians (FIGO). About 75% of patients present in stage I, 11% in stage II, 11% in stage III, and 3% in stage IV.

FIGO Surgical Staging for Endometrial Carcinoma

STAGE	GRADE	DESCRIPTION
Ia	1, 2, 3	Tumor limited to endometrium
Ib	1, 2, 3	Invasion to < 50% of myometrium
Ic	1, 2, 3	Invasion to > 50% of myometrium
IIa	1, 2, 3	Endocervical glandular involvement only
IIb	1, 2, 3	Cervical stromal invasion
IIIa	1, 2, 3	Tumor invades serosa and/or adnexa, and/or positive peritoneal cytology
IIIb	1, 2, 3	Vaginal metastases
IIIc	1, 2, 3	Metastases to pelvic and/or para-aortic lymph nodes
IVa	1, 2, 3	Tumor invasion of bladder and/or bowel mucosa
IVb	1, 2, 3	Distant metastases, including intra-abdominal and/or inguinal lymph nodes

12. How does endometrial cancer spread?

Endometrial cancer spreads most commonly by direct extension to adjacent organs, such as by invasion through the myometrium to the serosa of the uterus and to the cervix. Malignant cells may also be shed through the fallopian tubes to implant on the ovaries and other abdominal surfaces. Tumor may commonly spread by lymphatic channels to pelvic and para-aortic lymph nodes. Lung metastases are the result of hematogenous dissemination, which may less commonly cause liver and brain lesions as well.

13. What is the treatment for early-stage endometrial cancer?

The initial approach to treatment involves total abdominal hysterectomy and bilateral salpingo-oophorectomy whenever possible. All patients with grade 3 tumors, large grade 2 tumors (> 2 cm in size), deep myometrial invasion, cervical extension, or high-risk histologies should also undergo pelvic and para-aortic lymph node sampling and washings. Occasionally, an omental biopsy is taken, especially in the presence of a papillary serous histology. After surgery, selected high-risk patients may be offered adjuvant radiation. Occasionally, patients may be offered progestin therapy, but its benefit is unclear in the adjuvant setting.

14. How is late-stage endometrial cancer treated?

Advanced-stage endometrial cancer presents a difficult problem. Several chemotherapy combinations have been used in recurrent or advanced endometrial cancer. Agents such as doxorubicin and cisplatin have been shown to have some activity against the tumor. One clinical trial demonstrated a 66% response rate when the two drugs were combined.

15. What is the role of hormonal therapy for endometrial cancer?

Progestins have been evaluated in the adjuvant setting as a possible therapy to prevent recurrence. Studies comparing progestin with placebo in stage I patients demonstrated no benefit in overall survival. In the context of recurrent disease, only about 15–30% of patients may respond to progestin therapy, but side effects of treatment are minimal.

16. What are the prognostic indicators in endometrial cancer?

Stage of disease at diagnosis is the most significant prognostic factor in patients with endometrial cancer. Younger women have a better prognosis than older women. Some histologic subtypes also confer a worse prognosis, such as papillary serous and clear cell. Histologic grade and myometrial depth of invasion correlate strongly with prognosis. High-grade tumors and deep invasion are associated with increased risk for lymph node metastasis, positive washings, and local recurrence. Other factors, such as the presence of lymph-vascular space invasion and the lack of estrogen or progesterone receptor expression, have been shown to confer a worse prognosis. Tumors larger than 2 cm have a greater risk of lymph node metastasis.

17. What is the survival for patients with endometrial cancer?
The overall 5-year survival for patients with endometrial cancer is about 60–70%. However, patients with early-stage disease fare much better than those with late-stage disease.

Five-Year Survival by Stage at Diagnosis

STAGE	SURVIVAL
I	75%
II	60%
III	30%
IV	10%

BIBLIOGRAPHY

1. Barakat RR, Grigsby PW, Sabbatini P, Zaino RJ: Corpus: Epithlelial tumors. In Hoskins WJ, Perez CA, Young RC (eds): Principles and Practice of Gynecologic Oncology, 3rd ed. Philadelphia, Lippincott, Williams & Williams, 2000, pp 919–960.
2. DiSaia PJ, Creasman WT: Adenocarcinoma of the uterus. In DiSaia PJ, Creasman WT (eds): Clinical Gynecologic Oncology, 5th ed. St. Louis, Mosby, 1997, pp 134–167.
3. DiSaia PJ, Creasman WT: Endometrial hyperplasia/estrogen therapy. In DiSaia PJ, Creasman WT (ed): Clinical Gynecologic Oncology, 5th ed. St. Louis, Mosby, 1997, pp 107–133.
4. Hacker NF: Uterine cancer. In Berek JS, Hacker NF (eds): Practical Gynecologic Oncology, 2nd ed. Baltimore, Williams & Williams, 1994, pp 285–326.
5. Kurman JR, Kaminski PF, Norris HJ: The behavior of endometrial hyperplasia: A long-term study of "untreated" hyperplasia in 170 patients. Cancer 56:403–412, 1985.
6. Lewis GC, Slack NH, Mortel R, et al: Adjuvant progestogen therapy in primary definitive treatment of endometrial cancer. Gynecol Oncol 2:368–376, 1974.
7. Thigpen T, Blessing J, Homesley H, et al: Phase III trial of doxorubicin +/– cisplatin in advanced or recurrent endometrial carcinoma. (abstract) Proc Am Soc Clin Oncol 12:26, 1993.

29. BENIGN ADNEXAL MASSES

Yu-Hsin Wu, M.D.

1. How are adnexal masses diagnosed? Why do they need to be evaluated?

Bimanual examinations are recommended on a yearly basis to detect adnexal masses. Detection and evaluation of these masses is important because of the possibility of malignancy. Although most adnexal masses are physiologic or benign neoplasms, especially in young menstruating women, a physician must consider the worst scenario and rule out ovarian cancer. While ovarian cancer is the second most common malignancy of the female genital tract, it is the leading cause of death from gynecologic neoplasm in the United States. This high mortality is associated with late diagnosis, because patients usually do not become symptomatic until the disease is widespread.

2. What is the differential diagnosis for adnexal masses?

Benign	*Malignant*
Physiologic (Functional) Ovarian Cysts	Ovarian Malignancies
Follicular cyst	Epithelial cell
Corpus luteum cyst	Sex cord
Theca lutein cyst	Germ cell
Nonfunctional Ovarian Cysts	Fallopian tube cancers
Endometrioma	Nongynecologic Cancers
Polycystic ovaries	GI tumors
Inflammatory cyst	Lymphoma
Ovarian torsion	
Benign Ovarian Neoplasms	
Mature cystic teratoma	
Fibroma, adenofibroma, cystadenofibroma	
Serous cystadenoma, mucinous cystadenoma	
Brenner tumor	
Fallopian Tube Origin	
Ectopic pregnancy	
Paratubal cyst	
Hydrosalpingx, hematosalpingx	
Tubo-ovarian abscess	
Tubal torsion	
Nongynecologic	
Diverticulitis	
Appendiceal abscess	
Pelvic kidney	
Leiomyomata	

3. What are the most important patient characteristics to consider when creating the differential diagnosis for an adnexal mass?

The patient's age and menstrual status are the most important characteristics to consider when creating the differential diagnosis. Adnexal masses in women who are menstruating regularly frequently are physiologic in nature (follicular, corpus luteum, theca lutein cysts). The majority of the malignant adnexal masses occur in women over the age of 45, with the exception of germ cell tumors, which occur in younger women.

Other factors to consider are: (1) the patient's symptoms (e.g., weight loss, abdominal distention, and pulmonary, GI, or GU complaints are more likely associated with malignancy; (2)

nulliparity, which is associated with increased risk for ovarian neoplasm (use of oral contraceptive is protective); and (3) family history of gynecologic and breast cancers.

4. What characteristics of adnexal masses help differentiate between benign and malignant masses?

CHARACTERISTIC	BENIGN	MALIGNANT
Size	Usually < 8 cm	Usually > 8 cm
Number and Consistency	Unilocular simple cyst	Multilocular complex cyst with solid components present
Borders	Smooth, regular, well-defined borders	Vague borders with nodularity, excrescences, studding, papillary projections
Laterality	Unilateral	Bilateral
Mobility	Mobile	Fixed or adherent to other structures
Growth Rate	Slowly enlarging	Rapidly growing

Additional factors:
• Very large masses tend to be of borderline (low-grade) malignant potential.
• Mucinous tumors are notorious for reaching very large sizes (up to 40 pounds!).
• Malignant lesions are more likely to have areas of necrosis and hemorrhage than benign masses. (Hemorrhagic corpus luteum cysts and endometriomas are exceptions to this rule.)
• The presence of ascites usually indicates a malignant process.

5. How are follicular cysts created? What physical characteristics do they have?
Failed rupture of the dominant follicle or failed atresia of secondary follicles results in follicular cysts. Follicular cysts are simple cysts that average about 2 cm in size, but they can vary from a few millimeters to 8 cm. They are thin-walled and filled with clear, straw-colored fluid. When and if these cysts rupture, they can occasionally cause pain, and, more rarely, intraperitoneal hemorrhage.

6. How should cysts that are detected on bimanual exam or ultrasound be managed?
In menstruating women, cysts that have benign appearance on ultrasound and are less than 8 cm in size should be observed for one to two cycles. Almost all of these physiologic cysts resolve spontaneously during this observation period. Suppression with oral contraceptives to prevent additional cysts may be helpful, so that when the ultrasound is repeated, new cysts are not mistaken for a persistent ovarian cyst.

7. What is polycystic ovary syndrome (PCOS)? What characteristics do patients with this syndrome possess?
While the definition of PCOS is somewhat controversial, most experts would use the working definition of "ovulatory dysfunction with evidence of hyperandrogenism, clinically or by laboratory means, without other causes of hyperandrogenism identified." Ovulatory dysfunction is clinically manifested as abnormal menstrual cycles, usually oligomenorrhea or amenorrhea, or more subtlely as infertility. Androgen excess is clinically manifested as hirsuitism, acne, and signs of virilization such as clitoromegaly, voice changes, frontal baldness, and increased muscle mass. Obesity and insulin resistance are also common findings in women with PCOS.

8. How are the follicular cysts associated with PCOS different from other follicular cysts?
The follicular cysts in PCOS are usually bilateral and more numerous, but smaller in size than other physiologic follicular cysts. When a state of anovulation persists for a prolonged

period of time, numerous small follicles form, producing the classic polycystic ovary or "**pearl necklace**" appearance on ultrasound. However, multiple cysts on ultrasound are not required for the diagnosis of PCOS, nor do the ultrasound findings alone make the diagnosis in the absence of other PCOS characteristics.

9. What are endometriomas?

Endometriomas are endometrial implants on the ovary. Although the pathogenesis of endometriosis and endometriomas is unclear, the leading theory suggests **retrograde menstruation** as the cause of endometrial implants in the pelvis and adnexa. If symptomatic, endometriomas can cause chronic pelvic pain, dysmenorrhea, dyspareunia, or infertility.

10. How are endometriomas managed?

Because they often appear as complex adnexal masses on ultrasound, treatment is commonly surgical, to rule out malignancy. At the time of surgery, the endometrioma(s) should be resected, and pelvic implants suspicious for endometriosis should be laser or electrocautery ablated. Laparoscopic resection and ablation is preferred to laparotomy. If a patient is suspected to have residual disease, Lupron (a GnRH agonist) can be given postoperatively. A few studies have shown that surgery in conjunction with postoperative Lupron for 3–6 month prolongs a patient's pain-free interval. Medical management of endometriomas with oral contraceptive and depoprovera injections is minimally effective.

11. Why do theca lutein cysts develop? How are they managed?

Theca lutein cysts develop with prolonged or excessive ovarian stimulation by exogenous or endogenous gonadotropins. They are seen in association with molar pregnancies, choriocarcinomas, multiple gestations, pregnancies associated with large placentas, and with the use of ovulation induction agents. Gonadotropins cause luteinization of mature, immature, and atretic follicles, resulting in bilateral ovarian enlargement. These cysts are usually managed expectantly because they resolve spontaneously.

12. What are benign cystic teratomas?

Benign cystic teratomas, or dermoid cysts, are ovarian lesions that contain mature tissue of ectodermal, mesodermal, and/or endodermal origin. The most common elements are ectodermal derivatives such as skin, hair follicles, teeth, bone, and sebaceous or sweat glands.

13. What is the most frequent complication associated with benign cystic teratomas?

Ovarian torsion, which occurs typically in children and young women, is the most common complication of these dermoid cysts. Severe, acute abdominal pain is usually the initial symptom of torsion. While these cysts can reach very large dimensions and twist, they rarely rupture. If rupture does occur spontaneously or iatrogenically, a chemical peritonitis can occur due to spill of cholesterol-laden debris.

14. How are patients with ovarian torsion managed?

Ovarian torsion is a *gynecologic emergency* and requires prompt surgical management. Most cases of torsion can be managed with laparoscopy. In young women for whom fertility and preservation of ovarian function are important issues, conservative treatment with untwisting of the adnexa and ovarian cystectomy is preferred. However, this mode of surgical management requires prompt diagnosis and intervention to avoid strangulation and necrosis of torsed tissue. If strangulation and necrosis do occur, **adnexectomy** should be performed.

15. What laboratory tests are useful when evaluating an adnexal mass?

- CBC with differential, to rule out infection (gynecologic or nongynecologic)
- Beta hCG, to rule out cysts associated with pregnancy or ectopic pregnancy. If levels are unusually elevated, there is an increased suspicion for molar pregnancy or choriocarcinoma.

- Gonorrhea and chlamydia cervical cultures, when tubo-ovarian abscess or pelvic inflammatory disease is suspected
- Tumor markers:
    CA-125 is elevated in epithelial ovarian cancer
    Alpha-fetoprotein is elevated in germ cell tumors (endodermal sinus tumors, embryonal cell cancer, mixed germ cell malignancies)
    Beta hCG is unusually elevated in molar pregnancy and choriocarcinoma
    Lactate dehydrogenase is elevated with dysgerminomas

16. Are CA-125 levels more useful in premenopausal or postmenopausal women? Why?

Cancer antigen 125 levels are more useful in evaluating postmenopausal women with adnexal masses. The CA-125 antigen is expressed by epithelial ovarian tumors, and therefore its levels are markedly elevated in women with epithelial ovarian malignancies. However, the CA-125 determinant is also expressed by various other pathologic and normal tissues of mullerian origin, such as endometriosis, uterine leiomyomas, pregnancy, pelvic infections, and menstruation. Given that these conditions are more likely to occur in menstruating women, CA-125 levels are less specific for ovarian cancer in the premenopausal age group.

17. Adnexal masses of what size warrant surgical exploration?

Any patient with an adnexal mass > 10 cm in size requires surgical exploration, because functional cysts rarely exceed 7–8 cm. *Women of reproductive age* with adnexal masses < 10 cm can be followed up clinically in 1–2 months, with expected resolution of functional cysts during this time period. If the cyst persists or enlarges, surgical evaluation is warranted. *Postmenopausal women* with complex adnexal masses or masses > 5 cm require surgical exploration because of the increased risk of malignancy. In addition to the size of the adnexal mass, ultrasound characteristics that help differentiate between benign and malignant masses should also be factored into the equation when determining whether or not surgery is indicated.

BIBLIOGRAPHY

1. American College of Obstetricians and Gynecologists, Committee on Technical Bulletins: Medical Management of Endometriosis. ACOG Practice Bulletin No. 11. Washington, DC, ACOG, 1995.
2. DiSaia P, Creasman W: Clinical Gynecologic Oncology, 5th ed. St. Louis, Mosby-Year Book, Inc., 1997, pp 253–281.
3. Goldstein S: Postmenopausal adnexal cysts: How clinical management has evolved. Am J Obstet Gynecol 175(6):1498–1502, 1996.
4. Lewis V: Polycystic ovary syndrome: A diagnostic challenge. Obstet Gynecol Clin North Am 28(1):1–20, 2001.
5. Mishell DR, Stenchever MA, Droegemueller W, Herbst AL: Comprehensive Gynecology, 8th ed. St. Louis, Mosby-Year Book, Inc., 1997, pp 905–912.
6. Pfeifer S, Gosman G: Evaluation of adnexal masses in adolescents. Pediatr Clin North Am 46(3):573–592, 1999.
7. Speroff L, Glass RH, Kase NG: Clinical Gynecologic Endocrinology and Infertility, 6th ed. Baltimore, Lippincott Williams & Wilkins, 1999, pp 493–511.

30. OVARIAN CANCER

Christina S. Chu, M.D.

1. What is the incidence of ovarian cancer?

A woman's lifetime risk of ovarian cancer is about 1 in 70. Approximately 26,000 cases are diagnosed each year in the U.S. Only 23% of all gynecologic cancers are ovarian in origin, but ovarian cancer is responsible for more than half of gynecologic cancer deaths, with about 14,000 deaths per year in the U.S.

2. What are the different types of ovarian cancer?

Ovarian cancer is a diverse term describing several different histologies. Each type has a different natural history. The majority of ovarian cancer is epithelial in origin (70%). Other histologies include germ cell (15%), sex-cord/stromal (10%), and metastatic tumors to the ovary (5%).

3. How is ovarian cancer staged? Describe the staging system.

Ovarian cancer is surgically staged. The International Federation of Gynecology and Obstetrics uses the following staging system:

Stage I—Growth limited to the ovaries

IA   one ovary, no malignant ascites, no surface involvement

IB   both ovaries, no malignant ascites, no surface involvement

IC   IA or IB, with malignant ascites, capsule rupture, surface involvement, or positive washings

Stage II—Growth involving one or both ovaries with pelvic extension

IIA   extension of disease to uterus and/or tubes

IIB   extension to other pelvic tissues

IIC   IIA or IIB with malignant ascites, capsule rupture, surface involvement, or positive washings

Stage III—Tumor involving one or both ovaries with spread to the abdomen and/or positive retroperitoneal lymph nodes

IIIA   microscopic seeding of abdomen

IIIB   macroscopic implants < 2 cm in abdomen

IIIC   > 2 cm implants in abdomen, or any positive lymph nodes

Stage IV—Distant spread, such as parenchymal liver metastases or malignant pleural effusion

4. Which procedures may be included in the staging process?

Surgical staging is performed to assess the extent of disease spread, and may include careful inspection of all peritoneal surfaces, pelvic and abdominal washings, random peritoneal biopsies, biopsy of suspicious lesions, pelvic and para-aortic lymph node sampling, total abdominal hysterectomy, and bilateral salpingo-oophorectomy. Procedures are only performed as necessary to accurately assign a stage to describe the patient's disease.

For example, in a patient with large tumor implants in the upper abdomen, lymph node sampling, washings, and biopsies are unnecessary because the patient is classified as having stage IIIC disease on the basis of gross examination alone. A patient with no gross disease outside the ovary (apparent stage I disease) needs a complete staging procedure to rule out microscopic disease in the lymph nodes, pelvis, or abdomen, which would raise the stage. This is particularly important because up to 30% of patients who appear to have disease limited to the ovary will have positive lymph nodes.

EPITHELIAL OVARIAN CANCER

5. How do patients with epithelial ovarian cancer present?

More than 80% of patients with ovarian cancer are diagnosed after menopause. The median age at diagnosis is about 62. Most patients with ovarian cancer experience no symptoms, particularly in the early stages of the disease. When symptoms do arise, they are often nonspecific. Early in the disease, patients may complain of abnormal bleeding, urinary frequency, constipation, lower abdominal distension, or discomfort. Later in the disease, symptoms are related to the mass-effect of tumor spread or ascites. Patients may experience abdominal distension, dyspepsia, bloating, early satiety, weight change, anorexia, nausea, constipation, or abnormal vaginal bleeding. Consider the diagnosis of ovarian cancer in any woman over the age of 40 with persistent gastrointestinal symptoms of unknown etiology.

6. What are the different types of epithelial ovarian cancer?

Most epithelial cancers are serous (42%). Other types include mucinous (12%), endometrioid (15%), clear cell (6%), undifferentiated (17%), and Brenner (< 1%).

7. What are the risk factors associated with the development of epithelial ovarian cancer?

The greatest risk factor for developing ovarian cancer is a **family history** of disease. Patients with one first-degree relative with ovarian cancer have three times the baseline risk for developing the disease. Having two or more first-degree relatives increases the risk to 4 to 15 times baseline. The risk for developing ovarian cancer also increases with **age**. The highest incidence of ovarian cancer is found in the seventh decade. Some speculate that ovarian cancer is associated with "**incessant ovulation**." Accordingly, nulliparity, late menopause, and early menarche are associated with increased risk for ovarian cancer. In addition, factors that suppress ovulation such as oral contraceptives, pregnancy, and breastfeeding appear to be protective.

8. How does ovarian cancer spread?

Epithelial ovarian cancer primarily spreads by peritoneal dissemination. Cells exfoliated from the initial tumor site implant on various peritoneal surfaces, such as the cul-de-sac, paracolic gutters, hemidiaphragms, liver surface, mesentery, omentum, and bowel. Lymphatic spread occurs when tumor cells are disseminated to the pelvic and para-aortic lymph nodes. About 80% of patients with stage III disease have positive pelvic lymph nodes. Hematogenous spread at the time of diagnosis is rare. Only 2–3% of patients have lung or parenchymal liver metastasis at diagnosis. Most patients with spread outside of the abdomen have malignant pleural effusions.

9. Which studies are typically part of the work-up of a patient with suspected ovarian cancer?

When the diagnosis of ovarian cancer is suspected, a careful history and physical examination are the first steps in evaluation. While routine laboratory tests such as blood chemistries, CBC, and urinalysis are not helpful in the diagnosis of ovarian cancer, they may serve to rule out other disorders. A CA-125 level can be checked, though an elevated level does not necessarily guarantee the diagnosis of cancer; nor does a normal level exclude the diagnosis.

Radiologic imaging may include ultrasound or MRI to better characterize an ovarian mass. A CT scan can help define the extent of spread of the tumor and help to rule out primary tumors of other organs that have metastasized to the ovary, such as the bowel or pancreas. If a patient displays gastrointestinal signs and symptoms such as a change in bowel habits or heme positive stool, an upper GI series or barium enema can be performed to rule out a primary gastrointestinal tumor. A chest x-ray may be checked to detect a pleural effusion or lung metastases.

10. What is the typical stage at presentation?

The majority of patients are diagnosed in late stages, because the symptoms of ovarian cancer are nonspecific. Here is the percentage of patients in each stage upon presentation:

Stage I	27
Stage II	12
Stage III	40
Stage IV	21

11. What is the treatment for epithelial ovarian cancer?

The primary treatment of epithelial ovarian cancer is surgical. Laparotomy is the definitive method for diagnosis, staging, and treatment. After staging is performed, treatment consists of surgical cytoreduction, or debulking. Unlike all other solid tumors, survival is strongly related to the amount of residual tumor present at the conclusion of surgery. Every judicious effort is conducted to excise as much tumor as possible. Occasionally, even bowel resection is performed in the attempt to achieve minimal residual disease.

12. What is the role of chemotherapy?

After cytoreductive surgery, patients with high-risk stage I disease and all patients with stage II, III, and IV disease are treated with adjuvant chemotherapy. First-line regimens consist of combination treatment with paclitaxel and platinum. The overall response rate is about 70–80%. Many of these patients experience complete remission, though most patients recur and eventually die of chemotherapy-resistant disease. When patients recur, treatment may include second-line chemotherapy agents such as topotecan, liposomal doxorubicin, and gemcitabine.

13. What are some of the prognostic factors?

The most important prognostic factors are initial stage at diagnosis and extent of residual disease after primary surgery. Clinical factors such as age and performance status also have been shown to be independent prognostic factors. Pathologic factors such as tumor grade and histology are also important. Clear cell carcinomas are associated with a worse prognosis than other types of cancer. While several proto-oncogenes, such as HER-2/neu, have been identified as playing a role in the development and progression of ovarian cancer, their significance in predicting prognosis is controversial.

14. What is the survival rate for epithelial ovarian cancer?

The overall 5-year survival for epithelial ovarian cancer is about 30%. Survival is strongly related to stage at diagnosis.

	% 5-yr Survival
Stage I	79
Stage II	60
Stage III	22
Stage IV	14

15. Is there any cost-effective screening available?

There is *no cost-effective screening* available for ovarian cancer. Routine yearly physical examination is not reliable for early detection. While **transvaginal ultrasound** is promising (> 95% sensitivity to detect ovarian cancer), the false-positive rate is very high. **CA-125** is a serum marker that is expressed in over 80% of non-mucinous ovarian cancers, and it is elevated in patients with early ovarian cancer. However, many benign conditions such as pelvic inflammatory disease, endometriosis, benign ovarian cysts, infertility, hepatitis, cirrhosis, congestive heart failure, and even renal failure have been associated with elevated CA-125 levels. Because of the high false-positive rate for both CA-125 determination and transvaginal ultrasound, these tests are *not* recommended for routine screening. Even when screening only high-risk patients, no study has been able to identify any screening modality that improves survival.

16. How is CA-125 determination helpful?

For a patient with known ovarian cancer, CA-125 determination can be very useful to follow response to treatment, or as an early detector of disease recurrence. All patients with a complete response to adjuvant chemotherapy require office evaluation combined with CA-125 testing every 3 months to assess potential recurrence.

17. Is epithelial ovarian cancer hereditary?

About 5–10% of all ovarian cancers are familial. The genes responsible for hereditary ovarian cancer are transmitted in an autosomal dominant fashion with variable penetrance. There are three different syndromes of hereditary ovarian cancer: site-specific familial ovarian cancer, breast/ovarian familial cancer syndrome, and Lynch II syndrome.

Hereditary breast/ovarian cancer syndrome is the most common, accounting for 75–90% of all hereditary cases of ovarian cancer. Families usually exhibit multiple cases of breast and ovarian cancer diagnosed before 50 years of age. Almost all families with this syndrome display mutations in the BRCA1 and BRCA2 genes. There is evidence that these patients present at earlier ages and have better prognoses than patients with sporadic ovarian cancer.

Site-specific ovarian cancer accounts for about 5% of cases of familial ovarian cancer, and is thought to be a variation of hereditary breast/ovarian cancer syndrome. In this syndrome, only ovarian cancer is demonstrated in the family: the lack of breast cancer may be secondary to chance, incomplete family histories, or differences in the cancer risk associated with each specific gene mutation. BRCA1 and BRCA2 mutations are responsible for the overwhelming majority of these cases.

Finally, the **Lynch II syndrome**, also known as hereditary nonpolyposis colon cancer syndrome, is associated with mutations in the DNA mismatch repair genes, and accounts for about 2% of hereditary ovarian cancers. Lynch II families display nonpolyposis colorectal cancer as well as adenocarcinomas of the endometrium, ovary, stomach, skin, small bowel, and urinary tract.

18. What are low malignant potential (LMP) tumors?

Ovarian tumors of low malignant potential are also called borderline tumors. These lesions are characterized by epithelium that displays characteristics of malignant carcinomas, but no invasion is identified. About 15% of all ovarian malignancies are LMP. Most patients are young (mean age 45) at diagnosis. Pregnancy, oral contraceptives, and breastfeeding appear to be protective. These tumors have an excellent prognosis, with 5-year survival rates ranging from 95–100%. Twenty-year survivals have been reported to be 90% for stage I tumors, and 70% for stage III tumors. Though about 10–20% of patients experience late recurrence, more patients die *with* disease than *of* disease. There is no proven benefit to adjuvant chemotherapy either for early- or advanced-stage disease. Patients with invasive metastatic implants identified may be at higher risk for recurrence and warrant adjuvant chemotherapy.

MALIGNANT GERM CELL TUMORS

19. Who is a typical patient with a germ cell cancer of the ovary?

Most germ cell malignancies of the ovary are diagnosed in young women in their teens and twenties. Patients often present with acute pain, or a palpable, rapidly enlarging abdominal mass. Patients may have abnormal vaginal bleeding, as well as abdominal distension.

20. What are the different types of germ cell tumors?

Germ cell tumors of the ovary are a diverse group of neoplasms encompassing several histologic types. Each has different characteristics.

Dysgerminomas are the most common type of germ cell malignancy, comprising 50% of all germ cells cancers. In contrast to other germ cell tumors, the opposite ovary is involved in about 15% of patients. These tumors are sometimes associated with elevated serum lactate dehydrogenase or human chorionic gonadotropin (hCG). Dysgerminoma is one of the most common ovarian tumors to be diagnosed during pregnancy. Sometimes the neoplasm is discovered in patients who present with primary amenorrhea. In these cases, the diagnosis is often associated with gonadal dysgenesis and gonadoblastoma.

Endodermal sinus tumors (yolk sac tumors) are the second most common germ cell malignancy of the ovary, comprising about 25% of all tumors. A common histologic finding is the Schiller-Duval body, an isolated papillary projection lined with tumors cells surrounding a single central blood vessel. Most endodermal sinus tumors secrete alpha-feto-protein (AFP), making it a useful tumor marker. Only 5% of cases are bilateral.

About 20% of germ cell malignancies are **immature teratomas**. These tumors arise from all three embryonic germ cell layers. Immature teratomas are differentiated from their benign counterpart the mature cystic teratoma (or dermoid cyst) by the presence of immature or embryonal structures. The histologic grade is determined by the quantity of immature neural tissue present. These tumors are rarely bilateral (< 5% of cases).

Mixed germ cell tumors comprise about 8% of all germ cell malignancies. By definition, these cancers include at least two different malignant germ cell components. The most common components are dysgerminoma and endodermal sinus tumors.

Embryonal carcinoma is a very rare, aggressive tumor in the pure form and is most commonly seen as a component of a mixed tumor. These tumors may secrete estrogen and be associated with precocious puberty or irregular bleeding. These tumors often secrete hCG and AFP.

Choriocarcinoma of the ovary is also very rare. In children, these tumors present with signs of precocious puberty. Adults may have signs similar to an ectopic pregnancy because the cells secrete hCG.

Polyembryomas are very rare tumors characterized histologically by numerous structures resembling normal embryos. Only a few have been reported in the literature, and most are associated with mixed tumors. At the time of diagnosis, tumor has often metastasized to other structures in the pelvis and abdomen.

Gonadoblastomas are rare tumors sometimes associated with dysgerminomas. Most gonadoblastomas are diagnosed in the course of the work-up of abnormal external genitalia, virilization, or primary amenorrhea. Karyotyping of the patient often reveals either a single X chromosome (45, X) or a mosaic pattern (45, X/46, XY). Eighty percent of patients are phenotypic women; the rest are phenotypic men with hypospadias, cryptorchidism, and internal female sexual organs. Of the phenotypic women, approximately half are normal in appearance, and half are virilized with primary amenorrhea or abnormal external genitalia.

21. How are germ cell tumors treated?

Treatment for germ cell tumors is primarily surgical. Because patients with germ cell malignancies are often young and future reproduction is a concern, if no disease is apparent outside the affected ovary, a unilateral salpingo-oophorectomy may be performed leaving the uterus and contralateral ovary intact. Any suspicious lesions should be biopsied and a thorough staging procedure should be performed. In the setting of advanced disease, surgical cytoreduction is recommended. Patients with stage IA dysgerminomas or stage IA grade 1 immature teratomas may be treated with surgery alone. All other patients require adjuvant chemotherapy. Currently, treatment with bleomycin, etoposide, and cisplatin (BEP) is recommended.

22. What is the survival of patients with malignant germ cell tumors?

Most patients present in early stages with disease limited to the ovary. Dysgerminomas have an excellent prognosis, and most are cured. Patients with stage IA disease have greater than 95% 5-year survival. Even patients with advanced disease have 5-year survival rates of 85–90%. Patients with non-dysgerminomatous tumors in advanced stages have a 5-year survival of about 60–80%.

MALIGNANT SEX-CORD AND STROMAL TUMORS

23. How do patients with stromal tumors present?

These tumors often present in children and young women. Stromal tumors often produce sex steroids; thus presenting symptoms may include precocious puberty or virilization.

24. What are the different types of sex-cord and stromal tumors?

Granulosa cell tumors secrete estrogen, but virilization occasionally occurs. Granulosa cell tumors have two variants, juvenile and adult. Adult granulosa cell tumors account for 95% of these lesions. They occur most often in postmenopausal women and produce estrogen, resulting in hyperplasia or carcinoma of the endometrium, abnormal bleeding, and breast swelling. Histologically, Call-Exner bodies are common. Juvenile granulosa cell tumors usually present under the age of 30. Children may show signs of precocious puberty. Older women may have amenorrhea or irregular bleeding.

Thecomas and **fibromas** are rarely malignant. These tumors are rare before puberty and usually present in peri- or postmenopausal women. Thecomas may also produce estrogen.

Sertoli-Leydig cell tumors (androblastomas) are rare. Most are virilizing, some are estrogenic, and some produce no hormonal effects. Isosexual precocity may result from estrogen production, and signs of pregnancy may be simulated by progesterone production. The average age of presentation is about 25.

25. Describe the treatment of sex-cord and stromal tumors.

Treatment is primarily surgical. Surgical staging is important for patients with both granulosa cell and Sertoli-Leydig cell tumors. Young patients may have a wedge biopsy of the contralateral ovary in the absence of gross disease to attempt to preserve fertility. Any disease identified outside of the ovary should be debulked if possible. Adjuvant chemotherapy is controversial, but several different regimens may be employed including BEP, VAC (vincrisitine, dactinomycin, and cyclophosphamide), and PVB (cisplatin, vinblastine, and bleomycin). Thecomas and fibromas are treated with unilateral salpingo-oophorectomy.

26. What is the survival rate?

Overall, granulosa cell tumors have an excellent prognosis. Ten-year and 20-year survivals have been reported at 90% and 75%, respectively. Sertoli-Leydig cell tumors also have a good prognosis. Overall, the 5-year survival is approximately 70–90%. Recurrences are uncommon after 5 years.

27. Are stromal tumors associated with other cancers?

Because stromal tumors often produce estrogen, they are commonly associated with endometrial hyperplasia and carcinoma. Up to 13% of patients with granulosa cell tumors have a synchronous, well-differentiated endometrial adenocarcinoma.

28. What is Meigs syndrome?

Meigs syndrome is a triad of findings which includes ascites, pleural effusion, and benign ovarian fibroma. The cause is unknown, but after the ovarian lesion is removed, the ascites and pleural effusion resolve spontaneously.

OTHER OVARIAN CANCERS

29. What tumors are commonly metastatic to the ovary?

About 5% of ovarian tumors are metastases. The most common tumor metastatic to the ovary is breast cancer. Metastases from the gastrointestinal tract, particularly from the colon, are also common. Endometrial cancer may also metastasize to the ovary.

30. What is a Krukenberg tumor?

The term Krukenberg tumor describes metastatic adenocarcinoma of the ovary that contains significant numbers of signet ring cells in a cellular ovarian stroma. Almost all metastasize from the stomach, but some arise in the breast, colon, or biliary tract. Rarely, these tumors spread from the bladder or cervix.

31. List some other types of ovarian cancer.

Neoplasms may arise from the nonspecific mesenchymal tissue of the ovary as well. These tumors include benign lesions such as fibromas, hemangiomas, leiomyomas, and lipomas, but also encompass rare malignancies such as sarcoma and lymphoma.

BIBLIOGRAPHY

1. Berek JS: Epithelial ovarian cancer. In Berek JS, Hacker NF (eds): Practical Gynecologic Oncology, 2nd ed. Baltimore, Williams & Williams, 1994, pp 327–376.
2. Berek JS, Hacker NF: Nonepithelial ovarian and fallopian tumbe cancers. In Berek JS, Hacker NF (eds): Practical Gynecologic Oncology, 2nd ed. Baltimore, Williams & Williams, 1994, pp 377–402.
3. Chu CS, Randall TC, Mikuta JJ: Low malignant potential tumors of the ovary. Postgraduate Obstetrics and Gynecology 18:1–6, 1998.
4. DiSaia PJ, Creasman WT: The adnexal mass and early ovarian cancer. In DiSaia PJ, Creasman WT (eds): Clinical Gynecologic Oncology, 5th ed. St. Louis, Mosby, 1997, pp 253–281.
5. DiSaia PJ, Creasman WT: Epithelial ovarian cancer. In DiSaia PJ, Creasman WT (eds): Clinical Gynecologic Oncology, 5th ed. St. Louis, Mosby, 1997, pp 282–350.
6. DiSaia PJ, Creasman WT: Germ cell, stromal, and other ovarian tumors. In DiSaia PJ, Creasman WT (eds): Clinical Gynecologic Oncology, 5th ed. St. Louis, Mosby, 1997, pp 351–374.
7. Hurteau JA, Williams SJ: Ovarian germ cell tumors. In Rubin SC, Sutton GP (eds): Ovarian Cancer, 2nd ed. Philadelphia, Williams & Williams, 2001, pp 371–382
8. Schilder JM, Holladay DV, Gallion HH: Hereditary ovarian cancer: Clinical syndromes and management. In Rubin SC, Sutton GP (eds): Ovarian Cancer, 2nd ed. Philadelphia, Williams & Williams, 2001, pp 181–200.
9. Schwartz PE, Price FV, Snyder MK: Management of ovarian stromal tumors. In Rubin SC, Sutton GP (eds): Ovarian Cancer, 2nd ed. Philadelphia, Williams & Williams, 2001, pp 383–398.
10. Rubin SC, Benjamin I, Behbakht K, et al: Clinical and pathological features of ovarian cancer in women with germ-line mutations of BRCA1. N Engl J Med 335:1413–1416, 1996.

31. GESTATIONAL TROPHOBLASTIC DISEASE

Christina A. Bandera, M.D.

1. What is a gestational trophoblastic disease (GTD)?

GTD is an abnormal proliferation of placental-type tissue resulting from a union of egg and sperm with abnormal DNA content. Histologic findings may include vesicular chorionic villi and proliferative trophoblast. GTD refers to a variety of diseases, including complete and partial molar pregnancy and gestational trophoblastic tumors (GTT) such as invasive mole, choriocarcinoma, and placental-site trophoblastic tumor. Untreated, GTD may result in life-threatening bleeding, systemic disease, and metastatic cancer.

2. How common is GTD?

One in 1500 pregnancies in the United States is a molar pregnancy. Women less than 20 years old appear to have a slightly higher incidence of GTD. Women older than 40 years have a 10-fold higher risk of GTD. Furthermore, the prevalence of GTD is 10 times higher in Asia than in North America and Europe.

3. What is the origin of complete and partial molar pregnancy?

A *complete* mole results when an "empty egg" lacking maternal DNA is fertilized by one sperm (which then duplicates its DNA), or by two sperm simultaneously. The karyotype of a complete mole is paternally derived 46XX in 90% of cases, and paternally derived 46XY in 10% of cases.

A *partial* mole is the result of a haploid egg fertilized by two sperm. The karyotype is usually 69XXX or 69XXY, with two-thirds of the DNA of paternal origin.

4. What is the clinical presentation of a complete mole vs. a partial mole?

Abnormal bleeding in the first trimester of pregnancy is the most common presenting symptom for both complete and partial moles. Work-up is likely to include an ultrasound showing a "grape-like" collection of small cystic spaces in the uterus. A complete mole is commonly associated with a human chorionic gonadotropin (β-hCG or hCG) level > 200,000 mIU/ml, compared to a typical peak of 50,000–100,000 mIU/ml in a normal pregnancy. Symptoms that are more commonly seen when diagnosis is delayed until the second trimester include uterine size enlarged for gestational age, anemia, theca lutein cysts of the ovary, hyperemesis, hyperthyroidism, pre-eclampsia, and respiratory insufficiency.

These symptoms are rarely seen in conjunction with a partial mole, and β-hCG levels tend to be lower. Partial moles may be associated with a fetus, but the fetus is rarely viable.

5. How should a molar pregnancy be managed?

Dilatation and evacuation (D&E) of molar tissue should be performed in the operating room. If future fertility is not desired, a hysterectomy may be considered. Following treatment, check β-hCG levels weekly until undetectable for 3 consecutive weeks. Regular monthly β-hCG screening should continue for 1 year. During this surveillance period, encourage patients to use birth control. If the β-hCG level plateaus or rises, consider chemotherapy.

6. What is a gestational trophoblastic tumor (GTT)?

GTT refers to invasive or metastatic forms of gestational trophoblastic disease. There are three types of GTT:
- Invasive or persistent mole characterized by molar tissue invading the uterine myometrium
- Choriocarcinoma, which is a malignant epithelial cancer that is frequently associated with distant metastases
- Placental-site trophoblastic tumor, a rare and highly aggressive neoplasm.

7. Does a molar pregnancy always precede GTT?

No. Only two-thirds of GTT follow a molar pregnancy. The remaining one-third of cases follow miscarriage, therapeutic abortion, or ectopic pregnancy.

8. What is the risk of developing gestational trophoblastic tumor following dilation and evacuation for a molar pregnancy?

The risk of developing malignant GTT is 15–20% following a D&E for a *complete* mole. For a woman > 40 years old, or with a uterine size > 20 weeks, or a β-hCG level > 100,000 at the time of diagnosis, the risk is 40%. After a D&E for a *partial* mole, the risk of GTT is 2%.

9. How is GTT classified?

When the diagnosis of GTT is made the patient should have a complete work-up, including chest x-ray and CT or MRI of the abdomen and pelvis. Also consider imaging of the brain. Based on the radiologic studies, GTT is classified as non-metastatic or metastatic. Metastatic GTT is further subdivided into high-risk and low-risk categories according to the World Health Organization (WHO) Prognostic Scoring System (see table).

WHO Scoring System for Metastatic GTT Based On Prognostic Factors

PROGNOSTIC FACTORS	SCORE			
	0	1	2	3
Age (years)	≤ 39	> 39	—	—
Antecedent pregnancy	Mole	Abortion	Term	—
Interval since antecedent pregnancy (months)	4	4–6	7–12	> 12
HCG (U/l)	< 10^3	10^3–10^4	10^4–10^5	> 10^5
Blood type	—	O or A	B or AB	—
Largest tumor	< 3 cm	3–5 cm	> 5 cm	—
Site of metastases	—	Spleen, kidney	Gastrointestinal tract, liver	Brain
Number of metastases	—	1–3	4–8	> 8
Prior chemotherapy	None		Single drug	> 2 drugs

hCG = human chorionic gonadotropin, GTT = gestational trophoblastic disease
Scoring: ≤ 4 is low risk; 5–7 is intermediate risk; ≥ 8 is high risk

10. Describe the appropriate treatment for GTT.

For *non-metastatic* or *low-risk* GTT, single-agent chemotherapy with methotrexate or actinomycin-D is appropriate. Treatment is repeated until β-hCG falls to undetectable levels. Eighty percent of these patients are cured by one treatment, and nearly 100% are cured within three treatments.

High-risk GTT must be treated with combination chemotherapy such as EMA-CO (etoposide, methotrexate, actinomycin-D, cyclophosphamide, vincristine). Treatment continues for two to three courses beyond an undetectable β-hCG level. Survival is approximately 70%.

Regardless of the treatment, all patients with molar pregnancies or GTT should be followed with regular β-hCG screening for 1 year.

11. What is the mechanism of methotrexate treatment? What are the side effects?

Methotrexate is an anti-metabolite that kills cells in the S-phase of the cell cycle by binding dihydrofolate reductase and thus preventing the reduction of dihydrofolate to tetrahydrofolic acid. This in turn inhibits thymidylate synthetase and purine production, leading to decreased DNA, RNA, and protein production. The most common side effect is mucositis (patients typically complain of mouth sores).

Less common side effects include nausea, vomiting, anorexia, thinning of hair, leukopenia, hepatotoxicity and renal toxicity. Leucovorin "rescue" (calcium folinate) is commonly administered several hours following methotrexate to replenish folate and minimize side effects.

12. How should a woman with a history of GTD be counseled regarding subsequent pregnancies?

It is generally recommended that a woman avoid pregnancy for 1 year following a molar pregnancy to prevent misdiagnosis of recurrent disease.

The majority of pregnancies following treatment for a molar pregnancy or GTT result in normal, healthy babies. The risk of a second molar pregnancy is only 1%. A woman who has two molar pregnancies has a 15–28% chance of having a third. The risk following three molar pregnancies is nearly 100%. This elevated risk appears to persist even when the woman has a different male partner.

BIBLIOGRAPHY

1. Benson CB, et al: Sonographic appearance of first-trimester complete hydatidiform moles. Ultrasound Obstet Gynecol 2000;16(2):188–191.
2. Berkowitz RS, et al: Gestational trophoblastic disease: Subsequent pregnancy outcome, including repeat molar pregnancy. J Reprod Med 1998;43(1):81–86.
3. Blaustein A, Kurman RJ: Blaustein's Pathology of the Female Genital Tract, 5th ed. New York, Springer, 2002.
4. Hoskins WJ, et al: Principles and Practice of Gynecologic Oncology, 3rd ed. Philadelphia, Lippincott Williams and Wilkins, 2000.
5. Sand PK, et al: Repeat gestational trophoblastic disease. Obstet Gynecol 1984;63(2):140–144.
6. Semer DA, Macfee MS: Gestational trophoblastic disease: Epidemiology. Semin Oncol 1995;22(2):109–112.
7. Soto-Wright V, et al: The changing clinical presentation of complete molar pregnancy. Obstet Gynecol 1995;86(5):775–779.

III. Social/Health Issues

32. DOMESTIC VIOLENCE

Janice B. Asher, M.D.

1. Why is domestic violence a medical issue?

Just as physicians now recognize that social behaviors such as tobacco, alcohol, and substance abuse have enormous medical implications, we have also come to appreciate that domestic violence is an epidemic that has to be addressed by clinicians.

2. What are the characteristics of domestic violence?

Whether the violence is psychological, physical, or sexual, all violent relationships are characterized by the exertion of power and control by the perpetrator against the victim. Of particular importance for obstetrician/gynecologists to bear in mind are tactics such as refusing to permit negotiation of safer sex and contraceptive practices.

3. Why don't abused women just leave their abusers?

A woman may stay in an abusive relationship because she is even more fearful about what will happen to her and her children if she leaves. In fact, this fear is justified: abused women are at *highest risk for serious injury and death when leaving or after leaving* an abuser. She may be economically dependent on her partner and not be able to support herself and her children or have access to medical care if she leaves. She may feel a religious or cultural obligation to keep the family "intact." Finally, she may blame herself for the abuse, since her partner has blamed her for his inability to "control himself."

4. Who needs to be screened?

Since domestic violence crosses racial, socioeconomic, and cultural lines, and since it is so common, *all* **women** should be screened periodically for violence. While women do not generally spontaneously disclose abuse, there is ample evidence that they will respond when asked and that they are grateful for the opportunity.

Many studies have demonstrated that the incidence of domestic violence increases during pregnancy and the postpartum period. This fact, along with frequent doctor visits during pregnancy and a woman's concern for the safety and well-being of her child, make pregnancy a particularly important time for domestic violence assessment.

5. True or false: Dating violence is very common.

True. Therefore, all women—especially adolescents and younger women, who are more likely to be dating—should be screened. Most perpetrators of violence in dating relationships first display signs of excessive jealousy and controlling behavior. As many as 25% of college women report a history of attempted or completed "acquaintance rape." It is important to stress safety behaviors, including not drinking alcohol to a point of impaired judgment and not going off alone with someone a woman neither knows well nor trusts. However, this is not to say that the responsibility for sexual assault or violence rests with anyone other than the perpetrator.

6. What if there isn't time for domestic violence screening?

In addition to being standard of care practice, screening for violence may actually save time in the long run. Abused women have more physician visits, more sexually transmitted diseases, more adverse pregnancy outcomes, more unintended pregnancies, more pelvic pain and dyspare-unia, and more psychological symptoms, particularly depression, than do women who are not abused. Clearly, evaluation of such symptoms requires a great deal of time and resources.

7. How do I screen for domestic violence?

Interviewing the patient alone and asking direct, simple questions is recommended. Useful questions include:

- Are you in a relationship in which you've been threatened, hit, or forced to have sex?
- Is there anyone you're afraid of?

8. What do I do if a patient says she's being abused?

Simply asking a woman about domestic violence and then offering the patient a nonjudg-mental, compassionate response can, in itself, be a powerful form of intervention. The physician must resist the impulse to urge the patient to leave her abusive partner at once. Abused women are more likely to be seriously injured or killed at the time they attempt to leave their partner than at any other time. Furthermore, leaving an abusive relationship is a process, not an event (see ref. 4). We expect lifestyle changes, such as smoking cessation, to take time and to require multiple messages and strategies, and this is the case with addressing violence, as well.

Instead, assure the patient that she does not deserve to be abused and help is available. Recommend that she take measures to ensure the safety of herself and her children. Getting the patient to leave a violent relationship is not the goal; helping the patient to be safer, on the other hand, is of paramount importance.

9. Must I report domestic violence to police authorities?

In the U.S., 48 of the 50 states do not have laws mandating physician reporting of domestic violence involving competent adults. There is evidence that mandatory reporting, in addition to further eroding a victim's autonomy, may even increase her risk for additional violence in the future.

10. How do I document domestic violence?

Use the patient's own words whenever possible. Include the name of the perpetrator and a description of the nature of the violence and any weapons used. Ideally, take a photograph of any injuries. A standard consent form is adequate for taking photographs to document violence. Good documentation may provide crucial evidence for the patient at a later time, particularly if there are child custody issues, since there seldom are witnesses to corroborate abuse.

Note: While domestic violence belongs on the problem list and in the body of a medical record, it should not be included as a diagnosis for billing purposes if the patient is on her partner's medical plan.

11. But I'm not a domestic violence expert . . .

No one is a domestic violence expert. However, as is the case when their patients have other medical problems, physicians need to be aware of in-house and community resources available to victims of domestic violence.

12. How do I refer a patient who's been abused?

First, assure the patient that she does not deserve to be abused, that the situation is likely to get worse, and that if she is being hurt, her children are being hurt as well. Social workers may be able to offer counseling and help with information regarding "protection from abuse" (restrain-ing) orders, shelters, etc. Virtually every community has a domestic violence advocacy organiza-tion, as well, many of which print information that may be kept in clinicians' offices. *All violence-related materials should be available in patient restrooms*. If the patient has a partner who refuses to leave the examining room, the restroom may be the only site in the office where she has privacy.

Routine referral for couples counseling is *not* recommended. If the patient discloses feelings of anger, for example, in a counseling session, her partner's abusive behavior may escalate. After the violence and the threat of violence has ceased, joint counseling—in some cases—may then be an option.

While clinicians are not expected to be domestic violence experts, they should have access to names and phone numbers of local hot lines, shelters, and other resources. There is also a national number offering 24-hour information, counseling, and referral for victims of domestic violence and caregivers: 1-800-799-SAFE.

BIBLIOGRAPHY

1. Gazmararian JA, Adams MM, Saltzman LE, et al. The relationship between pregnancy intendedness and physical violence in mothers of newborns. Obstet Gynecol 85:1031–1038, 1995.
2. Gerbert B, Abercrombie P, Caspers N, et al: How health care providers help battered women: The survivor's perspective. Women & Health 29(3):115–135, 1999.
3. Lampe A, Solder E, Ennemoser A, et al: Chronic pelvic pain and previous sexual abuse. Obstet Gynecol 96:929–933, 2000.
4. Mayer L, Liebschutz J: Domestic violence in the pregnant patient: Obstetric and behavioral interventions. Obstet Gynecol Survey 53(10):627–635, 1998.
5. Petersen R, Gazmararian JA, Spitz AM, et al: Violence and adverse pregnancy outcomes: A review of the literature and directions for future research. Am J Prev Med 13:366–373, 1997.
6. Plichta S, Duncan M, Plichta L: Spouse abuse, patient-physician communication, and patient satisfaction. Am J Prev Med 12:297–303, 1996.
7. Rickert VI, Wiemann CM: Date rape among adolescents and young adults. J Ped Adolesc Gynecol 11(4):167–175, 1998.
8. Stewart DE: Incidence of postpartum abuse in women with a history of abuse during pregnancy. Can Med Assoc J 151(11):1601–1604, 1994.
9. Stewart DE, Cecutti A: Physical abuse in pregnancy. Can Med Assoc J 149:1257–1263, 1993.
10. Wingood GM, DiClemente RJ: The effects of an abusive primary partner on condom use and sexual negotiation practices of African American Women. Am J Public Health 87:1016–1018, 1997.
11. Wisner CL, Gilmer TP, Saltzman LE, Zink TM: Intimate partner violence against women. Do victims cost health plans more? J Fam Prac 48(6):439–443, 1999.

IV. Prenatal Care

33. PRECONCEPTION COUNSELING

Emmanuelle Paré, M.D., FRCSC

1. Why is preconception counseling important?

Preconception counseling plays multiple roles:

- Most interventions to **decrease birth defects** need to be in place prior to or at conception to be effective. By the time of the first prenatal visit, generally at 6–8 weeks' gestation, organogenesis has started and some irreversible teratogen effects might have already occurred.
- Preconception counseling allows **identification, assessment, and possible alteration of risk factors** that may influence maternal and fetal outcomes during pregnancy. Medication number and dosage should be kept to a minimum during pregnancy, and drugs in class X—those deemed unsafe in pregnancy—should be discontinued, but those adjustments should ideally be done before conception.
- Education about a woman's specific risk factors may affect her **decision to become pregnant or the timing of pregnancy**. For some women, their risk of maternal or fetal complications may be too high to attempt pregnancy. Women with chronic medical conditions should try to conceive when their disease is under optimal control. Some couples may want to complete screening for some genetic disorders to determine their risk more precisely and explore the possibility of prenatal diagnosis. Finally, it is a good occasion to assess and reinforce folic acid supplementation and to review the importance of seeking early (first-trimester) and regular prenatal care.

2. When should preconception counseling be performed?

Even though preconception counseling offers benefits to all women considering pregnancy, a minority of women will request or be referred for preconception counseling. Up to 50% of pregnancies in the U.S. are unplanned. Therefore, preconception counseling should be discussed with all women of childbearing age, especially if they are considering pregnancy in the next 1–2 years. Occasions to perform preconception counseling include an annual routine visit, consultation for contraception, or consultation for infertility.

3. Who can perform preconception counseling?

Preconception counseling can be performed by family physicians, internists, general obstetrician-gynecologists, maternal-fetal medicine (MFM) specialists, or geneticists. General preconception counseling and screening for risk factors can be done by primary care givers, with referral to an obstetrician-gynecologist, an MFM specialist, or a geneticist for further counseling when specific risk factors are identified.

4. What information should be obtained during preconception counseling?

- Medical and surgical history
- Gynecologic and reproductive history, with attention to potentially recurrent obstetrical complications
- Familial history, focusing on ethnic background, congenital anomalies and genetic disorders
- Medication
- Social and nutritional assessment

• Review of systems
• Physical examination, including a pelvic exam

5. Which laboratory tests may be indicated in preconception counseling?

Hematocrit—iron deficiency anemia, lowered mean corpuscular volume as a screen for hemoglobinopathies if appropriate

Rubella titer—immunization if nonimmune in the nonpregnant state

Hepatitis B antigen—women at risk by lifestyle or occupation should consider active immunization before pregnancy.

Screening for human immunodeficiency virus (HIV)—with appropriate counseling and consent

Screening for other sexually transmitted diseases—in particular, syphilis, which unrecognized can result in fetal complications

Screening for specific genetic disorders—according to the family history and to ethnic origin. Examples include Tay-Sachs, Canavan's disease, and cystic fibrosis for Ashkenazi Jews; hemoglobinopathies for African-Americans, Africans, Southeast Asians and Mediterraneans; and cystic fibrosis for Caucasians.

Routine preventative health care—Pap smear, mammogram if appropriate, cholesterol screening, and immunizations should be current.

6. What nutritional disorders should be recognized?

The following nutritional disorders or practices carry potential risks to the fetus and should be recognized and addressed during preconception counseling: pica, bulimia and/or anorexia, strict vegetarianism, and certain vitamin and mineral imbalances (deficiencies as well as excessive use).

7. Why is folic acid supplementation recommended before conception?

Folic acid supplementation for primary and secondary prevention of **neural tube defects** (NTDs) has been supported by randomized controlled trials. In women who had a *previous child with an NTD*, **high-dose folic acid (4 mg per day) decreased the risk by 70%**. In the U.S. this decreases the risk of recurrence from approximately 2–3% to less than 1%. The Centers for Disease Control and Prevention recommends that women who had a previous NTD-affected pregnancy take 4 mg of folic acid per day beginning at least 1 month prior to conception and continuing through the first trimester.

In women with *no history of an NTD-affected pregnancy*, supplementation with a multivitamin containing 0.4 mg (400 µg) folic acid will **prevent at least 50% of NTDs** when taken before conception and continued throughout the first trimester. Since up to 50% of pregnancies in the U.S. are unplanned, the U.S. Public Health Service recommends that all women of child-bearing age consume 0.4 mg (400 µg) of folic acid daily.

Risk factors for NTD, other than a previous NTD-affected pregnancy, include maternal diabetes (pre-gestational); maternal intake of valproic acid or carbamazepine; and patient, partner, or close relative who has an NTD. Unfortunately, no studies have addressed prevention of NTDs in those specific situations. Therefore, there is no evidence to support periconceptional high-dose folic acid (4 mg [4000 µg]) supplementation for women with these risk factors. They should definitely take at least 0.4 mg of folic acid daily, and consideration can be given to increasing their daily periconceptional folic acid intake to 4 mg. The potential risks of this higher dose of folic acid include masking the hematologic signs of vitamin B12 deficiency (pernicious anemia) without preventing its irreversible neurologic effects.

8. How much folic acid on average do American women consume in their daily diet?

Although the recommended dietary allowance (RDA) for folic acid is 400 µg for adults and 600 µg for pregnant women, the average U.S. diet contains about only 200 µg of naturally occurring food folate. Foods with high folate content include green, leafy vegetables; fruits; and fortified cereals.

9. How can the requirements for daily folic acid intake be met?

Additional intake of foods rich in folate can raise the average intake, but *naturally occuring folate* is less readily absorbed than *synthetic folic acid* in supplements or fortified foods. Since 1996, following the Food and Drug Administration (FDA) recommendations, enriched cereal-grain products are fortified with 140 µg of folic acid per 100 g of flour. However, this measure increases the average consumption of folic acid by only 100 µg/day and increases the proportion of women consuming the recommended daily dosage of 400 µg by only 3%.

Folic acid supplements are the only method of folic acid supplementation that has been tested and shown to decrease the primary and secondary incidence of NTD. The majority of multivitamin over-the-counter preparations contain 0.4 mg of folic acid. Most prescription prenatal vitamins contain 0.8 mg. Mutivitamin preparations containing 0.4 mg of folic acid should not be used to increase folic acid intake up to 1 mg or more, since they contain other vitamins that could have adverse effects when taken in large quantities, such as vitamin A.

10. What concerns have been raised about vitamin A and pregnancy?

Vitamin A is an essential vitamin, with an RDA in pregnancy of 5000 IU. An average balanced diet supplies 7000–8000 IU per day; thus additional supplementation is usually not needed. Daily vitamin A intakes **> 25,000 IU/day**, as with diets rich in liver and cod oil as well as supplemental vitamin A intake, **increase the risk of birth defects**. Recent concern has focused on an increased incidence of craniofacial, central nervous system (CNS), thymic, and cardiac defects with even lower levels of vitamin A supplementation, > 10,000 IU/day. Vitamin A supplementation in pregnancy is not necessary and may have harmful effects. It should therefore be discontinued.

11. What are the effects of caffeine during pregnancy?

Animal studies have shown an increased rate of birth defects with extremely high amounts of caffeine (at levels greater than reasonably consumed by a person, 15–25 cups of coffee/day). However, teratogenicity in humans has never been documented. There is some suggestion that heavy caffeine intake (> 300 mg/day; 3–4 cups coffee/day) is associated with increased risk for spontaneous abortions and decreased fetal growth.

When assessing caffeine intake, it is important to ask patients about their coffee consumption as well as their chocolate, tea, and carbonated beverages consumption.

12. What is the recommended maximum level of caffeine intake during pregnancy?

No standard recommendations currently exist as to caffeine ingestion during pregnancy. It seems prudent to recommend that pregnant women limit their intake to < 300 mg/day. For women who have a history of recurrent spontaneous abortions, intake should be limited to 150 mg/day (1–2 cups of coffee/day) during the first trimester.

13. What are the effects of alcohol during pregnancy?

Alcohol is a teratogenic agent and adversely affects fetal growth and CNS development. Alcohol and its metabolite, acetaldehyde, impact cell growth, number, and differentiation. The classic fetal alcohol syndrome (FAS) consists of intrauterine and post-natal growth restriction, facial dysmorphology, and CNS anomalies, ranging from hypotonia to developmental delay to mental retardation. In addition, excessive alcohol consumption is associated in some studies with congenital anomalies (especially cardiac defects, the most frequent being ventricular septal defects), increased risk of first- and second-trimester abortions, and placental abruption.

The teratogenicity of alcohol, as well as its other adverse effects, are dose dependent. The full FAS occurs in 30–40% of neonates born to women who consume more than 2 oz of absolute alcohol/day during the first trimester. Individual features of FAS, as well as other congenital anomalies, have been reported with consumption of 1 oz of absolute alcohol daily and with binge drinking.

14. How should I address the subject of alcohol use?
The importance of questioning women contemplating pregnancy and who are already pregnant about their alcohol consumption cannot be overstated. The physician must counsel them about the adverse fetal effects of alcohol. Several non-threatening, time-efficient screening tools are available to assess the level of alcohol consumption in the outpatient setting.

15. Is there a safe level of alcohol consumption during pregnancy?
No level of alcohol consumption has been proven safe. Therefore, total abstinence is recommended during the pregnancy.

16. Are any drugs of abuse safe in pregnancy?
No. No drug of abuse is absolutely safe to use during pregnancy.

17. Describe the effects of cocaine on the pregnant mom and the fetus.
Cocaine is probably the most deleterious drug in pregnancy, for both the fetus and the mother. Cocaine is a vasoconstrictive agent causing increased vascular resistance and decreased blood flow. *Maternal effects* from cocaine include hypertension, myocardial and cerebral infarction, intracranial hemorrhage, seizures, pulmonary complications, and sudden death. *Fetal effects* include congenital anomalies (cardiac defects, CNS anomalies, limb reduction defects, genitourinary malformations, and gastrointestinal anomalies), spontaneous abortions, intrauterine growth restriction (IUGR), placental abruption, preterm premature rupture of membranes, preterm delivery, intrauterine fetal death (IUFD) and intraventricular hemorrhage.

18. Describe the effects of narcotics abuse on mother and fetus.
Dependence on narcotics, such as heroin and methadone, is associated with IUGR, preterm delivery, IUFD, and neonatal withdrawal. Both overdose and withdrawal can be fatal to the fetus. Therefore, narcotic withdrawal is discouraged during pregnancy. However, heroin-dependent patients should be encouraged to enroll in narcotic maintenance programs using methadone since those programs improve perinatal outcome.

19. What other risks do drug abusers face?
Women who are abusing drugs are at increased risk for hepatitis B and C, HIV, syphilis, and other sexually transmitted diseases. Screening for these diseases should be offered in the preconception period, at the first prenatal visit, and repeated later in pregnancy if the risk factors are still present. At-risk women who are negative for hepatitis B antigen should be immunized; hepatitis B vaccine is safe in pregnancy.

20. What are the effects of smoking during pregnancy?
Cigarette smoking is associated with increased risks of spontaneous abortion, perinatal mortality, placenta previa, placental abruption, IUGR, preterm delivery and low birthweight. Neonates born to smokers weigh on average 200 g less than neonates born to nonsmokers. Smoking is also associated with increased risks of sudden infant death syndrome (SIDS) and childhood asthma. Recommend smoking cessation to smokers and offer assistance. Smoking cessation by the end of the first trimester can substantially reduce most of the smoking-associated risks.
Passive smoke exposure is associated with a small decrease (50 g) in mean birth weight as well as increased risk of SIDS and childhood respiratory disorders.

21. What relatively common medical conditions should be identified and addressed during preconception counseling?
Pre-gestational diabetes: Associated with an increased risk of birth defects (cardiac defects and neural tube defects are the most frequent). Risk further increased if glycemic control suboptimal.

Ideally, optimal blood sugar control, assessed by glycosylated hemoglobin (HbA_1C), achieved before conception. Assessment of overall health, including blood pressure and renal, cardiac, and retinal evaluation, useful in counseling patient about both impact of pregnancy on her disease and risks of fetal and pregnancy-related complications due to her diabetes.

Seizure disorders: Some seizure medications may be teratogenic. In conjunction with neurologist, consider trial of different or possibly no medication.

Hypertension: Assessment of cardiac and renal function probably best gauge for complications during pregnancy. Assess current medications; avoid angiotensin-converting enzyme inhibitors.

Connective tissue disorders (e.g., systemic lupus erythematosus): Evaluate current renal function, hypertension, and pericardial/pleural involvement to assess risk of pregnancy to underlying disease as well as potential for pregnancy complications. Studies can identify antibodies, including anticardiolipin antibody, lupus anticoagulant, anti-Ro, and anti-La, that may increase risk of adverse pregnancy outcome and congenital heart block. Some women without significant history may test positive for antibody. For these women with isolated laboratory finding but no history of thrombosis, adverse pregnancy outcome, or previous child with congenital heart block, there is no evidence that treatment affects outcome of pregnancy.

22. How should the family history be assessed?

Pay particular attention to family members (including the woman and her partner) with recognized Mendelian disorders (either recessive, dominant, or X-linked), multifactorial disorders (neural tube defect, cardiac anomaly, cleft lip or palate), and chromosomal disorders. A first-degree family member, either male or female, or multiple family members with mental retardation of unknown cause should initiate screening for fragile X syndrome.

23. What are the risks associated with advanced maternal age (≥ 35 years)?

- **Fertility** decreases as maternal age increases.
- **Chromosomal anomalies** increase with advancing maternal age, and this increase is mainly due to an increase in trisomies (the most frequent being trisomy 21 or Down's syndrome), due to an increase in non-disjunction associated with maternal age.
- The **spontaneous abortion** rate is increased with maternal age, mainly secondary to the increase in chromosomal anomalies.
- Note that other birth defects (non-chromosomal) are *not* increased with maternal age.
- Maternal complications such as **pre-eclampsia**, **gestational diabetes**, and **placenta previa** are more frequent in women age 35 or older. It is controversial how much of this increase is due to maternal age and how much is due to the fact that predisposing medical conditions (such as chronic hypertension and diabetes) are more frequent with advancing maternal age.
- The **cesarean section** rate is higher in older women. It is unclear if this effect is actually due to maternal age or to confounding factors associated with maternal age, such as medical and obstetrical complications and higher incidence of multiple gestation.

24. For which preconception patient should cardiac testing be undertaken?

Women with the following conditions should received a cardiac assessment (e.g., electrocardiogram, echocardiogram) prior to conception:
- Pre-gestational diabetes
- Chronic hypertension (longer than 10 years, or over age 40)
- Congenital heart disease
- Signs or symptoms suggestive of cardiac disease

25. What are the absolute contraindications to pregnancy?

Risk has to be individualized for every patient, but cardiac conditions associated with marked maternal mortality (50% or more) include Eisenmenger syndrome, primary pulmonary hypertension, Marfan syndrome with marked dilation of the aortic root, complicated coarctation of the aorta, uncorrected tetralogy of Fallot, and dilated cardiomyopathy.

BIBLIOGRAPHY

1. American Academy of Pediatrics. Folic acid for the prevention of neural tube defects. Pediatrics 104(2):325–327, 1999.
2. American College of Obstetricians and Gynecologists: Preconception Care. ACOG Tech Bull 205, 1995.
3. Burrow GN, Duffy TP: Medical Complications During Pregnancy, 5th ed. Philadelphia, W.B. Saunders, 1999.
4. Centers for Disease Control and Prevention: Recommendations for the use of folic acid to reduce the number of cases of spina bifida and other neural tube defects. MMWR 41:1–8, 1992.
5. Creasy RK, Resnik R: Maternal-Fetal Medicine, 4th ed. Philadelphia, W.B. Saunders, 1999.
6. Marchiano D: Prenatal nutrition. eMedicine 2(7), 2001.

34. NORMAL PHYSIOLOGY OF PREGNANCY

Gretchen Frey, M.D.

DIAGNOSIS OF PREGNANCY

1. How soon after fertilization can beta human chorionic gonadotropin (hCG) be detected?

By 7 days after fertilization (4–5 days after implantation), hCG can be found at levels above 25 mIU/ml and thus is detected with the most sensitive test (serum immunoassay). Levels of hCG peak at about 100,000 mIU by 60 days after conception, and then decrease to around 5000 mIU/ml by 100–130 days.

2. How does the pattern of hCG rise differ in normal and abnormal pregnancies?

In a normal intrauterine gestation, the hCG level should double roughly every 48–60 hours in the first 8 weeks. In an ectopic (tubal or otherwise extrauterine) gestation, the levels often rise more slowly or may plateau. In an impending miscarriage (spontaneous abortion), levels often fall before passage of the fetal tissue. Complicating these guidelines is the fact that in 15% of normal gestations, doubling is slower than usual; and in 17% of ectopic pregnancies, levels rise normally.

3. At what hCG level can fetal viability be confirmed by ultrasound?

With modern endovaginal imaging equipment, most experienced technologists can image a fetal pole with cardiac activity at a level of 1000–1500 mIU/ml hCG. This corresponds to 5 weeks after the last menstrual period, or < 24 days post conception (in cases of precise timing such as in vitro fertilization).

4. How accurate are most home pregnancy tests?

Most home urine pregnancy tests are now nearly as accurate as a laboratory test on serum, with a sensitivity of 25 mIU/ml of hCG.

5. What are the most common causes of false-positive pregnancy tests? False-negative tests?

With current immunoassay methods, only hCG-producing tumors, hemolysis, or lipemia should produce *false-positive* results. Of course, human errors in mislabeling samples or performing the assay are possible. *False-negative* tests generally result when the gestation is below the sensitivity for the test. In most cases, this involves a normal early gestation, although blighted ova and ectopic pregnancies also may cause a false-negative result.

6. What is pseudocyesis?

False pregnancy. In rare cases, increased weight, amenorrhea, and a subjective appreciation of fetal movement lead some women (usually those with an underlying psychiatric disorder) to convince themselves of pregnancy despite negative pregnancy testing.

PHYSIOLOGIC CHANGES OF PREGNANCY

7. By what mechanism is the uterus able to distend to 1000 times its normal volume?

Stretching and hypertrophy of uterine muscle, not new cell development, are responsible. Estrogen and progesterone initiate changes in the uterine muscle until 14 weeks of pregnancy, after which time the enlarging fetus exerts a direct stretching effect.

8. What is hyperemesis gravidarum? What causes it?

Hyperemesis gravidarum is an extreme manifestation of the common symptom of nausea in early pregnancy ("morning sickness"). It is usually seen in the first trimester. Women with this

- hCG   4-5 days implantation

$$\frac{7}{7}$$ after fertilization

- serum immunoassay
levels > 25 mIU/ml detectable

$$> 100,000 \text{ mIU/ml} \quad \frac{60}{7}$$

$$\sim 5000 \text{ mIU/ml} \quad \frac{100-130}{7}$$

(N) IUG
double q 48-60 hrs in first $\frac{8}{52}$ 15% Not true
ectopic / other   rise slowly / plateau   17%
miscarriage   fall

$$NP \male < 5.0 \text{ mIU/ml}$$
$$PM \male < 9.5 \text{ mIU/ml}$$

Follow up care of Ectopic &
Miscarriage

Is β HCG tested
when do they return for OP A

condition may be unable to keep down even fluids and sometimes require intravenous hydration and/or nutrition for a time. It is important to be vigilant for electrolyte imbalance, as cardiac arrhythmia and other serious side effects can result.

The cause is not well understood and may represent an unusual sensitivity of some individuals to hCG (believed to be the cause of normal first-trimester nausea). Another theory suggests subclinical hypoadrenalism, which self-corrects by the second trimester. Nonprescription measures that may be helpful include vitamin B6, 30–75 mg/day, and powdered ginger, 250 mg, 4 times daily.

9. Why is the uterus often dextrorotated, producing right lower quadrant pain as it enlarges?

The presence of the rectosigmoid colon in the left lower quadrant physically deviates the uterus slightly to the right. This is also the reason why the mild hydroureter of pregnancy (due to the smooth-muscle relaxing effect of progesterone) is often more pronounced on the right, because the mechanical pressure of the uterus at the pelvic brim is greater there than on the left.

10. What is the source of the progesterone that maintains the pregnancy during the first weeks?

The corpus luteum of the ovary. After 7–9 weeks, the placenta takes over the main production of progesterone.

11. What is Hartman's sign? How may it confuse the gestational age based on last menstrual period?

Some women experience several days' spotting as the blastocyst implants into the endometrium. Because this "light period" typically occurs 1 week after ovulation and fertilization (i.e., 3–3.5 weeks after last menses), it is sometimes mistakenly used for calculation of gestational age.

12. What changes typically occur in the pulmonary system as pregnancy progresses?

Mild, compensated, respiratory alkalosis is often present, primarily as a result of increased minute volume. An increase of 10–20% in baseline O_2 consumption is also seen.

13. What is characteristic about the cardiovascular system of pregnant women?

Typically a hyperdynamic state is caused by the 50% increase in blood volume, resulting in a slightly increased resting pulse, increased cardiac output, and flow murmurs. A progressive decrease in peripheral vascular resistance accounts for the slight decrease in blood pressure noted in normal second-trimester pregnancies.

14. What produces the inferior vena cava (supine hypotension) syndrome of pregnancy?

Compression of the inferior vena cava by the gravid uterus when the mother is supine can significantly decrease venous blood return to the heart, and therefore cardiac output. The supine hypotension syndrome is signaled by maternal complaints of dizziness upon lying supine; even fainting may occur. This effect can be avoided by having the mother lie in the left lateral position.

15. What is physiologic anemia of pregnancy?

The combination of increased plasma volume and less pronounced increase in red blood cell mass produces a dilutional anemia.

16. Can glycosuria be seen in normal pregnancies?

Yes. The glomerular filtration rate is increased during normal pregnancy; as a result, a glucose load may not be reabsorbed sufficiently. For this reason, urinary glucose is a poor indicator of control in the pregnant diabetic.

17. How does progesterone affect the gastrointestinal system?
Delayed gastric emptying time, poor esophageal sphincter tone, increased gallbladder stasis, and decreased gut motility are the sources of many bothersome but normal complaints of pregnancy, including esophageal reflux and flatulence.

18. Which hormone has the greatest effect on the ligaments during pregnancy?
Relaxin. In particular, the ligamentous symphysis pubis undergoes softening and partial separation at about 28–32 weeks, often resulting in a dull pain in this area, especially in multiparas.

19. What are common neurologic complaints during pregnancy?
Carpal tunnel syndrome. Bilateral or unilateral median nerve entrapment, perhaps secondary to fluid retention, may result in pain, decreased sensation, and weakness of predominantly the first three fingers. Splinting provides symptomatic relief, but rare cases may require surgical decompression.
Sciatica. Because of shifting of the pelvic bones and their relaxed ligaments, many women have classic sciatic nerve compression pain (felt in one buttock, radiating down the back of the leg to the lateral side of the foot). Fluid retention also may play a role.

20. Describe some common skin changes in pregnancy.
Increased pigmentation from increased estrogen and progesterone is seen in the areola, linea nigra, and perineum and also may cause chloasma (the facial pigmentation sometimes referred to as the "mask" of pregnancy). Pruritus gravidarum, or itching without skin changes, is also common (about 15% of pregnant women) and is probably secondary to elevation of bile salts due to changes in liver function. Symptomatic relief (with lotions, topical antipruritic agents, or oral antihistamines) usually suffices. When associated with specific types of skin changes, pruritis may be referred to as pruritic and urticarial papules and plaques of pregnancy (PUPPP). This more severe form usually requires topical or systemic steroids.

21. What changes occur in thyroid function in pregnancy?
Basal metabolic rate increases. Though free thyroxine (T4) and triiodothyronine (T3) levels remain unchanged, the total amounts of both hormones rise, along with thyroid-binding globulin. This can lead to confusion in interpreting thyroid function tests in pregnancy.

22. How is carbohydrate metabolism affected by pregnancy?
Carbohydrate utilization is enhanced, resulting in lower fasting blood glucose levels and greater carbohydrate (CHO) mobilization with exercise. When this adaptation mechanism fails, the entity known as gestational diabetes may result.

23. What changes can be seen in coagulation parameters in pregnancy?
Pregnancy is known as a hypercoagulable state, with a fivefold risk of venous thromboembolism over the nonpregnant condition. This is due to changes such as increases in factors I, VII, VIII, IX, and X; decreases in protein S and fibrinolytic activity; and increases in platelet activation and venous stasis.

24. What is the current maternal mortality rate in the United States? How does it differ from worldwide maternal mortality rates?
In 1999, national maternal mortality was recorded as 10.2/100,000 live births. This is five times less than in 1960. Worldwide mortality, however, currently equals one maternal death every minute of every hour, 365 days a year (comparative ratio of 550/100,000 live births). Women in the US and Europe have about a 1/1000 lifetime chance of pregnancy-related death, whereas women in some areas of Africa face a 1/25 chance of obstetric-related death.

25. What is the most common cause of maternal mortality in the U.S.?
Pulmonary embolism, followed closely by hypertensive disease, then hemorrhage.

EXERCISE IN PREGNANCY

26. What changes in physiologic parameters are seen in exercising pregnant women compared to the nonpregnant state?

Heart rate changes are not uniformly greater, but stroke volume and cardiac output are increased, as is hemoconcentration. Interestingly, a 12% incidence of ST segment depression on ECG has been reported, but is not felt to be related to ischemia and has no clinical sequelae.

27. What maximal pulse rate should be observed by exercising pregnant women?

A specific target rate is no longer recommended. Pregnant women are advised to continue whatever regimen they have been following, with appropriate modifications for decreased stamina and less available oxygen reserve (which translates, for most, to cutting back on the intensity and perhaps duration of exercise). Pregnancy is not a good time to begin an intensive fitness program, and episodic exercise is tolerated more poorly than a regular routine.

28. Are certain types of exercise to be avoided in pregnancy?

Yes. Because of increased ligamentous laxity, pregnant women are theoretically more subject to sprains and other ligamentous injury; and the shift in center of gravity as pregnancy progresses makes balance more difficult. Hence ballistic types of motion (jumping or bouncing), such as high-impact aerobics, should be undertaken with caution. Some sports such as water or snow skiing and horseback riding, are discouraged because of the potential for abdominal trauma; and scuba diving is not recommended, because of the unknown effect that breathing a compressed air mixture might have on the fetus.

29. Does exercise cause miscarriage?

No. Even vigorous exercise (such as daily running) in the first trimester has no effect on the rate of spontaneous abortion.

30. Why are pregnant women told not to exercise in the supine position after 20 weeks' gestation?

Because of the supine hypotension effect (see Question 14). Even if the woman is asymptomatic, the decrease in placental blood flow due to the combination of (1) caval compression and (2) shunting to the working skeletal muscle is believed to be potentially detrimental to the fetus.

BIBLIOGRAPHY

1. American College of Obstetrics and Gynecology (ACOG): Practice Bulletins—Ectopic Pregnancy. No. 3, December 1998; Exercise During Pregnancy and the Postpartum Period. No. 189, February 1994; Postpartum Hemorrhage. No. 243, January 1998.
2. Cunningham PG, McDonald P, Gant N (eds): Maternal adaptations to pregnancy. In Williams Obstetrics, 18th ed. Norwalk, CT, Appleton & Lange, 1989.
3. Grimes D: The morbidity and mortality of pregnancy: Still risky business. Am J Obstet Gynecol 170:1489–1494, 1994.
4. Gaby A: Nutritional Protocols for Treatment of Pregnancy Nausea. In Nutritional Therapy in Medical Practice. Seattle, Washington, Nutrition Seminars Inc, 2001.
5. Love TW, Cunningham GF: Thyroid Disease in Pregnancy. In Williams Obstetrics Supplement, no.9, Dec/Jan 1991.
6. Maine D: Maternal mortality: Helping women off the road to death. WHO Chron 40:175–183, 1986.
7. National Center for Vital Statistics: National Vital Statistics Report. Washington DC, 50 (5), Feb 12, 2002.
8. Parisi V, Creasy R: Maternal biologic adaptations to pregnancy. In Reece E, Mebbins J, Mahoney M, Petrie R (eds): Medicine of the Fetus and Mother. Philadelphia, Lippincott, 1992.
9. Rapini R, Jordon R: The skin and pregnancy. In Creasy R, Resnick R (eds): Maternal-Fetal Medicine: Principles and Practice, 3rd ed. Philadelphia, W.B. Saunders, 1994.
10. Yen S: Endocrinology of pregnancy. In Creasy R, Resnick R (eds): Maternal-Fetal Medicine: Principles and Practice, 3rd ed. Philadelphia, W.B. Saunders, 1994.

35. COMPREHENSIVE PRENATAL CARE

John G. McFee, M.D.

1. What does prenatal care encompass?

Prenatal care is the careful, systematic assessment and follow-up of a pregnant patient to assure the best possible health of the mother and her fetus. This care is threefold:

- To prevent, identify, and/or ameliorate maternal or fetal abnormalities that adversely effect pregnancy outcome, including socioeconomic and emotional factors as well as medical and obstetric
- To educate the patient about pregnancy, labor-delivery, and parenting as well as about ways she can improve her overall health
- To promote adequate psychological support from her partner, family, and caregivers, especially in the first pregnancy, so she can successfully adapt to the pregnancy and the challenges of raising a family.

Prenatal care therefore is a continuum from the preconceptional period through the first postpartum year. Prenatal care commences with an extensive initial history and physical examination. Estimated gestational age and estimated date of confinement (EDC) are determined. Routine laboratory tests are drawn. In subsequent visits the physician explores any problems, documents fetal growth, and identifies potential complications. Assessment for risk factors is done at the initial visit and on each revisit. Weight gain and nutritional well-being are evaluated at the outset and as the pregnancy progresses. Patient education is provided on a timely basis.

2. What are the goals and benefits of prenatal care?

Prenatal care is a preventive service and has been shown to be beneficial and cost effective. As a group, women receiving no or inadequate prenatal care have far more complications and poorer outcomes of pregnancy. The costs of care for "no-care" patients are also substantially higher, with increased rates of preeclampsia, low-birth-weight infants (both premature and growth retarded), and perinatal deaths.

3. How often should patients be seen?

The American College of Obstetricians and Gynecologists (ACOG) recommends that pregnant women be seen for an extensive initial visit in early pregnancy and then every 4 weeks until 28 weeks, every 2–3 weeks to 36 weeks, and then weekly until delivery. This may be too many visits for healthy women. For low-risk pregnancies, a national panel has suggested seven visits for parous women (6–8, 14–16, 24–28, 32, 36, 39, and 41 weeks) and nine for nulliparas (additional visits at 10–12 and 40 weeks). One clinical trial comparing these two approaches in initially low-risk patients (9 vs. 14 visits) showed similar, good outcomes. For high-risk patients, the schedule should be individualized and will usually require more visits.

4. How should prenatal care be recorded?

Good record keeping is important during pregnancy, and various forms are available. Whatever form is chosen should: (1) compel the obtaining of information, examinations, and diagnostic tests at appropriate times; (2) allow easy recognition of significant risk factors and problems; and (3) detail management plans. It is important to document all recognized problems *legibly* both for ease of giving care at future encounters and for medical-legal reasons. During the later months of pregnancy, a copy of the prenatal record should be sent to the obstetrical unit of the anticipated delivery hospital.

5. What historical information should be recorded at the initial visit?

Medical—Many chronic medical conditions have an effect, often adverse, on pregnancy outcome; conversely, pregnancy usually has a distinct effect on the course of the condition itself.

Surgical—In particular, note any prior surgical or anesthetic complications and need for transfusion.

Obstetric/gynecologic—Some events in the patient's obstetric history often recur in subsequent pregnancies (e.g., fetal and neonatal deaths, low-birth-weight infants, preterm deliveries, intrauterine growth restriction, fetal macrosomia [over 4000 g at birth], birth defects, abruptio placentae, preeclampsia or hypertension, and postpartum hemorrhage). A history of recent infertility treatment, pelvic inflammatory disease, or ectopic pregnancy is also important for identifying early pregnancy complications such as tubal pregnancy or multiple gestations. A history of past sexually transmitted diseases should also be taken.

Family history—Delving into inherited disease is important because, with time, progressively more of these conditions are becoming amenable to prenatal diagnosis. The history should focus on family members and relatives with cerebral palsy, mental retardation, neural tube defects, and other congenital malformations, as well as specific conditions such as cystic fibrosis, muscular dystrophy, and hemophilia.

Social—Psychosocial background and lifestyle are also important, as they frequently affect pregnancy and neonatal outcome. Ask questions about smoking, use of alcohol and illicit drugs, use of prescription and over-the-counter medications, employment and type of occupation, and the existence of problems at home such as domestic violence.

6. What history should be obtained at revisits?

A brief interval history should be obtained for all patients at each revisit to uncover any new problems as well as to provide follow-up on existing ones. Every patient should be asked about pain, contractions or cramping, pelvic pressure, bleeding, discharge, dysuria, gastrointestinal problems, presence and adequacy of fetal movements, and whether any new or other problems have arisen since the last visit. Smokers should be asked each time about number of cigarettes per day and progress in smoking cessation. Patients with medical conditions or known complications should be asked specific questions regarding those problems. Women desiring sterilization should be counseled well ahead of delivery

7. Describe the findings that should be noted at the initial visit.

Perform a **general physical examination** on all prenatal patients at the first visit. This exam may be the only one over a several-year period for many women, and thus it is important for health maintenance. Recording blood pressure and weight, listening to the heart and lungs, and palpating the breasts and abdomen are the principal components.

Examination of the pregnant uterus is vital. The fundal height is measured in centimeters from the symphysis pubis to the top of the uterus. Serial measurements over the course of pregnancy provide an excellent assessment of fetal growth with a rough approximation between centimeters and weeks gestation from 18–34 weeks in a patient with a normal body habitus. Fetal heart tones should be auscultated, and fetal position and estimated weight determined during the last trimester. Lastly, uterine contractions can be easily palpated during a routine exam and, if frequent and many weeks before term, may point to the possibility of preterm labor.

A routine pelvic examination can detect abnormalities of the vulva, vagina, cervix, uterus, and adnexa. It is important to estimate the size of the early gravid uterus in weeks and to assess the cervix for length. A Pap smear is taken, and cultures for sexually transmitted infections and wet preparations for any vaginal discharge can be done. Finally, clinical pelvimetry should be carried out to determine pelvic adequacy in first pregnancies and for multiparas who have experienced a previous abnormal labor or difficult delivery.

8. What are Leopold's maneuvers?

In the third trimester the uterus should be examined in four steps for fetal lie, presenting part, and position: (1) What fetal part lies in the fundus? (2) On which side is the fetal back? (3) What fetal pole is headed toward the pelvis, and is it engaged? (4) How far has the fetal presenting part descended into the pelvis?

9. What is important in the physical exam on revisits?

At each revisit, record the patient's weight and blood pressure. Then examine the gravid uterus, measure fundal height, determine fetal position by Leopold's maneuvers (last trimester), estimate fetal weight, and auscultate fetal heart tones.

The importance of this exam is illustrated by the following examples: (1) Failure of the fundal height growth may indicate intrauterine growth restriction and require extra fetal surveillance until delivery. (2) Recognition of a breech presentation at 36 weeks may require external version to vertex if spontaneous version does not occur by 37–38 weeks (successful external version can often prevent a cesarean section at term). (3) Fetal weight is estimated to identify small-for-date and large-for-date babies.

Other examinations, including vaginal, are done as indicated by the patient's interval history of problems.

10. How is gestational age determined?

An accurate last menstrual period (LMP) should be recorded at the first prenatal visit, along with the woman's normal menstrual cycle length and recent use of oral contraceptives. Careful determination of the EDC is needed so that therapeutic decisions at each stage of pregnancy are appropriately made. The EDC is initially calculated on the basis of the first day of the LMP: subtract 3 months and add 1 year and 7 days. This assumes that a term gestation is 280 days or 40 weeks from the start of the last period, and that menstruation is regular, occurring once every 28 days. Frequently, however, variations in the cycle and the timing of ovulation, use of oral contraception in the month preceding the LMP, and the appearance of menstrual-like bleeding during early pregnancy render the EDC inaccurate.

Other parameters that confirm or indicate a different EDC are:
• Date of a positive urine (about 4–5 weeks after the LMP) or serum (8th–10th postconceptional day) pregnancy test
• Uterine size during the first half of pregnancy
• Time of quickening (16–20 weeks)
• Time that fetal heart tones are first heard with electronic Doppler equipment (10–12 weeks) and nonelectronic fetoscope (18–20 weeks)
• Ultrasound—using the crown-rump length in the first trimester (error of 7 days) and the biparietal diameter, femur length, head and abdominal circumferences, and other measurements later on (error of 10–14 days up to about 22 weeks). Ultrasonic estimates of gestational age are much less accurate in the third trimester.

11. Why are the patient's weight before pregnancy and her weight gain during pregnancy important?

Women with a weight before pregnancy of < 110 lbs (50 kg) are at increased risk for preterm delivery. Additionally, many past reports have shown an association of pre-pregnant weight and/or pregnancy weight gain, with birth weight. There is a high risk for a low-birth-weight infant among underweight women who gain poorly, and for a macrosomic baby in overweight patients or those gaining excessively. This is in contrast to women with a normal habitus and weight gain who have, as a group, the most optimal pregnancy outcomes. (See table.)

Recommended Weight Gain During Pregnancy

PREPREGNANT WEIGHT	BMI (Kg/M^2)	WEIGHT GAIN (LBS)
Underweight	< 19.8	28–40
Normal weight	19.8–26.0	25–35
Overweight	26.0–29.0	15–25
Obese	> 29.0	15

BMI = body mass index; includes both weight and height
From the Food and Nutrition Board, Institute of Medicine, National Academy of Sciences, Washington DC, 1990

12. Describe the management of weight gain or loss in the pregnant patient.

At the initial visit, ascertain the pre-pregnant weight (as much as it is possible to do so), and record the patient's height and current weight. Nutritional assessment and guidelines should be discussed with each woman. Record the weight at each revisit, and evaluate over time for adequacy. This may best be done graphically. Those gaining poorly or excessively, as pregnancy progresses, need further investigation. Some with poor weight gain have nausea and vomiting, or esophageal reflux, which often responds to medical therapy. Others have poor eating habits or they smoke.

Gaining excessively often points to lack of physical activity or an increased consumption of high-caloric foods. It is important that initially overweight patients be allowed some weight gain (as described in the previous table) and that no attempt be made at weight reduction until postpartum. A sudden spurt of weight gain (> 2 lbs/week or 6 lbs/month) suggests fluid retention and should alert the caregiver to preeclampsia. The majority of patients lose almost all of their weight gain by 6 months postpartum. However, there are some who gain excessively and retain some of this weight, potentially contributing to a life-long excess weight problem.

13. Which laboratory tests should be ordered at the initial visit?

The number of laboratory determinations considered routine has increased with time. Certain routine tests should be done in all cases (see table). Additional tests at the initial prenatal visit are done for certain at-risk women only.

Prenatal Laboratory Tests

Routine	**In At-Risk Populations**
A. *Initial Visit*:	Gonorrhea culture
Hematocrit or hemoglobin	Chlamydia PDR
Urinalysis/dipstick, screen	Wet prep
for bacteriuria	Tuberculin skin test
Blood type and Rh	Sickledex
Antibody screen	Glucose screen
Serologic test for syphilis	
Rubella hemaglutination-	
inhibition titer	
Hepatitis B surface antigen	
HIV antibody (with consent)	
Pap smear	
B. *Later in Pregnancy*:	
Triple marker test (15–20 weeks)	
Glucose screen (24–28 weeks)	
Group B strep culture (35 weeks)	
Hematocrit (28, 36 weeks)	
Urine dipstick (each visit)	
Antibody screening test (Rh neg. patients at 28 weeks)	

Sickledex: see Questions 24 and 25

14. How are hematocrit determinations useful during pregnancy?

An adequate red blood cell (RBC) volume is of importance, especially after delivery that is associated with moderate (500–1000 cc) blood loss. Patients who are anemic need to be identified well ahead of delivery so that therapy can improve the hematocrit. Most anemia in pregnancy is due to iron deficiency, as it is often difficult to provide adequate iron in the diet to meet pregnancy requirements. Of equal importance is to identify those with unusually high hematocrits (over 40%), who are apt to have an inadequate plasma volume expansion and thus may be at risk for preeclampsia and other conditions.

15. How can urinalysis be best used?

All patients should have a complete urinalysis, including microscopic testing, and some means of screening for infection on the first visit. Testing for nitrites and leukocyte esterase, usually included in most urinalysis dipsticks, is a cost-effective way of screening for bacteriuria. A urine culture need be done only on positive screens to determine the organism and its antibiotic sensitivities. Detection of the approximately 5% of patients with asymptomatic bacteriuria can prevent progression to pyelonephritis.

16. What is the importance of the blood type and antibody screening test?

Rh-negative women must be identified so that they can be given Rh immune globulin (RhoGAM) at 28–30 weeks and within 72 hours of delivery in order to prevent Rh sensitization. The antibody screening test is done to detect antibodies, both Rh and other less common types (e.g., lesser Rh, Kell, Duffy, Lewis), some of which have the potential of causing hemolytic disease in the fetus and newborn infant.

17. Is serologic testing for syphilis (STS or rapid plasmin reagin) still important?

Both primary-secondary and congenital syphilis have substantially declined in the U.S. since 1990. However, the infection continues to be a problem in large urban areas, especially in the South, and among ethnic minorities. Women who test positive on the serologic test for syphilis (STS) should be given a fluorescent treponemal antibody (FTA) test; if the FTA is also positive, syphilis is diagnosed. If there is no history, or the treatment inadequate or unknown, the patient must be assumed to have syphilis and be treated with penicillin. The status of past treatment given anywhere in the U.S. can usually be ascertained by contacting the state health department's division of disease control. Follow-up of both mother and baby with serial Venereal Disease Research Laboratory titers is mandatory.

18. What is the purpose of the rubella hemagglutination-inhibition titer?

Congenital rubella syndrome is now rare because of vaccination of susceptible individuals, especially children, over the last 25 years. However, substantial numbers of adults (10–15%) continue to show susceptibility by serology. Therefore, to keep this highly contagious infection under control, continued surveillance and vaccination of susceptible individuals are indicated. Mothers who are seronegative should be immunized postpartum. In addition, the test is helpful for advising and for following-up a patient exposed to someone with a rash or mild febrile illness suggestive of rubella.

19. Why test for hepatitis B?

Mothers who are chronic carriers for the hepatitis B virus transmit this infection to a substantial proportion of their infants during or after birth. Many of these babies also become carriers and can develop various forms of chronic hepatitis; approximately 25% of those affected eventually die from cirrhosis or hepatocellular carcinoma. The Centers for Disease Control therefore recommends that all gravidas be screened for the hepatitis B surface antigen and that all newborn infants receive vaccination against hepatitis B. Infants delivered of antigen-positive mothers should be given hepatitis B immune globulin as well as the vaccine, both within the first 12 hours of life.

20. Are Pap smears interpreted any differently in pregnant women?

No. A Pap smear should be taken if one has not been done in the previous 6–12 months. Abnormal smears should be managed and followed as for nonpregnant women. Women with smears suggestive of inflammation or infection should be evaluated and treated for specific vaginal or cervical infection. Many low-grade (LSIL including ASCUS and CIN I) and all high-grade squamous intraepithelial lesions (HSIL including CIN II-III and CIS), as well as smears positive for carcinoma, require colposcopy and biopsy for further diagnosis. Endocervical curettage, which is usually a component of colposcopy for Pap smear abnormalities, is generally not performed during pregnancy. Treatment, except in cases of invasive cervical cancer, is usually postponed until after delivery.

21. Of what benefit are other tests for sexually transmitted disease?

A cervical culture for gonorrhea and test for chlamydia, usually polymerase chain reaction (PCR), should be obtained in at-risk patients, i.e., those under age 25, unmarried, or with multiple sexual partners. Many authorities recommend both as routine tests for all pregnant women; some also urge that the tests be repeated at 36 weeks' gestation.

In earlier times, gonorrheal transmission at birth caused eventual blindness in many newborn infants (gonococcal ophthalmia neonatorum). State laws mandate the use of eye prophylaxis in the infant at the time of birth, usually with an antibiotic. In addition, the gonococcus can cause chorioamnionitis after preterm rupture of membranes (PROM), resulting in a high rate of prematurity and infant morbidity. Pregnant women with a positive culture and their partners should be treated with ceftriaxone. Once treated, cervical cultures should be obtained for test of cure and repeated at 36 weeks' gestation.

Neonatal chlamydial infection occurs in 60–70% of babies passing though an infected birth canal. Conjunctivitis develops in 25–50% and chronic pneumonia in 10–20% of exposed infants. Whether this infection adversely affects the pregnancy in utero is controversial. Women who are positive should be treated with azithromycin or erythromycin (doxycycline or azithromycin for partners) and retested at 36 weeks' gestation. Because there is a high percentage of coinfections involving both gonorrhea and chlamydia, patients positive for gonorrhea should be treated for chlamydial infection as well.

22. Should prenatal patients have a wet prep of vaginal secretions at the initial visit?

Some forms of lower genital tract infections (e.g., bacterial vaginosis) are associated with spontaneous preterm birth. Because these lower tract infections are often asymptomatic, it may be helpful to screen and treat these infections to help reduce the incidence of preterm birth in high-risk populations.

23. Should pregnant women be screened for tuberculosis?

The incidence of tuberculosis nationwide has declined since 1992. However, this infection remains a problem for women born in foreign countries with high infection rates. Thus, a tuberculin skin test (purified protein derivative [PPD]) is a good idea for women who have immigrated from Asia, Africa, or Latin America, where the infection is not under good control. The same applies to some inner-city areas of this country. The newborn infant is especially susceptible to tuberculosis. Thus, women who are PPD-positive should be investigated for active disease, including a chest x-ray, and, if tuberculosis is found, treated with isoniazid (INH) and other appropriate therapy during pregnancy. If there is no evidence of active disease, the PPD positive mother is usually treated with INH after delivery.

24. Describe the Sickledex test.

This test is done to detect hemoglobin S, the predominant hemoglobin responsible for sickling of red blood cells in patients with sickle cell, sickle cell–hemoglobin C disease, sickle cell–thalassemia, and others. Because of different solubilities, blood containing hemoglobin S added to the Sickledex solution results in turbidity and red-cell lysis; this does not occur with hemoglobin A. Sickledex-positive patients should have a hemoglobin electrophoresis to identify the specific hemoglobinopathy.

25. Why perform a Sickledex in pregnant black women?

Women with sickle cell trait, which is seen in 8.5% of blacks, are well, have normal hematocrit levels, and do not have a chronic disabling condition, as do those with full-blown sickle cell anemia. However, under certain circumstances (e.g., physical stress, shock, dehydration, hypoxia) sickling can occur and result in thrombosis. Such women are also prone to urinary tract infections, believed to be due to minor degrees of sickling in small renal vessels, leading to infarction of surrounding renal parenchyma. If the partner also has the sickle trait, the risk of sickle cell anemia in the offspring is 25%. Prental diagnosis of the fetus is now possible.

26. Should pregnant women be screened for acquired immunodeficiency syndrome (AIDS)?

Yes! Perhaps the greatest progress toward the control of HIV infection has been the substantial reduction of viral transmission to the newborn infant in recent years. During this time, many new effective antiretroviral drugs have been developed which have contributed to the improved outlook. The ACOG and the American Academy of Pediatrics have now recommended offering HIV screening to all prenatal patients. Positive results from the initial ELISA test should be confirmed by Western blot analysis. Diagnosed women should then be assessed for viral load (PCR) and be counseled about the spread of HIV infection and how transmission can be prevented.

Most patients are offered treatment during pregnancy with a combination of drugs coupled with intravenous AZT during labor and oral medication to the newborn. More recently, elective cesarean section has been recommended to further reduce transmission in some cases. Altogether, these recent, more aggressive forms of therapy should result in further lowering of perinatal HIV transmission.

27. Should screening for group B streptococcus (GBS) be done during pregnancy?

GBS infection is a cause of neonatal sepsis and carries a high neonatal mortality and morbidity, especially in premature neonates. Although GBS is frequently cultured in mothers (5–30%), actual newborn sepsis occurs in only 0.1–0.5% of all births. Eradicating the organism with an antibiotic, usually penicillin or ampicillin, at the time of delivery is the best means of preventing early-onset neonatal GBS sepsis. Although this approach is costly and encourages the development of antibiotic resistance, treatment is less effective once bacteremia is established. A recent report has demonstrated a 65% reduction in early-onset GBS neonatal infection from 1993 to 1998 by this intrapartum therapy.

The Centers for Disease Control currently recommends one of two approaches to prevent early-onset GBS infection: (1) routine screening of all mothers for GBS at 35–37 weeks and treating positives in labor; or (2) giving intrapartum treatment for patients with known risk factors for neonatal GBS sepsis (e.g., < 37 weeks' gestation, ruptured membranes > 18 hours, or maternal fever in labor). In addition, intrapartum prophylaxis should be given to all patients with GBS bacteriuria or a history of a previous infant with GBS disease. For some situations (e.g., preterm PROM) there is often time before labor to make a definite diagnosis by taking a GBS culture on admission. Rapid tests for GBS, although available, are not very sensitive to light colonization.

28. Discuss the ramifications of gestational diabetes.

Pregnancy poses a diabetogenic stress, and about 4% of gravidas develop gestational diabetes. The primary perinatal effect of this is an increased risk of fetal macrosomia (> 4000 g birth weight). Long-term, however, roughly 30–50% of these women will become diabetic, usually type 2, later in life. Moreover, the offspring of these women are at increased risk for obesity and abnormal glucose tolerance. Many patients with hyperglycemia early in pregnancy may in reality have pre-existing diabetes.

29. Who should be screened for diabetes?

A glucose screen (a 1-hour blood sugar following 50 g of oral glucose load) should be done on most gravidas at 24–28 weeks' gestation. A glucose screen should also be done at the initial visit for patients at very high risk for gestational diabetes (e.g., morbid obesity, strong family history to type 2 diabetes, prior macrosomic infant or fetal death). Patients at low risk for gestational diabetes (see table) and those with no risk factors probably do not require testing. The American Diabetes Association has recommended 140-mg/dl plasma glucose as the upper limit of normal following a 50-g glucose load. Levels above this ultimately identify about 80% of women with gestational diabetes.

Many now recommend a lower threshold of 130 mg/dl, which will increase the sensitivity to about 90%. However, this results in a much larger group of women needing additional testing (20–25% of the population).

Patients with abnormal values should have a 3-hour oral glucose tolerance test with a 100-g glucose load; threshold values for a positive test currently recommended are any two values above 95 mg/dl fasting and 180, 155, and 140 for 1, 2 and 3 hours, respectively. Some advocate repeat diabetes screening at 32 weeks in high-risk women whose initial screen is negative.

Risk Factors for Gestational Diabetes

HIGH RISK (Any One)	LOW RISK (All Must Be Present)
Previous macrosomic infant	< Age 25
Previous stillbirth	No prior poor obstetric outcomes
Previous gestational diabetes	associated w/gestational diabetes
Strong family history of diabetes	Negative family history
Maternal obesity	Normal body habitus
Glucosuria	Ethnic background with low prevalence
Ethnic groups Hispanic,	
African-American, Native American,	
East and Southeast Asian	
Pacific Islanders	

30. What is the purpose of the triple marker-screening test?

This test should be offered to all pregnant women between 15 and 21 weeks' gestation. It identifies pregnancies at risk for certain fetal anomalies and chromosomal abnormalities. The test involves three components: maternal serum levels of alpha-fetoprotein (MSAFP), human chorionic gonadotropin, and estriol. It gives results in terms of an MSAFP level, and, using the levels of the three components together with other factors (age, weight, ethnic group, and diabetic status), it gives a risk for Down syndrome (and trisomy 18). Elevated MSAFP values (> 2.5 muliples of median) are seen with some congenital malformations (neural tube defects, abdominal wall defects, esophageal-duodenal atresia, some renal and urinary tract abnormalities, chromosomal abnormalities [Turner's syndrome]) and various less-specific poor pregnancy outcomes (fetal death, low-birth-weight infants, fetal-maternal hemorrhage). MSAFP screening detects about 85% of open neural tube defects. Use of amniocentesis or chorionic villus sampling for fetal karyotype in women 35 years or older at delivery and in those with a Down's risk of 1:270 or higher identifies 60–65% of fetuses with Down syndrome.

Patients who have a positive triple screen test should undergo further counseling and be offered testing for the identification of specific disorders. Additional markers currently under investigation, both in serum and on ultrasound, will no doubt improve the sensitivity of identifying fetuses with Down syndrome and other structural and chromosomal abnormalities.

31. Should a routine prenatal ultrasound scan be done?

Performing an ultrasound scan of the fetus as a routine part of prenatal care is controversial. Using rules of evidence-based medicine, The ACOG reviewed a number of investigations comparing patients who underwent routine ultrasound vs. those who were scanned only on indication. They found that: (1) the ability to identify specific fetal anomalies by routine scan has wide, often relatively low, sensitivity (17–74%), probably related to the skills of various ultrasonographers, but a very high specificity (> 99%); and (2) in low-risk populations, routine scans did not result in better pregnancy outcomes, either regarding mortality or certain forms of morbidity.

On the other hand, in prenatal populations who have higher overall risk and/or who usually enroll in prenatal care during late mid-pregnancy or later, after many gestational milestones have passed, routine screening may be valid for dating alone. In addition, although uncommon, serious congenital abnormalities can be identified early, allowing the option of pregnancy termination for some and time for future planning for others. Whether these advantages of universal ultrasonography have significant cost savings has not yet been determined.

32. Which laboratory tests are repeated during the prenatal course?

- The **hematocrit** is repeated in the third trimester, or more frequently in at-risk women, to identify women with anemia ($\leq$ 32%) or hemoconcentration (40% +).
- **Urine dipstick** is done on each revisit. Presence of significant proteinuria mandates investigation for preeclampsia, urinary tract infection, and renal disease. Glucosuria can point to gestational diabetes, although it may reflect normal decreased renal glucose absorbance during pregnancy. Presence of nitrites and/or leukocyte esterase mandates searching for urinary or genital tract infection.
- **Antibody screening test** is repeated at 28 weeks' gestation in Rh-negative women and, if negative, Rh immune globulin (RhoGAM) should be given.
- **Sexually transmitted disease testing**—including serologic test for syphilis (STS), gonorrhea culture, and chlamydia PCR—is repeated at 28 or 36 weeks' gestation in many offices caring for indigent women, in whom the prevalence of these infections is relatively high.
- **Glucose screen** is often repeated at 32 weeks' gestation in women with risk factors for diabetes but normal values at weeks 24–28.

33. How is a patient determined to be high risk?

At the conclusion of the initial prenatal exam, the patient should be evaluated for overall risk. Scoring systems for risk assessment have evolved in recent years and are available in the literature. Significant problems should be listed in a prominent part of the prenatal record, and a plan for management and follow-up should be proposed. Such high-risk charts should be easily identifiable by outpatient care providers and labor-delivery personnel. On each revisit, reassess risk; review old problems; remove resolved problems from the chart; and add any new problems to the patient's record.

34. Are there any routine medications that should be prescribed during pregnancy?

Most authorities recommend supplemental iron, as it is often difficult to meet iron requirements of pregnancy by diet alone, and in these cases iron-deficiency anemia can occur. Otherwise, there are no "routine" medications for a pregnant woman. Prenatal vitamins, most of which contain 40–65 mg elemental iron and 0.4–1.0 mg folic acid, are probably not necessary if the patient is eating a nutritious diet. For iron supplementation, patients can take these vitamins or, if enrolling initially in care late, they should be given a standard form of oral iron (ferrous sulfate, gluconate, or fumarate) two or three times a day.

35. How prevalent is domestic violence in the U.S.?

Domestic violence is a major public health problem in the U.S. It is estimated to involve 5 million women annually and pervades all socioeconomic strata. Furthermore, it is the most common cause of trauma to women, accounting for about one-third of all visits by women to an emergency room. Most importantly, spousal abuse is responsible for about one-third of homicides in women ages 15–45. Several reports have found that an average of 4–8% (up to 22% in some reports) of pregnant women are battered by their spouses or partners. As a group, victims of domestic violence are at high risk for poor pregnancy outcomes and are likely to commence prenatal care late in pregnancy. Although common, much domestic violence goes unrecognized by health professionals, and finding solutions for each family is difficult.

36. How do you identify a victim of domestic violence?

Identification of a battered woman is important because her life and the lives of her children are in danger. History-taking at the initial prenatal visit should include inquiry into the existence and extent of domestic violence. When trauma is present, and is not related to obvious other causes, such questioning is critical. In less acute circumstances, initial clues may involve various, often vague somatic symptoms such as headache, insomnia, hyperventilation, choking sensation, gastrointestinal symptoms, and pain in the chest, pelvis, or back.

A quick, effective way to screen for domestic violence is to ask the following three questions: (1) Have you been hit, kicked, punched, or otherwise hurt by someone within the past year? If so, by whom? (2) Do you feel safe in your current relationship? (3) Is there a partner from a previous relationship who is making you feel unsafe now? These simple questions can be included on the prenatal form for use on all patients.

37. What role should the obstetrician play if he/she suspects a pregnant patient is a victim of domestic violence?

Some states require reporting of domestic violence to the authorities. Because there are distinct pros and cons of this, the ACOG has taken the stand that such mandatory reporting is not yet justified and that statutes for such should not be implemented without provisions that enable women to override or veto reporting requirements.

Most battered women need prompt help from resources that are available in many communities. Depending on the urgency of the situation, the woman should be referred to family crisis centers, shelters for battered women, the local police department, hospital emergency rooms, legal aid services, and social service departments. These resources usually have expertise in providing urgent help for the woman and her children, dealing with the male batterer, and planning for the future. In addition, if the patient cannot or does not wish to leave home, she should formulate a plan of exit from her house for when the need arises. Long-term counseling is usually necessary by a social worker, psychologist, psychiatrist, or others who are experts in the management of battered women. Any children also require help, as they have often been abused as well—at the very least, they have suffered as observers of their mother's mistreatment.

38. What advice should be given to pregnant women regarding work outside of the house?

For the most part in the U.S., regular employment at one's usual occupation during pregnancy, with certain adjustments and exceptions, does not contribute to increased perinatal morbidity. Obviously, some women with specific medical or obstetrical conditions who are at high risk for poor outcomes will need to discontinue work early for therapy and rest. In addition, bodily changes that accompany pregnancy, especially late pregnancy—weight gain, fatigue, difficulty breathing, balance problems, backache—may make it difficult for some to continue working depending on the type of job and each patient's adjustment to it. There is also accumulating evidence that standing or walking for long periods on the job is a contributing factor to adverse pregnancy outcome.

In general, low-risk pregnant women can continue working at their regular jobs so long as the job is not dangerous (physically or environmentally), overly strenuous, or cause physical or mental exhaustion. Many women want to take leave or reduce their hours as the demands of pregnancy increase in the last trimester. Job requirements often can be modified to reduce the physical workload, or the woman can be transferred to less strenuous work. Frequent breaks, elevation of legs, and changes in position are good ideas for all working gravidas.

39. How should you advise mothers regarding occupational maternal leave and insurance coverage?

The patient should find out if there are maternity benefits offered by her employer. By federal law, employers offering medical disability compensation must treat pregnancy-related disabilities in the same way as temporary disabilities (illness or injury) suffered by non-pregnant employees. Such temporary disability can be due to pregnancy per se (e.g., musculoskeletal symtpoms), complications of pregnancy, or hazardous occupational exposure during pregnancy. If the employer offers this coverage, a pregnant employee can apply for benefits if the disability is certified by her obstetrician. If employee disability coverage is not available, the patient may be eligible for state unemployment benefits, or she must use sick leave or vacation time, or take an unpaid leave of absence. Regarding the latter, a federal statute (the Family and Medical Leave Act of 1993) provides that any pregnant woman working for a government or a company of over 50 employees is allowed up to 12 weeks of non-paid maternal leave, during which time the employer must continue her benefits and seniority, and retain her job position or equivalent when she returns after delivery.

40. Describe helpful education for the pregnant patient.

Educating the pregnant woman about her pregnancy, labor-delivery, care of her infant and parenting, common complications of pregnancy, and general improvement in her health is an integral part of prenatal care. Some of this should be discussed at each visit, in a logical sequence. Information can be presented on a one-to-one basis by the physician or nurse, via small group sessions, by videotape or posters (while the patient is sitting in the waiting room), over the internet, and in books and handouts to be read at home. Note that any reading material should be written in a manner appropriate for the individual patient's education level and in her primary language; otherwise, it will provide little or no benefit. Finally, Lamaze and other childbirth preparation classes are an excellent source of information about pregnancy and labor.

41. Can pregnant women exercise during pregnancy?

Most women can continue some form of exercise during pregnancy, although special consideration should be given to women with medical or obstetric complications. In otherwise healthy women, regular exercise (three times/week) should be encouraged over intermittent exertions. Supine positions after the first trimester should be avoided (due to vena caval obstruction by the enlarging uterus). Duration and intensity of exercise should be self-monitored; encourage cessation at early signs of fatigue, rather than attainment of rigid goals based on the nonpregnant state. Exercises requiring balance should be avoided during the third trimester in particular. Encourage careful fluid-dietary supplementation and heat dissipation.

42. How can prenatal care help prevent premature birth?

Preterm delivery accounts for 8–10% of births in the U.S., a rate that has not changed for decades. Roughly two-thirds of these are spontaneous, i.e., due to preterm labor, premature rupture of membranes, abruption, and other natural events leading to spontaneous active labor and delivery. Many factors have been found that increase the risk for spontaneous preterm birth. The major ones are:
- History of previous preterm birth
- Current obstetric problems (e.g., twins, incompetent cervix, bleeding)
- Low prepregnant weight and inadequate weight gain
- Lower genital tract infections
- Adverse psychosocial factors

Recognition of these factors—and correction, when possible—can be incorporated into prenatal care. Use of recently developed predictors, such as cervical length and fetal fibronectin or salivary estriol, can also be helpful.

43. List the danger signs during pregnancy of which the patient should be made aware.

Vaginal bleeding
Abdominal or pelvic pain or cramping
Frequent uterine contractions from weeks 20–36
Leaking of fluid from vagina
Significant decrease in fetal movements
Severe headache or blurring of vision
Persistent vomiting
Chills or fever
Swelling of hands or face

44. Which common complications of pregnancy can be prevented or minimized by good prenatal care?

Anemia due to iron or folic acid deficiency
Urinary tract infections and pyelonephritis
Pregnancy-induced hypertension (preeclampsia)
Preterm labor and delivery
Intrauterine growth retardation
Sexually transmitted diseases and their effect on the newborn infant
Rh isoimmunization
Fetal macrosomia
Breech presentation at term
Hypoxia or fetal death from post-term birth

BIBLIOGRAPHY

1. Abrams B, Pickett KE: Maternal nutrition. In Creasy RK, Resnik R (eds): Maternal-Fetal Medicine: Principles and Practice, 4th ed. Philadelphia, W.B. Saunders Co. 1999, pp 122–131.
2. American College of Obstetricians and Gynecologists: Exercise During Pregnancy and the Postpartum Period. ACOG Technical Bulletin No. 189, February 1994.
3. American College of Obstetricians and Gynecologists: Routine Ultrasound in Low Risk Pregnancy. ACOG Practice Patterns No. 5, August, 1997.
4. American College of Obstetricians and Gynecologists: Pregnancy Disability. Statement of Policy, September 1999.
5. Centers for Disease Control: 1998 Guidelines for Treatment of Sexually Transmitted Diseases. MMWR 47, RR1, 1998.
6. Cunningham FG, McDonald PC, Gant NF, et al (eds): Williams Obstetrics, 20th ed. Stamford, CT, Appleton & Lange, 1997, pp 227–250.
7. Eisenstat SA, Bancroft L: Domestic violence. New Eng J Med 341:886, 1999.
8. Gibbs RS, Sweet RL: Maternal and fetal infectious disorders. In Creasy RK, Resnik R (eds): Maternal-Fetal Medicine: Principles and Practice, 4th ed. Philadelphia, W.B. Saunders, 1999, pp 659–724.
9. Kios SL, Buchanan TA: Gestational diabetes mellitus. New Eng J Med 341:1749, 1999.
10. McGregor JA, French J, Parker R, et al: Prevention of premature birth by screening and treatment for common genital tract infections: Results of a prospective controlled evaluation. Am J Obstet Gynecol 173:157, 1995.
11. Schrag SJ, Zywcki S, Farley MM, et al: Group B streptococcal disease in the era of intrapartum antibiotic prophylaxis. New Eng J Med. 342:15, 2000.

36. NUTRITION IN PREGNANCY

Kirsten Lawrence, M.D.

1. How do maternal body weight and weight gain in pregnancy affect pregnancy outcome?

The optimal amount of prenatal weight gain is modified by a woman's pre-pregnancy weight for height (body mass index [BMI]). Recommended total weight gain ranges from 28–40 pounds for underweight women (BMI < 19.8) to 15–25 pounds for an overweight woman (BMI > 26). This translates to .5 kg/week for underweight women, .4 kg/week for normal weight, and .3 kg/week for overweight women. The impact of maternal weight gain on birth weight decreases with increasing pre-pregnancy weight. The pattern of weight gain through gestation is thought to be critical, in that maternal gain in the second trimester is most important for **fetal growth**, and is protective of fetal growth even if overall weight gain is poor.

Underweight women and women with low pregnancy weight gains are at higher risk for delivery of an infant weighing < 2500 grams, and the highest risk is for women with both risk factors. There is also a statistically significant relationship between low rate of maternal weight gain and **preterm delivery**.

Overweight women and women with high pregnancy weight gain are at increased risk for **macrosomia**, which has been variably defined as birthweight > 4000 grams, > 4500 grams, or > 90% for gestational age. Macrosomia is a risk factor for shoulder dystocia resulting in brachial plexus injury, as well as for cesarean section. Pre-pregnancy obesity is also associated with **hypertension** and **diabetes** in pregnancy, as well as postoperative wound infection in the case of cesarean delivery.

2. What is the average maternal weight gain?

The average weight gain at term is 28 pounds, which is attributable to fetal weight, placental weight, amniotic fluid, breast enlargement, increased volume expansion, and appropriate fat stores.

3. Describe the optimal diet in pregnancy.

Because energy requirements in pregnancy are increased by approximately 17% over the nonpregnant state, a woman of normal weight should consume an additional 300 kcal/day, and these calories should be concentrated in foods of high nutrient density, a value based on the percent protein, vitamins, and minerals per 100 kcalories. Generally, thin and undernourished women require higher energy intakes than other women.

Protein should comprise 20% of a normal pregnancy diet. The recommended daily allowance for a pregnant woman is 60 grams. As many animal protein sources are high in fat, these should be used sparingly so as to avoid excessive weight gain. Fat should comprise 30% of diet in pregnancy, and carbohydrates the remaining 50%.

A sample diet in pregnancy based on the food pyramid should include 6–11 servings of grains, 3–5 servings of vegetables, 2–4 servings of fruit, 3–5 servings of dairy, 2–3 servings of meats, beans, or nuts, and one serving of sweets. Total caloric intake will vary based on BMI, but the average recommendation is 2500 kcal/day.

4. Should the diet differ for multiple gestations?

Yes. Although the exact caloric requirement for multiple gestations has not been well described, it is thought to be significantly increased from singleton pregnancies, and recommendations of an additional 300 kcal and 10 grams of protein per fetus beyond singleton are standard.

5. How important is periconceptional nutrition?

It is well established that periconceptional supplementation with **folic acid** can reduce the incidence of neural tube defects by 50%, and this finding is the basis for the CDC's recommendation that women of childbearing age who have a chance of becoming pregnant consume 0.4 mg of folate/day. Women with a history of pregnancy complicated by a neural tube defect should consume 4 mg of folate/day from 1 month preconception until the end of the first trimester.

Women with **diabetes** should be counseled preconceptionally. The fourfold increase in the incidence of major congenital malformations in the offspring of women with pregestational diabetes has been related to poor control of diabetes during embryogenesis.

Women with **phenylketonuria** have an increased risk of fetal malformations, including cardiac defects and microcephaly. These risks can be significantly reduced if a phenylalanine-restricted diet is implemented 3 months before conception. The incidence of low birth weight (LBW) associated with maternal phenylketonuria is reduced if phenylalanine levels are normalized by 8 weeks of gestation.

6. Are vitamin and mineral supplements necessary during pregnancy?

The overall quality of a woman's diet affects her need for supplementation. If all the necessary nutrients can be consumed in the daily diet, then the answer is no. However, women with special needs should be addressed separately. Various categories of special need for vitamin and mineral supplementation include:

- **Dilantin therapy**. Animal studies have shown more favorable fetal outcomes when folate, vitamins, and amino acids are supplemented. Favorable outcomes include greater fetal weight and length, decreased subcutaneous bleeding, more ossification centers, and fewer malformations.
- **Increased risk of lead exposure**. Women working in manufacturing plants, recent immigrants from countries where lead-free gasoline is not mandated, and residents of old buildings undergoing renovations may benefit from supplementation with vitamins C and E. These antioxidant vitamins may play a role in the reduction of potentially adverse effects of lead during pregnancy, including protection of the fetus against lead toxicity and/or free radical change.
- **Multiple gestations**. Although the exact amount is not known, supplemental folate is recommended, given the increased red blood cell production.
- **HIV infection**. Supplemental selenium has been shown to inhibit reverse transcriptase activity in RNA of virus-infected animals. Selenium with antioxidant vitamins has been speculated as a measure to reduce the probability of placental transmission of HIV.
- **Alcohol consumption**. Moderate-to-high alcohol intake may deplete many nutrients, notably B complex, that should be repleted.
- **Hemoglobinopathies** may benefit from supplemental folate, given the increased red blood cell turnover.
- **Hypertension** may benefit from calcium supplementation.

7. What problems are associated with megadose vitamin and mineral therapy?

Large intakes of fat-soluble vitamins such as vitamin A and D have been shown to cause birth defects in both humans and animals. Megadoses of selenium have a similar risk. Large doses of zinc suppress the immune system. Large amounts of fluoride during pregnancy have been associated with mottled teeth. Dolomite from harvested clam shells is often used for calcium supplementation. At one point, dolomite was found to contain heavy minerals such as lead after shell contamination with industrial wastes. Many small manufacturers of vitamin and mineral supplements may not use the same quality control standards as large firms.

There are also issues of nutrient displacement. For example, excessive vitamin C appears to interfere with copper metabolism. Additionally, zinc competes with iron for absorption, and iron deficiency anemia may result.

8. True or false: All herbal remedies are safe in pregnancy.

False. Health food stores frequently advocate various herbal remedies and supplements for complaints ranging from headache to heartburn. Some of these may be dangerous during pregnancy.

Remedies marketed as calmatives or nervines may contain large amounts of alkaloids, shown to cause hepatic damage. Mate, a tea-like infusion commonly found in health food stores, has been reported to increase the risk of digestive tract cancers. An herbal tea, pleurisy root, has been shown to have digoxin-like factors. "Pregnancy tea," containing chamomile, mint, and raspberry leaves, appears to be safe when consumed in moderation.

9. What are the guidelines for fluid requirements during pregnancy?

Pregnancy is associated with increased fluid requirements. An average of 9 L of fluid gained during gestation translates into 30 ml/day requirement above the nonpregnant state. The calculation of maintenance fluids based on body weight—100 ml/kg for first 10 kg, 50 ml/kg for next 10 kg, and 25 ml/kg above 20 kg—provides a baseline assessment of fluid needs, although it overestimates the requirement in obese patients and underestimates it in underweight patients.

Maternal fluid status may affect the regulation of amniotic fluid volume, and there is data to demonstrate that acute changes in maternal osmolality alter fetal hydration.

10. Do all pregnant women need additional iron?

No. Women who eat carefully planned daily diets with maximal dietary iron probably do not need supplemental iron. However, numerous dietary surveys indicate that iron intake is suboptimal in a high percentage of the population. The heart-healthy move to less red meat has much to do with this change. Absorption of iron from heme sources is 10%; from non-heme sources it is approximately 2%. Thus large portions of non-heme foods are required to compensate. Iron-deficient persons, however, generally absorb twice as much iron from a meal as those without iron deficiency. Additionally, in a small study, iron absorption was observed to increase with gestational age: 7% at week 12, 36% at week 24, and 66% by week 36.

11. List the sorts of foods that should be encouraged, to increase iron in the diet.

High sources: oysters; lean red meats, especially liver; in vegetarian diets, tofu, legumes, and beans when consumed with an acidic beverage such as orange, grapefruit, or tomato juice.

Moderate sources: enriched grain products and cereals

Low sources: light and white meats, including chicken, salmon, and pork; dairy products

Iron, whether dietary or supplemented, should not be consumed within 1 hour of calcium intake. An insoluble complex can result in reduced iron absorption. Antacids taken for heartburn can also interfere with iron absorption. Tea and coffee can cut absorption of non-heme iron by more than half compared with water.

12. What special considerations apply to women with unusual diets due either to cultural diversity or food fads?

Most obstetric practices are multicultural, which makes it difficult to assess dietary adequacy without a trained perinatal nutritionist. In addition to the various ethnic foods that may make up a daily diet, some cultures have pregnancy taboos that alter nutritional intake. One example is the prohibition in some cultures against consumption of eggs by pregnant women. Asian women may have diets based on raw fish, which can reduce thiamine status because raw fish contains thiaminases. Raw fish also presents danger from parasites and is a potential source of food poisoning. In Bangladesh and other Asian countries, the chewing of betel nuts is a common practice.

13. What are the nutritional concerns for the pregnant vegetarian?

The specific restrictions of vegetarian diets should be explored. Ovolactovegetarians consuming milk products, eggs, fish, and poultry generally meet the suggested guidelines without further supplementation. More restrictive diets (lactovegetarian—no fish, eggs, or poultry; vegan—plants only) should prompt consideration of vitamin B complex, which includes B12, calcium, and additional iron supplementation. Highly restrictive diets (only fruits, Zen macrobiotic diets) are best avoided during pregnancy.

14. What are the nutritional concerns with adolescent pregnancy?

Girls under the age of 17 are at increased risk for preterm delivery, perinatal mortality, and LBW—outcomes correlated with sociocultural stress. In terms of nutrition, girls within 2 years of menarche are at highest risk for LBW, presumably because their own body growth demands compete with those of the fetus. These patients may require additional energy, protein, and calcium to meet their nutritional needs for maternal *and* fetal growth. Poor nutrition, with unbalanced diets, erratic use of vitamin supplements, preoccupation with body image and associated dieting, as well as the use of drugs and alcohol are important factors which contribute to poor weight gain and LBW.

15. What is pica?

Pica is the craving and eating of nonfoods, such as cornstarch, clay, and ice cubes. Risk factors for this behavior include family history of pica, rural residence, and African American race. The etiology is unknown, although iron deficiency anemia, cultural beliefs, and limited access to nutrition are thought to be possible etiologies. Dangers of this practice include the risk of ingestion of toxic substances and an increased risk of iron deficiency anemia due to the binding of dietary iron by nonfoods. Appropriate management is based on the detection of pica, and counseling as to its detrimental effects in pregnancy.

16. What role does a perinatal nutritionist play?

Perinatal nutritionists, a subgroup of the American Dietetic Association (ADA), specialize in the science of food and nutrition, from source to processing, digestion, and metabolism. In addition to assessing nutritional contribution, they are qualified to advise the obstetric client in various situations of nutritional risk. To obtain a list of perinatal nutritionists in a given area, call the ADA at 1-800-877-1600.

BIBLIOGRAPHY

1. Allen LH: Iron-deficiency anemia increases the risk of preterm delivery. Nutr Rev 51:49–52, 1993.
2. American College of Obstetricians and Gynecologists: Nutrition during pregnancy. ACOG Tech Bull 179, 1993.
3. Backton J: Ginger in preventing nausea and vomiting in pregnancy: A caveat to its thromboxane synthetase activity and effect on testosterone binding. Eur J Obstet Reprod Biol 42:163–164, 1991.
4. Barrett JF, Whittaker PQ, Williams JG, Lind T: Absorption of non-heme iron from food during normal pregnancy. BMJ 309:79–82, 1994.
5. Creasy RK, Resnik R: Maternal Fetal Medicine, 4th ed. Philadelphia, WB Saunders, 1999, pp 122–131.
6. Czeikel AE: Nutritional supplementation and prevention of congenital abnormalities. Curr Opin Obstet Gynecol 92:88–94, 1995.
7. Erick M: Vitamin B6, ginger in morning sickness. J Am Diet Assoc 95:416, 1995.
8. Franko DL, Walton BE: Pregnancy and eating disorders: A review and clinical implications. Int J Eat Disord 13:41–47, 1993.
9. Kilpatrick SJ, Safford KL: Maternal hydration and amniotic fluid index in women with normal amniotic fluid. Obstet Gynecol 81:49–52, 1993.
10. Wada L, King JC: Trace elements and nutrition in pregnancy. Clin Obstet Gynecol 37:754–786, 1994.
11. Worthington-Roberts B: Perinatal nutrition: General issues. In Worthington-Roberts B (ed): Nutrition in Pregnancy and Lactation, 6th ed. Madison, WI, Brown & Benchmark Publishers, 1997.

V. Complications of Pregnancy

37. NAUSEA AND VOMITING OF PREGNANCY

Kirsten Lawrence, M.D.

1. How common is nausea and vomiting in pregnancy (NVP)?

In multiple surveys, 60–70% of women experience symptoms of nausea and vomiting in pregnancy. In one large comprehensive study, investigators found that symptoms began between the 4th and 7th menstrual week in 70% of patients with NVP, but that 7% had symptoms prior to their first missed period. Resolution of symptoms varied: in 30% symptoms disappeared by 10 weeks; in 60% symptoms were gone by 12 weeks; and 99% of patients were symptom-free by 20 weeks gestation. Most commonly, women experienced symptoms between 6 AM and noon, but many reported nausea and vomiting throughout the day.

2. How is nausea and vomiting differentiated from hyperemesis gravidarum (HG)?

There is no universally accepted definition for HG, but most clinicians consider this diagnosis in the setting of compromised fluid, electrolyte, and nutritional status. Some use a maternal weight loss of 5% and persistent significant ketonuria to make the diagnosis. A wide range of laboratory abnormalities may be seen, but a patient with moderate to severe disease will present with hyperchloremic metabolic alkalosis. In the setting of longstanding volume depletion, acidosis will be present. Both liver function tests and pancreatic enzymes amylase and lipase may be elevated.

HG is much less common than nausea and vomiting, affecting approximately five per thousand pregnancies. Women most at risk are those with multiple gestations, obese women, and nulliparas. Women with a previous history of HG have an increased risk of recurrence in a subsequent pregnancy compared to women with no history.

3. What is the differential diagnosis of nausea and vomiting in pregnancy?

In terms of obstetric conditions, several disease states have been associated with an increased risk of NVP, including multiple gestation, gestational trophoblastic disease, and fetal aneuploidy (triploidy and trisomy 21). If a patient presents with symptoms in the third trimester, acute fatty liver of pregnancy and preeclampsia must be ruled out. Outside of direct obstetric-related complications, the differential diagnosis is broad, and other medical disorders should be considered if vomiting persists, if symptoms begin later than 9 weeks' gestation, or if symptoms acutely worsen.

Primary gastrointestinal disorders to consider are biliary tract disease, hepatitis, intestinal obstruction, peptic ulcer disease, pancreatitis, appendicitis, and gastroenteritis. Endocrine disorders include hyperthyroidism, diabetic ketoacidosis, and Addison disease. Genitourinary disorders include pyelonephritis, nephrolithiasis, ovarian torsion, and degeneration of uterine fibroids. Finally, the diagnosis of migraine headache and pseudotumor cerebri as well as primary CNS lesions may be entertained.

4. Are there fetal complications?

Both NVP and hyperemesis gravidarum have been associated with a *decreased* risk of spontaneous abortion in the first and second trimester. In terms of adverse outcome, there does not appear to be any significant risk of intrauterine growth restriction (IUGR) or stillbirth with mild to moderate symptoms. The literature on severe disease is mixed. In one study, 32% of infants born to mothers with weight loss in pregnancy had weights < 10% for gestational age at birth, compared to 6% incidence of IUGR in mothers with nausea and vomiting without weight loss. Other authors have not confirmed this risk, and the issue remains controversial. There does not, however, seem to be any increased risk of congenital anomalies with HG.

5. What are the maternal complications?

The most commonly reported serious complication associated with hyperemesis is Wernicke's encephalopathy due to thiamine deficiency, sometimes associated with central pontine myelinolysis. A classic triad of ataxia, confusion, and ocular motor signs characterizes this syndrome. Women with prolonged vomiting should receive supplemental thiamine to prevent this dangerous complication.

Other complications related to prolonged vomiting include Mallory-Weiss tear, esophageal rupture, splenic avulsion, and peripheral neuropathy secondary to vitamin B6 and B12 deficiency.

6. What is the etiology of hyperemesis?

The causes of NVP/HG remain poorly understood. The major theories of causation involve hormonal variables, abnormal gastric motility, and psychosocial stress.

Hormonal variables: Some women with hyperemesis appear to be hyperthyroid, which is associated with higher levels of circulating human chorionic gonadotropin (hCG) or higher biological activity of hCG. There has also been some association between progesterone and delayed gastric emptying. A more precise association has not been elucidated.

Gastric motility: Some studies have demonstrated decreased gastric motility by electrogastrography to be associated with higher levels of nausea, but others have shown no difference in motility between symptomatic and aymptomatic patients. There has also been discussion of central nervous system changes, especially in the "vomiting center"(including the dorsal motor nucleus of the vagus nerve) in response to hormonal triggers as the etiology.

Psychosocial stress: Theories describe three potential processes—conversion disorder/somatization, heightened perception of sensations by the mother resulting in vomiting as a conditional response, and an inability of the mother to respond to life stress. There is limited data to support any of these associations.

7. How should nausea and vomiting/hyperemesis be managed?

The mainstay of treatment is symptomatic therapy with close attention to fluid balance. Frequent small meals and avoidance of aggravating food sources are important. Ginger tea is a much touted anecdotal remedy, and powdered ginger has been proven effective when studied clinically. A randomized clinical trial of vitamin B6 versus placebo proved its efficacy in patients taking 30 mg of pyridoxine daily. Recent studies looking at acupressure bands and transcutaneous nerve stimulation have shown some efficacy.

Antiemetics are indicated for intractable symptoms despite adequate hydration: metoclopromide (Reglan), phenothiazines, and ondansetron (Zofran) are effective, and appear to be safe in pregnancy. Systemic steroids are an additional therapy of interest for patients who fail antiemetics; a randomized controlled trial of 40 patients comparing oral methylprednisolone to oral promethazine demonstrated a superior response to steroids, as no patients in the methylprednisolone group required readmission, compared to 5/17 in the promethazine group. No adverse fetal effects have been described with this treatment.

Finally, total parenteral nutrition is merited for patients who cannot sustain their weight and have persistent vomiting despite therapy.

BIBLIOGRAPHY

1. Abell T, et al: Hyperemesis gravidarum. Gastroenterol Clin North Am 21:835, 1992.
2. Creasy RK, Resnik R: Maternal Fetal Medicine, 4th ed. Philadelphia, WB Saunders, 1999, pp 122–131.

3. Gadsby R, et al: A prospective study of nausea and vomiting during pregnancy. Br J Gen Pract 43:245–248, 1993.
4. Goodwin, T Murphy: Hyperemesis gravidarum. Clin Obstet Gynecol 41:597–605, 1998.
5. Gross S, et al: Maternal weight loss associated with hyperemesis gravidarum: A predictor of fetal outcome. Am J Obstet Gynecol 160:906–909, 1989.
6. Safari, et al: The efficacy of methylprednisolone in the treatment of hyperemesis gravidarum: A randomized, double blind controlled study. Am J Obstet Gynecol 179:921–924, 1998.

38. HYPERTENSION IN PREGNANCY

Thomas J. Bader, M.D., and L. Dorine Day, M.D.

1. How is hypertension during pregnancy defined?

In a pregnant woman, a systolic blood pressure above 140 mmHg or a diastolic blood pressure above 90 mmHg is considered hypertension.

2. How are hypertensive disorders in pregnancy classified?

In 2000, the National High Blood Pressure Education Program Working Group revised the classification system for this set of conditions. Four categories are now recognized for hypertension in pregnancy: chronic hypertension, gestational hypertension, preeclampsia, and chronic hypertension with superimposed preeclampsia. The American College of Obstetricians and Gynecologists has adopted the Working Group's system.

3. What is the definition of chronic hypertension in pregnancy?

Hypertension (as defined in Question 1) that predates pregnancy or is identified before 20 weeks' gestation is classified as chronic hypertension. If a woman begins her prenatal care after 20 weeks, and if she has hypertension that persists more than 12 weeks post-partum, she is also considered to have chronic hypertension.

4. What is the definition of preeclampsia?

Preeclampsia is defined by hypertension and proteinuria. For women who do not have chronic hypertension, an elevation above 140 mmHg systolic or 90 mmHg diastolic meets the criteria. Proteinuria is defined by more than 300 mg of protein in a 24-hour urine collection.

In the past, an increase in blood pressure above baseline (a 30 mmHg increase in systolic or a 15 mmHg increase in diastolic) also met the blood pressure definition of preeclampsia, but this relative definition has been discarded in favor of the absolute definition of 140 mmHg or 90 mmHg.

Proteinuria is technically defined by the outcome of a 24-hour urine collection. In practice however, the consistent presence of more than trace protein on urine dipstick correlates well with proteinuria of 300 mg in 24 hours. Therefore the diagnosis is commonly made without a formal 24-hour evaluation.

Edema of the face and hands used to be a component of the diagnosis of preeclampsia. This criterion has been dropped because of its poor predictive value. Many pregnant women with normal blood pressure have hand and facial edema.

5. List other signs and symptoms that may be present in preeclampsia.

In addition to hypertension and proteinuria, women with preeclampsia may show evidence of the disease's effect on a number of systems. Women may have headaches, visual disturbances, and epigastric pain. There may be elevations in liver enzymes, elevated or decreased hematocrit, and decreased platelets.

6. What is gestational hypertension?

Hypertension occurring after 20 weeks' gestation but not accompanied by proteinuria is termed gestational hypertension. It was previously called pregnancy-induced hypertension.

7. What is the definition of chronic hypertension with superimposed preeclampsia?

If a woman with known chronic hypertension develops increased blood pressures along with proteinuria, this is defined as surperimposed preeclampsia.

It can be difficult to distinguish clinically between worsening of chronic hypertension and the development of superimposed preeclampsia. The development of proteinuria and the presence of other abnormalities associated with preeclampsia (e.g., headache, visual disturbances, elevated liver enzymes) assist with the diagnosis.

8. Are women with chronic hypertension considered high-risk pregnancies?

Yes. Because of poor placental vascular development and ongoing elevations of blood pressure, the pregnancy is at risk for intrauterine growth restriction, abruption, and stillbirth. From a maternal perspective, the patient may develop superimposed preeclampsia and all of the associated consequences.

9. Can anything be done to prevent complications in patients with chronic hypertension?

There is no apparent benefit to treatment of *mild* chronic hypertension (systolic blood pressure 140–179 mmHg, diastolic blood pressure 90–109 mmHg) in pregnancy. Patients who are newly diagnosed with mild disease during pregnancy can be monitored off medication for signs of worsening hypertension or superimposed pre-eclampsia. Patients with chronic hypertension should ideally have their blood pressure under control when they conceive and should continue blood pressure medications when they are pregnant.

If your patient has *more severe* chronic hypertension, remember that angiotensin-converting enzyme (ACE) inhibitors are contraindicated in pregnancy. If a pregnant woman is taking an ACE inhibitor, her medical regimen should be changed prior to attempting conception or as soon as the pregnancy is diagnosed. There are a number of effective medications that appear safe in pregnancy. Alpha-methyl dopa has been used safely for decades. Labetalol and calcium channel blockers also appear to be safe and effective. Beta blockers have been used, but there is a link between these drugs and small-for-gestational-age births.

Because of the risks associated with chronic hypertension, most clinicians follow pregnancies complicated by the disorder with serial ultrasounds for fetal growth and a schedule of fetal surveillance with non-stress tests or biophysical profiles. However, there is no data to support this approach. In general, these pregnancies are not allowed to continue past the due date and are induced at 40 weeks.

10. How often does preeclampsia occur? Which women are at greater risk?

Preeclampsia occurs in 6–8% of all live births. Risk factors include nulliparity, extremes of reproductive age (< 15 and > 35 years of age), African-American race, history of preeclampsia in a first-degree female relative, history of preeclampsia in a prior pregnancy, diabetes, chronic vascular or renal disease, chronic hypertension, and multiple gestations.

11. Do we know what causes preeclampsia?

No. Preeclampsia has been described since the time of the ancient Greeks. However, the cause remains unknown. We know that hypertension, proteinuria, and the other signs and symptoms of the illness are merely the outward manifestations of a systemic illness characterized by vasoconstriction and hypovolemia. All organs, including the fetoplacental unit, show evidence of poor perfusion.

12. What are some of the theories of the cause of preeclampsia?

Immunologic response. Inadequate maternal antibody response to the fetal allograft results in vascular damage from the circulating immune complexes. This theory is supported by an increased prevalence of the disease in pregnancies with limited prior antigen exposure (young nulliparas) and in situations with increased fetal antigen (twins, molar pregnancy, hydropic pregnancies, and diabetics with large placentas). Actual measurement of immune complexes has been inconsistent.

Circulating toxins. Vasoconstrictive substances reportedly have been extracted from blood, amniotic fluid, and the placenta in women with preeclampsia. Symptoms have been reproduced in some but not all animal studies.

Endogenous vasoconstrictors. Increased sensitivity to vasopressin, epinephrine, and norepinephrine have all been reported. Loss of normal third-trimester resistance to angiotensin II has also been noted.

Endothelial damage. Primary endothelial damage results in a decrease in prostacyclin production (potent vasodilator) and a relative increase in thromboxane A_2 (relative vasoconstrictor). Low-dose heparin or baby aspirin may play a role in prevention, but the cause of the endothelial damage and prostaglandin change is unclear.

Primary disseminated intravascular coagulation. Microvascular thrombin formation and deposition have been noted, producing vessel damage especially in the kidney and in the placenta.

13. What fetal and maternal risks are associated with preeclampsia?

Fetal risks include:
- Growth restriction
- Oligohydramnios
- Placental infarction
- Placental abruption
- Consequences of prematurity (when maternal disease necessitates delivery remote from term)
- Uteroplacental insufficiency
- Perinatal death

Maternal risks include:
- Central nervous system manifestations, including seizures and stroke
- DIC and its complications
- Increased likelihood of cesarean delivery
- Renal failure
- Hepatic failure or rupture
- Death

Preeclampsia is a leading cause of maternal mortality. However, most patients who survive, even those who suffer strokes, suffer no long-term sequelae.

14. Does preeclampsia recur in subsequent pregnancies?

Yes. If preeclampsia occurs in the first pregnancy there is a 25% chance of recurrence in subsequent pregnancies. The recurrence rate appears to be affected by gestational age at onset in the first pregnancy, severity, underlying maternal diseases, and underlying obstetric diseases. Women who develop preeclampsia early in pregnancy, or who develop severe preeclampsia; those with chronic medical conditions (e.g., chronic hypertension, renal disease); and those with no apparent fetal contribution (such as fetal aneuploidy) are at greater risk to develop preeclampsia in the future.

Multiparous patients who have had preeclampsia have a recurrence rate of up to 50% with subsequent pregnancies.

15. Does preeclampsia have ramifications later in life?

No. Preeclampsia does not increase the risk of hypertension later in life. An exception may be women who have recurrent preeclampsia, which may suggest unrecognized chronic hypertension or other underlying maternal diseases.

16. Is there a way to prevent preeclampsia?

Numerous interventions have been attempted. Dietary manipulation, with decreased sodium intake or increased calcium intake, and pharmacologic therapy, with prophylactic low-dose aspirin, have been extensively studied with randomized controlled trials. Unfortunately neither of these interventions has been able to reduce the incidence of preeclampsia.

17. Can women who have a pregnancy complicated by preeclampsia take birth control pills after delivery?

Yes. Preeclampsia, especially in a primiparous patient, does not contraindicate the use of oral contraceptives after delivery.

18. How is preeclampsia classified? What are the implications of the classification?

Preeclampsia is classified as mild and severe. Preeclampsia is considered severe if any one of a number of systems shows evidence of significant compromise. Any of the following parameters classify a woman's preeclampsia as **severe**:

- Systolic blood pressure > 160 mmHg or diastolic blood pressure > 110 mmHg on two occasions at least 6 hours apart
- Proteinuria ≥ 5 g/24 hr
- Oliguria < 500 cc/24 hr
- Cerebral or visual symptoms
- Epigastric or right upper quadrant pain
- Pulmonary edema or cyanosis
- Low platelets
- Elevated liver function tests
- Fetal growth restriction

The definition of **mild** preeclampsia is any preeclampsia that is not considered severe. There is no category of moderate preeclampsia.

The classification of severity is directly related to management and the decision about when to deliver the baby.

19. Describe the management of preeclampsia.

Delivery of the fetus "cures" preeclampsia. With delivery, signs and symptoms of preeclampsia resolve, although the time required for resolution is variable. The difficulty in therapy is deciding when to deliver the infant. Traditionally, all term pregnancies with preeclampsia—mild or severe—were delivered. For preterm pregnancies, those with severe disease were delivered and those with mild disease were managed conservatively with bedrest and close fetal and maternal surveillance.

Recently there have been efforts to extend preterm pregnancies complicated by severe preeclampsia rather than proceeding with immediate delivery. Administration of a short course (48 hours) of steroids to the mother confers significant benefit to premature newborns. Therefore, if preeclampsia develops before 32 weeks, even a short period of conservative management prior to delivery may be beneficial. Conservative management of severe preeclampsia in order to gain greater fetal maturity should only be attempted in carefully selected patients and should be managed by experienced physicians. These women should be hospitalized and must be observed closely for signs of worsening maternal disease or evidence of fetal compromise.

Obviously, at term the decision is easy to make, whether the preeclampsia is mild or severe. The difficulty arises when preeclampsia is remote from term. The degree of severity and the fetal gestational age are taken into consideration, and either the pregnancy is delivered or the patient is placed at bed rest. With bed rest therapy, close maternal and fetal surveillance is performed until the pregnancy reaches term or the degree of severity worsens, dictating the need to deliver.

20. How should delivery be accomplished in patients with preeclampsia?

There is no advantage to cesarean delivery over vaginal delivery for preeclampsia. Therefore, delivery route should be based on obstetric indications. An indication for cesarean section may be the inability to accomplish a vaginal delivery within a fixed, specified time, governed by maternal condition.

21. What special medicines are used in the delivery process?

A prophylactic agent against overt seizure activity is generally given during the labor process and for the first 24 hours of the postpartum period. The drug of choice in the U.S. is magnesium sulfate ($MgSO_4$). The usual dosing is a 4- to 6-g bolus, followed by a 2-g continuous infusion. If magnesium levels are monitored, the usual goal is a level in the 4–8 mg/dl range. Magnesium sulfate does not prevent all seizure activity. However, studies have demonstrated that magnesium is superior to other agents in the prevention of seizures in women with preeclampsia.

22. What is the role of antihypertensives in preeclampsia?

Mild elevations in blood pressure usually are not treated with anti-hypertensives. With more marked elevations (diastolic > 110 mmHg or a mean arterial pressure > 125 mmHg), medications with rapid onset, such as hydralazine and labetalol, are used intravenously. Generally such management is undertaken while also proceeding with delivery, due to the severity of the disease.

Diuretics are generally not used as a first-line treatment because preeclampsia is characterized by vasoconstriction and intravascular depletion, which are worsened by diuretics. As for other antihypertensive agents, work has shown that treatment of patients with mild-to-moderate hypertension (i.e., 90–110 mmHg diastolic pressure) does not decrease perinatal morbidity or mortality. Therefore, antihypertensive therapy is not usually used. Severe hypertension (> 110 mmHg diastolic pressure) is associated with severe preeclampsia. More than likely, delivery needs to be undertaken in this circumstance, and rapid-acting antihypertensive agents (i.e., intravenous hydralazine or labetalol) are used to control severe hypertension during labor.

In a patient with known chronic hypertension whose elevated blood pressure is believed to be due to underlying disease rather than preeclampsia, an increase in antihypertensive therapy may be appropriate

23. What is eclampsia?

Eclampsia is the clinical diagnosis given to patients who have seizure activity due to preeclampsia. Eclampsia is considered one of the most severe forms of preeclampsia, and delivery is undertaken after a seizure. About 1% of patients with preeclampsia have eclampsia. There are no recognized clinical determinants of who will experience seizure activity. Because we cannot predict which preeclamptic patients will have seizure activity, the majority (if not all) of these patients are treated with medicine for seizure prophylaxis.

24. How is delivery accomplished in eclamptic patients?

As with preeclamptics, obstetric indications are used to determine route of delivery. It is not unusual to encounter evidence of fetal compromise in eclamptic patients, but this is not necessarily an indication for cesarean delivery. In general, fetal resuscitation is best accomplished in utero by controlling the maternal state. Stabilizing the patient (i.e., airway, oxygen, circulation, and control of seizure activity) improves fetal status and subsequently neonatal outcome. Labor can then be initiated and vaginal delivery accomplished, assuming no obstetric indications for a cesarean delivery.

25. Is MgSO₄ used for eclamptic patients?

In the past there have been advocates for other agents, particularly phenytoin. However, a randomized controlled trial in women with eclampsia clearly favored $MgSO_4$ over phenytoin for recurrent seizure prophylaxis.

26. What is HELLP syndrome?

HELLP is an acronym for a syndrome of *h*emolysis, *e*levated *l*iver function, and/or *l*ow *p*latelets. HELLP syndrome is thought to be a subcategory of severe preeclampsia. Patients may or may not have other signs of preeclampsia. HELLP syndrome often has a rapidly accelerating downhill course. Most clinicians deliver infants expeditiously regardless of the gestational age.

27. What causes midepigastric pain in HELLP syndrome?

Liver capsule distention produces midepigastric pain, often with associated nausea and vomiting. Liver capsule distention can lead to hepatic rupture, with poor maternal and fetal outcomes.

28. What diagnoses should be considered in the patient who presents at 18 weeks' gestation with increased blood pressure?

Preeclampsia in the second trimester is a rare event. When this occurs, other diagnoses or fetal abnormalities should be considered.

Hydatidiform mole. A mole is a form of gestational trophoblastic disease. Increased blood pressure, hyperemesis, and fetal size greater than dates are characteristic clinical findings.

Hyperthyroidism and distant metastases may be associated with the clinical picture. Hydropic changes in the placenta can be seen on ultrasound.

Chromosomal abnormalities in the fetus. Triploidy is sometimes associated with preeclampsia in the second trimester.

Chronic hypertension. In some instances, chronic hypertension may have been previously diagnosed and treated. When previous evaluation has not been undertaken, care should be exercised to exclude secondary causes such as renal disease, pheochromocytoma, Cushing syndrome, or coarctation of the aorta.

Drug use. Cocaine use has been associated with increased blood pressure as well as poor perinatal outcome. In some cases, drug withdrawal (i.e., from heroin) has also been associated with hypertension.

CONTROVERSY

29. Should all women with gestational hypertension or preeclampsia be treated with magnesium for seizure prophylaxis?

The purpose of magnesium sulfate is to reduce the likelihood of seizures. Seizures occur less frequently in women with gestational hypertension and mild preeclampsia compared to women with more severe disease. In addition, like any medication, magnesium can have side effects, the most significant of which is respiratory compromise due to respiratory suppression and pulmonary edema. Because of this risk and given the lower risk of seizures in women with mild disease, many clinicians reserve anti-convulsive prophylaxis for women with severe preeclampsia, HELLP syndrome, or eclampsia.

BIBLIOGRAPHY

1. American College of Obstetricians and Gynecologists: Diagnosis and Management of Preeclampsia and Eclampsia. ACOG Practice Bulletin No. 33. Obstet Gynecol 99:159–167, 2002.
2. American College of Obstetricians and Gynecologists: Chronic Hypertension in Pregnancy. ACOG Practice Bulletin No. 29. Obstet Gynecol 98:177–185, 2001.
3. Berg CJ, Atrash HK, Koonin LM, Tucker M: Pregnancy-related mortality in the United States, 1987–1990. Obstet Gynecol 1996;88:161–167, 1996.
4. Caritis S, Sibai B, Hauth J, et al: Low-does aspirin to prevent preeclampsia in women at high risk. Natinoal Instituteof Child Health and Human Development Network of Maternal-Fetal Medicine Units. N Engl J Med 338:701–705, 1998.
5. Collaborative Eclampsia Trial Group: Which anticonvulsant for women with eclampsia? Evidence from the collaborative eclampsia trial. Lancet 345:1455–1463, 1995.
6. Knuist M, Bonsel GJ, Zondervan HA, Treffers PE: Low-sodium diet and pregnancy-induced hypertension: A mulit-centre randomized controlled trial. Br J Obstet Gynaecol 105:430–434, 1998.
7. Levine RJ, Hauth JC, Curet LB, et al: Trial of calcium to prevent preeclampsia. N Engl J Med 337:69–76, 1997.
8. Lubbe WF: Low-dose aspirin in prevention of toxemia of pregnancy: Does it have a place? Drugs 34:515, 1987.
9. Lucas MJ, Leveno KJ, Cunningham FG: A comparison of magniesuium sulfate with phenytoin for the prevention of eclampsia. N Engl J Med 333:201, 1995.
10. National High Blood Pressure Education Program: Working Group Report on High Blood Pressure in Pregnancy. Am J Obstet Gynecol 2000;183:S1–S22.
11. Repke JT: Preeclampsia and eclampsia. In Repke JT (ed): Intrapartum Obstetrics, New York, Churchill Livingstone, 1996.
12. Roberts JM: Pregnancy-related hypertension. In Creasy R, Resnik R (eds): Maternal-Fetal Medicine: Principles and Practice, 3rd ed. Philadelphia, W.B. Saunders, 1994, pp 804–843.
13. Sibai BM, Spinnato JA, Watson DL: Pregnancy outcome in 303 cases with severe preeclampsia. Obstet Gynecol 64:319, 1984.
14. Sibai BM, Mercer BM, Schiff E, Friedman SA: Aggressive versus expectant management of severe preeclampsia at 28–32 weeks gestation: A randomized controlled trial. Am J Obstet Gynecol 171:818, 1994.
15. Weinstein L: Preeclampsia/eclampsia with hemolysis, elevated liver enzymes, and thrombocytopenia. Obstet Gynecol 66:657, 1985.
16. Witlin AG, Sibai BM: Magnesium sulfate therapy in preeclampsia and eclampsia. Obstet Gynecol 92:883–889, 1998.

39. DIABETES IN PREGNANCY

Hyagriv N. Simhan, M.D.

GESTATIONAL DIABETES MELLITUS

1. What is gestational diabetes (GDM)?

GDM is defined as the state of carbohydrate intolerance that has its onset or first recognition during pregnancy.

2. Does the definition vary with severity?

No. The definition applies regardless of severity and whether or not insulin is required for treatment or the condition persists after pregnancy.

3. Does GDM include type I and type II patients?

Yes. GDM may include a small group of women with previously unrecognized overt diabetes mellitus type I or type II. However, usually the glucose intolerance is mild before pregnancy.

4. How is true GDM differentiated from unrecognized overt type I or type II diabetes mellitus?

- In GDM, the glycosylated hemoglobin (HbA1C) is normal.
- At 6 weeks after delivery, evaluation with 75-g oral glucose tolerance test reveals reversion to normal, nonpregnant carbohydrate tolerance in GDM.

5. List the similarities between GDM and noninsulin-dependent diabetes (NIDDM).

- The endocrine (impaired insulin secretion) and metabolic (insulin resistance) abnormalities that characterize both disease states are virtually identical.
- The risk factors for development of NIDDM are similar to those for development of GDM.
- In people with normal glucose tolerance, the metabolic abnormalities that indicate a high risk for developing NIDDM are similar to those that indicate an increased risk of GDM. Furthermore, women with GDM are at a markedly increased risk for developing NIDDM. GDM thus may represent an early stage in the natural history of NIDDM.

6. What is the importance of the GDM diagnosis?

The diagnosis of GDM identifies patients in whom aggressive glycemic control will prevent perinatal complications. The diagnosis also identifies patients who may benefit from early therapeutic interventions after pregnancy, such as improved nutrition, weight loss (if obese), and regular exercise program to prevent development of NIDDM and associated complications later in life.

7. What is the incidence of GDM?

Incidence varies from 0.15% to 15% of all pregnancies. Because GDM is such a heterogeneous entity, estimates of occurrence vary with ethnic diversity of the population under study, geographic area, screening frequency, and diagnostic criteria.

8. Describe the effects of GDM on pregnant women.

Pregnant women with GDM have an increased incidence of short-term maternal complications such as preeclampsia, preterm labor, pyelonephritis, polyhydramnios, and cesarean section. In the long term, such patients are at higher risk of developing NIDDM and associated complications, especially cardiovascular.

9. What are the effects of GDM on the fetus?

Short-term effects include increased perinatal morbidity and mortality. In addition, the incidence of fetal macrosomia, shoulder dystocia, operative delivery, stillbirth, and metabolic problems is similar to that in infants of an insulin-dependent diabetic mother. Long-term effects include an increased incidence of childhood obesity, early adulthood type II diabetes mellitus, and intellectual-motor impairment.

10. Is a patient with well-managed GDM and glucose in the recommended range (fasting plasma glucose < 105 mg/dl) and 2-hr postprandial glucose < 120 mg/dl) at the same risk for developing obstetric complications as the general population?

Yes. The cornerstone of management of GDM is glycemic control. Although other noncarbohydrate fuels are involved in fetal growth and metabolism, glucose and its effects on insulin and insulin-like growth factors is of primary concern.

11. Is there an increased rate of congenital malformations in women with GDM?

No. True GDM usually develops late, in the second trimester or early in the third trimester when organogenesis is already complete. If GDM is diagnosed in the first trimester, then it is imperative to confirm with the help of HbA1C whether it may be overt type I or type II diabetes, which may affect the incidence of congenital malformation.

12. What are the recommendations for GDM screening?

The American College of Obstetricians and Gynecologists (ACOG) recommends selective screening of women ≥ 30 years of age with 50-g oral glucose load between 24–28 weeks' gestation. ACOG acknowledges that some populations may benefit from earlier or universal screening. Patients with plasma glucose levels ≥ 140 mg/dl should be evaluated with a diagnostic 3-hour oral glucose tolerance test.

The American Diabetes Association (ADA) recommends screening for women who are ≥ 25 years old; have a family history of diabetes; are Hispanic, African-American, Native-American, Asian-American, or Pacific Islander; or were obese prior to pregnancy.

13. Which patients are at high risk for developing GDM?

The following patients are at high risk for GDM and should be screened at the first prenatal visit and again in each subsequent trimester:
- Previous history of GDM
- History of recurrent spontaneous abortions
- History of unexplained intrauterine fetal death
- Previous infant with major congenital anomalies (e.g., of the central nervous, cardiac, or skeletal systems)
- Previous macrosomic infant (> 4000 g)
- History of recurrent preeclampsia
- History of recurrent moniliasis
- Family history of DM in first-degree relatives
- History of polyuria, polydipsia, or glycosuria
- Maternal obesity (pregnancy weight > 150 lb or body mass index of > 27 kg/m2)
- Development of polyhydramnios and/or fetal macrosomia in present pregnancy
- Excessive weight gain (> 40 lb) during pregnancy
- Maternal age over 30 years

14. When can a 50-g glucose load be administered?

Randomly (i.e., either in fasting or fed state).

15. Can a reflectance meter be used for screening after 50-g glucose load?

No, because capillary values tend to be variable.

16. What is the rationale for recommending a particular threshold for screening?

The rationale is based on population studies, desired levels of sensitivity and specificity, and maintaining a favorable cost:benefit ratio. Using 130-mg/dl venous plasma levels by hexokinase method of glucose analysis, the sensitivity for diagnosis of GDM is 99%, but specificity is 50%. If a screening test threshold of > 135 mg/dl is used, sensitivity is 79% and specificity is 87% for all pregnant patients.

17. What diagnostic test is recommended for GDM?

The recommended test varies among countries and institutions. At present, the 3-hour oral glucose tolerance test (OGTT) is the definitive diagnostic test for GDM.

18. Describe the testing methodology for the 3-hour oral glucose tolerance test.

In the United States, the test is conducted with a 100-g glucose load. To standardize testing conditions, an overnight fast should be conducted for at least 8 hours, but not more than 14 hours. Adequate pretest loading with 150 g/day of carbohydrate for 3 days before testing is necessary to avoid false-positive responses. The patient should rest for approximately 30 minutes before starting the test and not smoke for 12 hours before the test. During the test the woman should not smoke and should remain seated with minimal physical exertion. After the fasting sample is drawn, the patient drinks 100 g of a glucose solution within 5 minutes. For consistency, the timing clock is started the moment the patient begins to drink. Subsequent blood samples are taken at 1, 2, and 3 hours. After the test, the patient may eat whole wheat bread and protein snacks to minimize rebound hypoglycemia.

19. What are the cut-off levels used for the diagnosis of GDM in a 3-hour OGTT?

The most recent criteria have been proposed by Coustan and Carpenter. An abnormal fasting glucose is ≥ 95 mg/dL. An abnormal 1-hour value is ≥ 180 mg/dL. An abnormal 2-hour value is ≥ 155 mg/dl. An abnormal 3-hour value is > 140 md/dl. An abnormal 3-hour OGTT is defined by two or more abnormal values.

A less rigorous standard with a lower sensitivity but fewer false positives uses values for fasting 1-hour, 2-hour and 3-hour of 105, 190, 165 and 145 mg/dl, respectively.

20. What factors regulate blood glucose levels?

- Stress: physical and emotional stress, infection, inflammation, hormonal imbalance of pregnancy, growth
- Time and type of insulin taken
- Diet: type and timing
- Exercise: type and duration

21. What are the dietary recommendations in GDM?

This author prescribes 30–35 kcal/kg of ideal body weight per day, with no patients receiving < 1800 or > 2800 calories/day. There is some controversy regarding use of hypocaloric diets in markedly obese women because of the hypothetical risks to the fetus from ketonemia due to starvation.

22. What role does exercise play in the management of GDM?

Exercise plays an important role in the management of GDM. Large skeletal muscles, depending on the type of exercise, increase glucose utilization. The effects may be immediate, as with brisk walking, or sustained for a few hours, as after swimming. The Third International Workshop Conference on GDM advocates exercise as a treatment modality in women who do not have a medical or obstetric contraindication. Upper body cardiovascular training has resulted in lower glucose concentrations than in women treated with diet only. The effects of exercise on glucose metabolism may become apparent after 4 weeks of training and involve both hepatic glucose output and glucose clearance. A cardiovascular conditioning program may obviate the need for insulin treatment in some women with GDM.

23. What are the recommendations for timing and frequency of blood glucose monitoring?

The recommendations are controversial. Usually it is recommended that fasting, 2-hour post-prandial, and bedtime plasma glucose levels be monitored with a reflectance meter at home. But there is evidence that monitoring of fasting and 1-hour plasma glucose level < 140 mg/dl decreases the risk of neonatal hypoglycemia, macrosomia, and cesarean delivery.

24. Describe the management of patients with one abnormal value on the 3-hour OGTT.

Management is controversial, and recommendations vary based on when the test value is obtained. If the test value is obtained before 28 weeks' gestation, the 3-hour OGTT should be repeated 4 weeks later and managed appropriately. If the test value is obtained after 34 weeks, management depends on the level and timing of hyperglycemia (i.e., fasting or postprandial).

This author's recommendation for women with a single abnormal fasting value is to introduce visual home glucose monitoring and appropriate dietary strategies to maintain euglycemia with fasting values < 105 mg/dl and 2-hour postprandial values < 120 mg/dl. This approach should help to decrease the incidence of maternal hyperglycemia, but it is not a universally accepted management plan.

25. When is insulin recommended in the management of GDM?

When to use insulin in GDM is rather arbitrary. If euglycemia is not achieved with an appropriate diet within 1–2 weeks, use of subcutaneous human insulin is recommended. The type of insulin employed is controversial. Some authorities recommend intermediate insulin such as NPH (human insulin isophane suspension) or Lente (insulin zinc suspension) forms in the evening or morning or both, whereas others recommend using a mixture of short-acting and intermediate-acting in both the evening and morning (mixture of regular with NPH or Lente). Either regimen is fine as long as euglycemia is achieved.

Patients treated with insulin should be reminded about the importance of diet at the time of initiation of therapy, especially the consistency with which the diet is followed. Several studies show the benefits of insulin therapy.

26. Describe the management of preterm labor in women with GDM.

Intravenous magnesium sulfate is used most commonly because beta-adrenergic agonists can cause maternal hyperglycemia. Steroid therapy to accelerate fetal lung may increase the insulin requirement, but it has significant fetal benefits.

27. Are women receiving terbutaline for preterm labor at higher risk for developing GDM?

Yes. Studies indicate that dose-independent, terbutaline-induced glucose intolerance is mediated by glucagon and caused by diminished insulin sensitivity. Body mass index directly correlated with postchallenge measures of insulin, insulin:glucose ratio, and pancreatic polypeptide, but not with other parameters.

28. When and how often should antepartum fetal surveillance be done in women with GDM?

Weekly antenatal surveillance should begin at 38–40 weeks' gestation. But if GDM is complicated with fetal macrosomia, polyhydramnios, pregnancy-induced hypertension, or insulin requirement, antepartum surveillance should begin at 32 weeks' gestation. Antepartum surveillance may consist of nonstress testing and/or biophysical profile, usually conducted weekly or twice a week.

29. When and how should a woman with GDM be delivered?

Delivery is recommended at no later than 40 weeks' gestation in patients requiring insulin therapy and at no later than 42 weeks for diet-controlled patients. No elective delivery should be performed prior to 39 weeks without establishing lung maturity because of the possibility that even mild GDM can delay lung maturity.

GDM is not an absolute indication for cesarean section, but complications related to diabetes may be. For example, if estimated fetal weight exceeds 4500 g, elective cesarean section is a viable option to avoid shoulder dystocia. Even among diabetic women, however, the risk of permanent brachial plexus injury after a shoulder dystocia is low. At lower estimated weights, previous obstetric history and clinical pelvimetry are useful tools in obstetric management.

30. Describe the management of labor in women with GDM.

Attempts should be made to avoid maternal hyperglycemia during labor, because acute fetal hyperglycemia and hyperinsulinemia may be associated with neonatal hypoglycemia. Maternal glucose levels should be checked every 1–2 hours during labor, and a continuous insulin infusion may be started if values exceed 100–120 mg/dl.

31. How should a woman with GDM be followed after delivery?

Between 5% and 20% of women with GDM continue to have diabetes or impaired glucose tolerance after they have delivered; presumably the same problem existed before pregnancy. Thus the ADA suggests a 75-g, 2-hour OGTT 6 weeks after delivery.

32. What percentage of women with GDM become diabetic later in life?

The incidence is variable based on the course of GDM and whether intervention such as weight loss was introduced. O'Sullivan has found that 36% of women diagnosed with GDM in an index pregnancy are diagnosed as diabetic within 15 years.

33. Once a woman has GDM, what specific risk factors increase her risk for GDM in subsequent pregnancies?

In general, women with GDM have a recurrence risk of 60–70%. But recurrence risk based on pre-pregnant body mass index and fasting plasma glucose level (from pregnant OGTT) plus time since the index pregnancy can predict the likelihood of subsequent glucose tolerance test abnormality.

34. What types of contraception are recommended for a patient with GDM?

There are no specific contraindications to available forms of contraception based on a history of GDM.

35. What are the rules of 15?

15% of the obstetric population have abnormal glucose load test
15% of patients with abnormal GLT have abnormal OGTT
15% of patients with abnormal OGTT require insulin
15% of all patients with GDM have infants > 4000 g
Capillary levels are about 15% higher than plasma levels after meals.

CONTROVERSY

36. Can oral hypoglycemic agents be used in pregnancy?

Most oral hypoglycemic agents cross the placenta and could potentially have fetal metabolic effects. In the second trimester they can increase fetal insulin production, leading to fetal growth abnormalities and severe neonatal hypoglycemia. The sulfonylurea **glyburide** does not cross the placenta in significant quantity. Initial human clinical studies of glyburide treatment for GDM suggest that it is safe and may have similar effectiveness as insulin with respect to glucose control.

There is insufficient safety and efficacy data to support the use of metformin in GDM.

INSULIN-DEPENDENT DIABETES

37. What changes in energy metabolism occur during the first trimester?

The hormonal milieu of the first trimester is dominated by estrogen and progesterone production by the corpus luteum and early placenta. Maternal serum amino acid levels go down, including the level of alanine, which is the amino acid chiefly used for gluconeogenesis. Hepatic glucose production decreases, whereas tissue glycogen storage and peripheral glucose utilization increase. These changes combine to decrease maternal fasting plasma glucose levels.

38. How does energy metabolism change as pregnancy advances?

Estrogen and progesterone production continue to rise throughout pregnancy, but during the second trimester, prolactin and human placental lactogen (hPL) (also known as human chorionic somatomammotropin [hCS]) of placental origin begin to appear in the maternal circulation. Both free and total cortisol levels also begin to rise during the second trimester. These hormones antagonize the actions of insulin, producing insulin resistance. Compared with the non-pregnant state, fasting glucose concentrations remain somewhat lower during later pregnancy. Conversely, postprandial glucose levels are higher and require more insulin to bring them down.

Pregnant diabetic women in good metabolic control respond to hypoglycemia less well than non-pregnant women. The counterregulatory hormones, glucagon and epinephrine, do not begin to rise until maternal glucose levels have fallen lower; they rise less quickly and to lower peaks than in non-pregnant women. These changes produce wider excursions in blood glucose throughout the day, with higher highs and lower lows.

39. What are the practical implications of the first-trimester physiologic changes for women with insulin-treated diabetes mellitus?

Some degree of anorexia, nausea, and vomiting is quite common, if not universal, in the first trimester. Nondiabetic women respond to the resulting decrease in metabolic fuel intake by decreasing insulin production. Diabetic women taking a fixed amount of insulin daily are at increased risk for hypoglycemia. Insulin reactions are common in early pregnancy, and many diabetic women first recognize that they are pregnant when reactions begin to occur for no obvious reason—most commonly, in the morning.

The appropriate response is to decrease the patient's insulin dose. Dietary manipulations, such as eating small meals frequently (every 2–3 hours), avoiding caffeine and fatty and spicy foods, and drinking fluids between meals rather than with meals, may also be helpful.

40. Are there any prophylactic measures that can prevent malformations among infants of diabetic mothers?

The only measure known to be effective in preventing malformations is good glycemic control during organogenesis. The vast majority of major malformations arise between 2 weeks of fertilization age and 7 weeks (9 weeks from last menstrual period). Because many women do not recognize their pregnancy, and the first visit to their obstetrician is 8 or more weeks after their last menstrual period, it may take several weeks of adjustment of diet and insulin to achieve good metabolic control. Therefore, it is critical for diabetic women to plan their pregnancies and *conceive* in good metabolic control.

Prophylactic dietary supplementation with **folic acid** has been shown to reduce the incidence of neural tube defects in the general population. Although folic acid dietary supplementation is prudent and appropriate for diabetic women too, it has not been shown to protect effectively against neural tube defects specifically in this population.

41. Given their increased risk for occurrence of major malformations, what is an appropriate strategy for screening diabetic patients for malformations?

Maternal **serum alpha-fetoprotein** (MSAFP) screening should be offered to diabetic patients as to any other patients. MSAFP levels tend to be about 20% lower for women with insulin-treated diabetes mellitus than for non-diabetic women; thus, it is important for the laboratory to know the patient's history of diabetes to interpret correctly the results of the assay. Most physicians who care for diabetic patients recommend an **ultrasound** examination, including careful study of cardiac anatomy (four-chamber and outflow tract views) at approximately 18 weeks' gestation to screen for major malformations. In many centers, fetal **echocardiography** is offered to all pregnant women with pre-gestational diabetes mellitus.

The success rate for diagnosing major malformations varies considerably among laboratories from 17% to virtually 100%. The response to an elevated MSAFP and the decision to perform an amniocentesis depend on both the degree of elevation and the confidence of the sonographer in ruling out major malformations.

42. What is the White classification of diabetes during pregnancy? How is it used?

More than 50 years ago Dr. Priscilla White proposed a classification system for women with diabetes prior to pregnancy based on factors that could be identified at the first prenatal visit. It was hoped that this classification could be used both to prognosticate how women would do during pregnancy and to provide guidance for treatment according to the degree of severity of the disease. Although treatment of patients in the various classes without nephropathy is not significantly different, the risks of hypertension and prematurity do vary by class. Most centers continue to use this classification for statistical purposes and to compare their outcomes with other centers. (Please see reference 18.)

43. Should patients be switched to continuous subcutaneous insulin infusion (CSII) pumps to obtain optimal metabolic control during pregnancy?

The single most important intervention to optimize metabolic control is undoubtedly **home capillary blood glucose monitoring**. Frequent self-monitoring of capillary blood glucose values with adjustments of diet, insulin, and exercise as necessary are the keys to good metabolic control. The types of insulin used (long-acting vs. intermediate-acting) and mode of delivery (standard injections vs. CSII pump) are less important. The published experience with the insulin pump has demonstrated that this therapy can achieve glucose control and perinatal outcomes comparable to that obtained with multiple-dose insulin injection therapy.

44. What are the goals of metabolic therapy in pregnancy?

The risks for spontaneous abortion and major malformation depend on the degree of control in the first trimester, whereas the risks for macrosomia and stillbirth are related to control in the second and third trimesters. Gradually improving glucose control prior to pregnancy can reduce the likelihood of deterioration of retinopathy, which has been observed when poorly controlled pregnant patients rapidly become euglycemic.

Minimizing the risks for major malformations and spontaneous abortions requires only fair-to-good control, whereas control must be nearly perfect to avoid macrosomia. The blood glucose goals should be fasting values < 105 mg/dl and 2-hour postprandial values < 120 mg/dl.

45. How should an insulin reaction be treated?

Ideally, treatment for an insulin reaction should restore a normal blood glucose level without resulting in hyperglycemia. If the reaction is mild to moderate and the patient is awake and alert enough to take something by mouth, any glucose-containing solution can be given. Four to six ounces of fruit juice or a soft drink should be adequate; more will cause hyperglycemia. If the patient is comatose or poorly arousable, a friend or relative on the scene can easily administer a dose of glucagon. All insulin-requiring diabetic patients should be given a prescription for glucagon to be filled and kept in the refrigerator for just such a possible circumstance. All diabetic women should be educated regarding the early symptoms of developing hypoglycemia such as nausea, irritability, fatigue, and diaphoresis.

46. What are the most important complications of late pregnancy among diabetic women?

Hypertension, prematurity, macrosomia, and late fetal demise occur with increased frequency among diabetic women compared with the general population. The incidence of preeclampsia has been reported to be 20–40% in diabetic women and as high as 60% among women with diabetic nephropathy. Prematurity is approximately twice as common among diabetic women and is due mostly to the development of hypertension. As many as 25% of infants of diabetic mothers are larger than 4000 g, and 60% may be larger than the 90th percentile for gestational age. This results in a higher incidence of operative delivery and an increased risk for birth trauma. Late near-term fetal demise has become much less common in the past 20 years but is still a risk to be kept in mind and avoided.

47. What is the mechanism of late fetal demise? How can it be avoided?

Glycosylated hemoglobin carries less oxygen, molecule for molecule, than native hemoglobin. It also binds oxygen more avidly and releases it less readily in areas of low oxygen tension, such as the placental bed. Acute maternal hyperglycemia causes fetal hyperglycemia, which stimulates the fetal pancreas to secrete more insulin. Fetal hyperinsulinemia causes an increased demand for oxygen in fetal tissues, potentially outstripping placental supply. Thus, both chronic and acute hyperglycemia contribute to a physiologic state that can result in a lethal degree of hypoxemia. The best prophylaxis is to keep the patient's diabetes under the best possible control at all times.

48. What fetal surveillance is indicated in late pregnancy?

The optimal scheme for routine antepartum surveillance of women with diabetes has not been established in a scientifically rigorous fashion. Nonetheless, most practitioners begin routine surveillance on a weekly basis at 32 weeks' gestation, using nonstress testing. At 36 weeks, the frequency is usually increased to twice weekly. Nonreactive nonstress tests can be followed with either contraction stress tests or biophysical profiles for reassurance of fetal well-being.

49. How should delivery be timed?

The decision about the timing of delivery should take into consideration the risk for respiratory distress syndrome (RDS), favorability of the cervix for labor, the size of the fetus, and ongoing exposure to the risk of stillbirth. RDS is more common among infants of diabetic mothers at relatively late gestational ages than among other infants. Generally, lung maturity studies should be obtained for any fetus to be delivered electively before 39 completed weeks of gestation. After 39 weeks, the risk is so small that it can be ignored.

Patients with *poorly controlled diabetes* and macrosomic fetuses are at greater risk for stillbirth and, generally, should be delivered somewhat earlier (37–38 weeks) if lung maturity can be assured.

Patients with *well-controlled diabetes* and normal-size fetuses are at lower risk for stillbirth and may be allowed to wait later into their pregnancies for cervical maturity. However, most U.S. obstetricians do not allow diabetic patients to go beyond 40 weeks under any circumstances.

50. How should the route of delivery be determined?

Macrosomic infants of diabetic mothers are at greater risk for shoulder dystocia during vaginal delivery than either nonmacrosomic infants or similar-weight infants of nondiabetic women. Most shoulder dystocias do not result in birth injury, and most birth injuries do not result in permanent disability. Nonetheless, the risk for traumatic birth injury is intimidating. It is difficult to predict accurately which fetuses are macrosomic and which are likely to suffer significant birth injury.

Despite this imprecision, most obstetricians give serious consideration to cesarean delivery for any infant of a diabetic mother estimated to be larger than 4500 g. Fetuses less than 4000 g deserve a trial of labor. Fetuses estimated to weigh 4000–4500 g may be delivered either way at the discretion of the physician and patient. Diabetes per se is *not* an indication for cesarean section.

51. How should the metabolic control of diabetes be managed during labor?

During labor, insulin requirements are generally relatively low because of reduced caloric intake and probably the work of labor. A patient scheduled for induction should receive a modest dose of intermediate-acting insulin (one-half to one-third of her usual morning dose) before beginning the induction. During labor, give a glucose-containing solution (D_5 in a solution of one-half normal saline) at approximately 125 ml/hr, strictly controlled on an infusion pump. Monitor capillary blood glucose values hourly. If the blood glucose rises above 120 mg/dl, give the patient a continuous intravenous infusion of regular insulin at a rate sufficient to bring the blood glucose down to 80–120 mg/dl.

Even with good glucose control during labor, it is important to follow the neonatal blood sugar by heel stick to evaluate for hypoglycemia. Neonates with persistently low sugars often require early feeds or intravenous glucose therapy.

BIBLIOGRAPHY

1. Anonymous. ACOG technical bulletin. Diabetes and pregnancy. Number 200, December 1994 (replaces No. 92, May 1986). Committee on Technical Bulletins of the American College of Obstetricians and Gynecologists. Int J Gyn Obstet 48:331–339, 1995.
2. Berkus MD, Langer O, Piper JM, Luther MF: Efficiency of lower threshold criteria for the diagnosis of gestational diabetes. Obstet Gynecol 86:892–896, 1995.
3. Brown FM, Hare JW: Diabetes complicating pregnancy. The Joslin Clinic Method, 2nd ed. New York, Wiley-Liss, 1995.
4. Combs CA, Gunderson E, Kitzmiller JL, et al: Relationship of fetal macrosomia to maternal postprandial glucose control during pregnancy. Diabetes Care 15:1251–1257, 1992.
5. Coustan DR, Carpenter MW, O'Sullivan PS, Carr SR: Gestational diabetes: Precursors of subsequent disordered glucose metabolism. Am J Obstet Gyecol 168:1139–1144; discussion, 1144–1145, 1993.
6. Coustan DR, Nelson C, Carpenter MW, et al: Maternal age and screening for gestational diabetes: A population-based study. Obstet Gynecol 73:557, 1989.
7. Foley MR, Landon MB, Gabbe SG, et al: Effect of prolonged oral terbutaline therapy on glucose tolerance in pregnancy. Am J Obstet Gynecol 168(Pt 1):100–105, 1993.
8. Gabbe S, Hill L, Schmidt L, Schulkin J: Management of diabetes by obstetrician-gynecologists. Obstet Gynecol 91:643–647, 1998.
9. Gabbe SG: New concepts and applications in the use of the insulin pump during pregnancy. J Matern Fetal Med 9:42–45, 2000.
10. Greene MF, Benacerraf BR: Prenatal diagnosis in diabetic gravidas: Utility of ultrasound and maternal serum alpha-fetoprotein screening. Obstet Gynecol 77:520–524, 1991.
11. Greene MF, Hare JW, Krache M, et al: Prematurity among insulin-requiring diabetic gravid women. Am J Obstet Gynecol 161:106–111, 1989.
12. Jovanovic-Peterson L, Peterson CM: Gestational diabetic women? Diabetes 40(Suppl 2):179–181, 1991.
13. Kitzmiller JL, Buchanan TA, Kjos S, et al: Pre-conception care of diabetes, congenital malformations, and spontaneous abortions. Diabetes Care 19:514–541, 1996.
14. Kuhl C: Etiology and pathogenesis of gestational diabetes. Diabetes Care 21:B19–26, 1998.
15. O'Sullivan JB: Long-term follow-up of gestational diabetes. In Camerini-Davalos RA, Cole HD (eds): Early Diabetes in Early Life. New York, Springer-Verlag, 1979, pp 425–435.
16. Rouse DJ, Owen J: Prophylactic cesarean delivery for fetal macrosomia diagnosed by means of ultrasonography—A Faustian bargain? Am J Obstet Gynecol 181:332–338, 1999.
17. Tam WH, Rogers MS, Yip SK, et al: Which screening test is the best for gestational impaired glucose tolerance and gestational diabetes mellitus? Diabetes Care 23:1432, 2000.
18. White P: Pregnancy complicating diabetes. Am J Medicine 7:609–616, 1949.

40. THYROID DISEASE IN PREGNANCY

Anthony O. Odibo, M.D., MRCOG

1. Describe the normal physiological changes in thyroid function during pregnancy.

Test	Pregnancy Change
Thyroid-stimulating hormone (TSH)	None
Thyroid-binding globulin (TBG)	Increases
Total thyroxine (T_4)	Increases
Total tri-iodothyronine (T_3)	Increases
T_3 total resin uptake (T_3RU)	Decreases
Free T_4	None
Free T_3	None

2. Explain the increase in T_4 and T_3 seen during normal pregnancy.

Approximately 70% of circulating T_4 and T_3 is bound to thyroxine-binding globulin (TBG). Pregnancy results in an estrogen-mediated increase in TBG and hence increased T_4 and T_3. However, the free thyroid hormone levels remain unchanged.

3. List the indications for thyroid function testing during pregnancy.

The most common indications for ordering a thyroid panel are: women on thyroid hormone, family history of autoimmune thyroiditis, presence of goiter, past history of radiation to thyroid, and type 1 diabetes.

4. What is the incidence of hyperthyroidism in pregnancy? What are the most common causes?

Hyperthyroidism affects 1:2000 pregnancies. Causes of hyperthyroidism in pregnancy include Graves' disease, toxic adenoma, subacute thyroiditis, iatrogenic ingestion of thyroxine, transient hyperthyroidism secondary to hyperemesis gravidarum, and gestational trophoblastic disease.

5. What is Graves' disease? How does it affect the mother, fetus, and newborn infant?

Graves' disease results in maternal hyperthyroidism secondary to autoantibodies capable of stimulating thyroxine synthesis. Maternal symptoms include weight loss or poor weight gain, tachycardia, and heat intolerance. Laboratory studies reveal increased T_4 and T_3 levels, an increased free thyroid index, and a low TSH. Untreated maternal hyperthyroidism results in an increased risk of pre-eclampsia and congestive heart failure.

The thyroid-stimulating antibodies can cross the placenta readily to stimulate the fetal thyroid. Fetal complications include in utero demise, prematurity, intrauterine growth retardation, a widespread fetal autoimmune reaction with lymphatic hypertrophy and thrombocytopenia, fetal goiter, and fetal exophthalmos.

Affected newborns can be expected to have a transient course over 1–5 months as the maternal autoantibodies are slowly cleared from their systems.

6. Should diagnostic iodine studies be performed to confirm the diagnosis of Graves' disease during pregnancy?

No. Such iodine studies are performed with radioactive tagging. Radioactive iodine crosses the placenta and is concentrated in the fetal thyroid after 10 weeks' gestation. Iatrogenic fetal hypothyroidism can result.

7. What are the treatment options for Graves' disease during pregnancy?

Prophylthiouracil (PTU) is the treatment of choice. It generally decreases both T_4 and the symptoms by 4 weeks after initiating therapy. PTU is gradually decreased thereafter to maintain the mother's T_4 at upper limits of normal and to prevent overtreatment and hypothyroidism. Some advocate continuing to decrease PTU and even discontinuing it during the third trimester. Some women experience temporary remission of disease possibly secondary to the relative immunosuppression of pregnancy.

Methimazole is an alternative treatment. It is not the first-line drug due to reports of scalp defects (aplasia cutis) in newborns exposed to methimazole. Beta blockers such as propranolol may diminish the symptoms of thyrotoxicosis. Failure of medical therapy to alleviate the symptoms may necessitate a subtotal thyroidectomy.

Radioactive iodine therapy for gland ablation is contraindicated for the same reasons that diagnostic studies with radioactive iodine should not knowingly be undertaken.

8. Describe the fetal effects of therapy with prophylthiouracil.

PTU crosses the placenta and iatrogenic fetal hypothyroidism can be produced, with the long-term effects not clearly established. There is some evidence for delayed bone age and central nervous system effects in exposed infants.

9. How can an infant still develop neonatal Graves' disease when the mother's hyperthyroidism is well controlled with PTU?

Transplacental passage of thyroid-stimulating antibodies can result in neonatal Grave's disease. These antibodies remain in the maternal circulation regardless of the treatment of the mother. Even mothers with hypothyroidism secondary to subtotal thyroidectomy or radiation therapy for Graves' disease are at risk for a fetus with thyrotoxicosis. Neonatal Graves' disease occurs in about 1% of women with Graves' disease regardless of their history of treatment. Treatment of the mother who has had a subtotal thyroidectomy and is on thyroid replacement therapy may be necessary and require PTU for the sole purpose of treating fetal hyperthyroidism caused by autoantibodies.

10. How does pregnancy affect Graves' disease?

Patients tend to have aggravation of symptoms during the first half, followed by amelioration during the second half of pregnancy and postpartum recurrence. This is thought to be due to the relative immunosuppression of pregnancy.

11. Can women on PTU breastfeed?

Yes. PTU is excreted in small quantities in breast milk and can theoretically suppress the infant's thyroid function. However, because the amount excreted is small, breastfeeding is generally permitted in conjunction with monitoring of the newborn's thyroid function.

12. What is "thyroid storm"? When does it usually present?

Thyroid storm is characterized by a hypermetabolic state, fever, and change in mental status. This life-threatening complication can occur during labor or cesarean section, or in conjunction with an antepartum or postpartum infection. Thyroid storm can also occur in patients with gestational trophoblastic disease. Most often it manifests itself in the woman with unrecognized hyperthyroidism.

13. How is thyroid storm managed?

By symptomatic and supportive treatment of the pyrexia, tachycardia, and severe dehydration. Thionamides, PTU, beta-blocking agents, steroids, iodines, or ipodate (to block thyroid hormone release) are the mainstays of therapy. It is important to treat any associated hypertension, infection, or anemia.

14. What are the common causes of maternal hypothyroidism?

Common etiologies include: Hashimoto's thyroiditis, previous treatment of Graves' disease by radioactive iodine or subtotal thyroidectomy, and excessive doses of PTU for the treatment of Graves' symptomatology.

15. What are the maternal, fetal and newborn effects of untreated hypothyroidism?

Most women with untreated hypothyroidism are subfertile, since marked hypothyroidism usually results in increased prolactin levels (secondary to increased thyrotropin-releasing hormone) and anovulation. In women with overt hypothyroidism who do become pregnant, there is a significantly higher incidence of anemia, preeclampsia, abruption, postpartum hemorrhage, and cardiac dysfunction. Likewise, fetal complications, including low birth weight and perinatal demise, are increased. Lesser degrees of untreated hypothyroidism may be associated with pregnancy loss and prolonged gestation. Women with subclinical disease (increased TSH but normal T_4) and women receiving adequate replacement therapy have better outcomes.

16. How should the hypothyroid mother be treated?

Treatment consists of 1.6 mcg/kg of Synthroid, Levothroid, or Levoxyl, with variation on an individual basis. Assessment of TSH in the first trimester seems reasonable, because up to 45% of treated women with hypothyroidism require higher doses during pregnancy. Postpartum, preconception doses are appropriate, with assessment of TSH 6–12 weeks after delivery.

17. Should women with hyperemesis gravidarum have thyroid function tests?

Hyperemesis gravidarum in the presence of a viable gestation has been associated with abnormal values on thyroid studies. It is thought that elevated HCG seen in these patients has TSH-like effects. The majority of these women have no other clinical signs of hyperthyroidism, and treatment is not advocated. In a small number of cases, hyperthyroidism exists clinically, and treatment of thyrotoxicosis can help to alleviate hyperemesis gravidarum. Use of free T_4 by equilibrium dialysis may help to clarify thyroid status.

18. What is postpartum thyroiditis?

Occurring 1–8 months postpartum, this condition may affect 5% of parturients. Initial hyperthyroidism (1–4 months) is followed by hypothyroidism (5–8 months), with thyroid antibodies often present. Spontaneous recovery occurs, but during the intervening period may be misdiagnosed as postpartum depression or psychosis. In 10–30% hypothyroidism is permanent. Postpartum thyroiditis tends to recur with subsequent pregnancies.

19. What diagnostic tests would you order for a woman with a thyroid nodule during pregnancy?

An ultrasound exam can disclose if the nodule is cystic or solid. Solid nodules are more likely to be malignant. Confirmation is by fine-needle aspiration or tissue biopsy. Avoid radioactive iodine, especially in the first trimester.

BIBLIOGRAPHY

1. American College of Obstetricians and Gynecologists: Thyroid Disease in Pregnancy. ACOG Tech Bull 181, 1993.
2. Mestman JH: Hyperthyroidism in pregnancy. Clin Obstet Gynecol 40:45–64, 1997.
3. Mestman JH: Endocrine diseases in pregnancy. In Gabbe SG, Niebyl JR, Simpson JL (eds): Obstetrics: Normal and Problem Pregnancies, 4th ed New York, Churchill Livingstone, 2002.

41. SEIZURES IN PREGNANCY

Dominic Marchiano, M.D.

1. How does epilepsy affect conception?

Epilepsy, in itself, has no impact on fertility. However, the *treatment* of epilepsy can impact conception. Phenobarbital, phenytoin, and carbemazepine are metaboized in the hepatic P450 system. Their metabolism increases the production of sex hormone–binding globulin, which can decrease the unbound, active fractions of hormonal contraceptive agents. Therefore, hormonal contraception with combination estrogen-progestin pills or progestin only is much less reliable in women taking these anticonvulsant medications. Unintended pregnancy may result. Non-hormonal contraceptive choices should be emphasized to these women.

2. How does pregnancy affect the frequency of seizures?

Seizure disorders are the most common neurological problem in pregnancy. Between 25% and 50% of women with idiopathic epilepsy have an increase in seizure fequency during pregnancy, usually during the first trimester. Of the remainder, most have no change in seizure pattern. Patients with frequent seizures *before* pregnancy are likely to experience worsening of seizure control *during* pregnancy. Likewise, good seizure control before pregnancy usually correlates with a lower risk of exacerbation during pregnancy.

3. What is the cause of increased seizure frequency during pregnancy?

The etiology is often unclear. Possible causes include not only poor seizure control before conception, but also little or no prepregnancy counseling, poor compliance, and lower serum levels of anticonvulsants during pregnancy. Note that increased seizure activity during one pregnancy does not predict a similar response in future pregnancies.

4. What is gestational epilepsy?

Occasionally, idiopathic epilepsy is diagnosed for the first time during pregnancy. Twenty-five percent of these newly diagnosed epileptics are known as gestational epileptics—individuals who only manifest symptoms during pregnancy. Gestational epilepsy in one pregnancy is not predictive of recurrence in future pregnancies.

5. How do seizures affect the course of pregnancy?

Several studies have suggested mildy increased risks for a multitude of obstetric complications. Included among these are preeclampsia, preterm labor, and stillbirth. However, other studies have failed to duplicate these associations. Vaginal bleeding is more common in epileptics, probably secondary to anticonvulsant therapy–induced vitamin K deficiency.

6. Which anticonvulsants are commonly used during pregnancy?

Phenytoin, phenobarbital, and carbemazepine are used more frequently than either primidone (a structural analogue of phenobarbital) or valproic acid. Each medication, however, is associated with specific fetal and neonatal risks. Therefore, monotherapy is preferred over polytherapy.

Anticonvulsants Commonly Used During Pregnancy

MEDICATION	THERAPEUTIC LEVEL (MG/L)	NON-PREGNANT DOSE	USUAL HALF LIFE	PROTEIN-BOUND FRACTION
Carbamazepine	4–10	600–1200 mg/day in 3–4 divided doses	16–36 hours	76%

(Table continued on next page.)

Anticonvulsants Commonly Used During Pregnancy (cont.)

MEDICATION	THERAPEUTIC LEVEL (MG/L)	NON-PREGNANT DOSE	USUAL HALF LIFE	PROTEIN-BOUND FRACTION
Phenobarbital	15–40	90–180 mg/day in 2–3 divided doses	100 hours	Variable
Phenytoin	10–20 total, 1–2 free	300–500 mg/day single or divided doses (for > 300)	24 hours	90%
Primidone	5–15	750–1500 mg/day in 3 divided doses	8 hours	Metabolized to phenobarbital
Valproic acid	50–100	550–2000 mg/day in 3–4 divided doses	6–16 hours	90%

7. How does pregnancy affect blood levels of anticonvulsants?

Subtherapeutic levels of phenytoin, carbemazepine, and phenobarbital can occur as a result of the increased maternal plasma volume, delayed gastrointestinal absorption, and increased hepatic clearance associated with pregnancy. In addition, folic acid supplementation may lower plasma levels of phenytoin. Even though total levels of these medications may fall, the active (nonprotein-bound) levels often increase as serum albumin decreases during pregnancy. Therefore, anticonvulsant levels should be monitored periodically and adjusted as needed.

8. What metabolic abnormalities associated with anticonvulsant therapy should be corrected during pregnancy?

Folic acid is known to reduce the risk of neural tube defects (NTDs). Women at high risk of having a fetus affected by an NTD, including those on antiepileptic medications, should supplement their diet with 4 g of folic acid per day. However, it has not been firmly established that folic acid reduces the rate of anticonvulsant-associated NTD.

Folic acid can decrease plasma levels of phenytoin. Therefore, serum anticonvulsant levels should be closely monitored throughout the pregnancy in women concurrently taking both folic acid and phenytoin.

9. Which anticonvulsants are safe during pregnancy?

Anticonvulsants in general should not be considered "safe" during pregnancy. Nevertheless, uncontrolled seizures are dangerous for both the woman and the fetus, supporting their judicious use when needed. Tailor the choice of medicine to the individual.

10. Are any anticonvulsants absolutely contraindicated during pregnancy?

Yes. Most physicians avoid trimethadione. "Trimethadione syndrome" consists of developmental delay, low-set ears, palate anomalies, irregular teeth, speech disturbances, and V-shaped eyebrows. Intrauterine growth retardation, short stature, cardiac anomalies, ocular defects, simian creases, hypospadias, and microcephaly are also often present. Up to two-thirds of exposed fetuses will manifest congenital defects. Because trimethadione is associated with a greater risk of anomalies compared with other anticonvulsants, its use should be abandoned.

11. What neonatal complications have been associated with phenytoin, phenobarbital, carbamazepine, and valproic acid?

- The fetal hydantoin (phenytoin) syndrome consists of various combinations of craniofacial and limb abnormalities. Because this pattern is also associated with other anticonvulsants, the combination of major anomalies, microcephaly, growth retardation, midface hypoplasia, and digital hypoplasia is also known as "anticonvulsant embryopathy."
- Although phenobarbital has been associated with some birth defects, its major risk is neonatal addiction and withdrawal syndrome.

- Carbamazepine used to be considered among the safest anticonvulsants for use during pregnancy. However, more recent data suggest that carbamazepine may be associated with an increased incidence of craniofacial defects, developmental delay, and neural tube defects.
- Valproic acid should be considered a human teratogen. It has been implicated in cardiac, orofacial, and limb abnormalities, but the major concern is with neural tube defects. When exposure occurs between 17 and 30 days after conception, the risk of an NTD is 1–2%. Women exposed during the critical period should be closely screened.

12. What are the recommendations regarding some of the newer anticonvulsants?

Felbamate, gabapentin, and lamotrigine are new anticonvulsant medications. There is little information regarding their use in pregnancy. Although their manufacturers have described these three medications as belonging to pregnancy category C, their routine use cannot be recommended without more supporting evidence.

13. With anticonvulsant therapy, what is the overall risk for congenital malformations?

In epileptic women on anticonvulsant medication, the risk of congenital anomalies is two to three times greater than that of the general population. However, it remains unclear whether this increased risk is due solely to the medications. It is possible that idiopathic epilepsy itself is associated with a risk of fetal anomalies. Accordingly, it also remains unclear whether epileptic women not on seizure medication are at increased risk of congenital malformations. It is known that seizure control with anticonvulsant monotherapy poses a lower risk than polypharmaceutic treatment.

14. Describe the role epoxide hydrolase plays in the development of congenital malformations.

Epoxide hydrolase is an enzyme within a metabolic pathway common to many anticonvulsant medications. Genetic heterogeneity within this enzyme can affect its overall efficacy. Homozygosity in the fetus for the genes producing lowered efficacy of this enzyme is associated with the highest development rate for features of congenital phenytoin syndrome.

15. What about hemorrhagic disease of the newborn?

Phenytoin, phenobarbital, and primidone may cause hemorrhagic disease of the newborn. The exact mechanism is unknown, but is related to vitamin K deficiency, which results in suppression of factors II, VII, IX, and X. Therefore, it is recommended that exposed infants receive vitamin K in the delivery room and be closely observed for signs of a clotting abnormality.

Carbemazepine and valproic acid are not associated with this effect.

16. Should a woman with seizures stop her medications when she becomes pregnant?

Stopping anticonvulsant therapy during the first trimester can result in uncontrolled seizures which may be more harmful to the fetus than the therapy. Some suggest a trial off anticonvulsants prior to pregnancy if the woman has been seizure-free for at least 2 years. Once successfully withdrawn from her medication, a woman may be followed expectantly during a pregnancy.

17. What is the risk of epilepsy in the child if a parent has seizures?

In general, the child has a 3% risk of epilepsy. The risk may be higher if the parental seizure etiology is unknown, the mother is the affected parent, or the child has febrile seizures.

18. Is breastfeeding contraindicated for women taking anticonvulsants?

No. Anticonvulsants are excreted minimally in breast milk and generally do not harm the infant. However, accumulation of phenobarbital (and primidone, which is metabolized to phenobarbital) can cause lethargy, poor feeding, and inadequate weight gain. If this occurs, bottle feeding may need to be substituted. Breastfeeding does not increase the frequency of seizures.

Note that felbamate, gabapentin, and lamotrigine are not recommended during lactation because of the paucity of evidence supporting their safety.

BIBLIOGRAPHY

1. Aminoff MJ: Neurologic disorders. In Creasy RK and Resnick R (eds): Maternal-Fetal Medicine, 4th ed. Philadelphia, W.B. Saunders Company, 1999, pp 1091–1095.
2. Briggs GG, Freeman RK, Yaffe SJ: Drugs in Pregnancy and Lactation, 5th ed. Philadelphia, Lipincott, Williams, and Wilkins, 1998.
3. Holmes LB, et al: The teratogenicity of anticonvulsant drugs. N Engl J Med 344:1132–1138, 2001.
4. Seizure disorders in pregnancy. ACOG Educational Bulletin 231. Washington DC, American College of Obstetricians and Gynecologists, 1996.
5. O'Brien TJ, Vadja FJ: Contemporary management of epilepsy in pregnancy. Aust N Z J Obstet Gynecol 40:413–415, 2000.
6. Yerby MS: Special considerations for women with epilepsy. Pharmacotherapy 20(8 Pt 2): 159S–170S, 2000.

42. CARDIOVASCULAR DISEASE IN PREGNANCY

Sally Segel, M.D.

1. What are the normal changes in cardiac physiology during pregnancy?

The normal physiologic changes of pregnancy include: increased blood volume, increased cardiac output, increased heart rate, and decreased blood pressure.

In general, maternal **blood volume** increases up to 50% above nonpregnant levels. Blood volume begins to increase in the first trimester and continues until approximately 32 weeks' gestation; it then remains constant until delivery. Maternal plasma volume increases by 50% while maternal red blood cell mass increases by 20%. This discrepancy is responsible for the dilutional anemia of pregnancy. The hormonal mechanisms responsible for this increase include: steroid hormones of pregnancy, increased plasma renin activity, and hyperaldosteronism.

Cardiac output begins to increase in the first trimester and peaks at 30–50% above nonpregnant levels by 20 weeks' gestation; it then remains constant until term. At 38–40 week's gestation, cardiac output decreases. This change is more pronounced in the supine position due to vena caval compression by the enlarged uterus. Early in pregnancy an increased stroke volume is responsible for the changes in cardiac output, while later in pregnancy an **increased heart rate** is responsible.

In a normal pregnancy there is a slight decrease in systolic **blood pressure** and a moderate decrease in diastolic. The nadir occurs in mid-trimester, and then there can be a slow increase to the patient's nonpregnant blood pressure.

2. What are the normal changes in cardiac physiology during labor and delivery?

During a uterine contraction, 300–500 cc of blood is shifted from the uterus to the maternal systemic circulation. As a result of this auto-transfusion, systemic venous pressure and right ventricular pressure increase. Maternal mean arterial pressure rises and is followed by a reflex bradycardia. Maternal pain and anxiety result in increased adrenaline, which increases maternal blood pressure and heart rate. Following delivery, vena caval compression is decreased and blood volume is increased. These changes cause a 10–20% increase in circulating cardiac output.

3. Describe the hemodymanic changes caused by regional anesthesia.

Both spinal and epidural anesthesia cause peripheral vasodilation. Peripheral vasodilation can cause a significant decrease in preload. The changes may produce a decrease in cardiac output and blood pressure. In an attempt to diminish the hemodynamic changes of regional anesthesia, most patients are hydrated prior to its administration.

4. What symptoms merit a cardiac evaluation during pregnancy?

During a normal pregnancy it is not unusual for women to experience fatigue, shortness of breath, orthopnea, and peripheral edema. However, progressive limitation of physical activity by shortness of breath, chest pain accompanying exercise or physical activity, and syncope preceded by palpitations or physical exertion should cause the physician to suspect an underlying cardiac condition.

5. How do you take care of a woman with a congenital ventricular or atrial septal defect (VSD, ASD)?

Women with an ASD and a left-to-right shunt usually do well in pregnancy. Peripheral vasodilation of pregnancy decreases the left to right shunt. A small percentage of women have paroxysmal atrial flutter, which recurs when the heart rate is difficult to control. The recommended treatment is catheter ablation—after completion of the pregnancy, since the procedure requires extensive radiation exposure. Women with these defects are not at risk for bacterial endocarditis and do not need antibiotic prophylaxis in labor.

Women with a VSD and a left-to-right shunt also do well in pregnancy. These patients are less prone to arrhythmia, but are at significant risk for bacterial endocarditis. As a result, they need antibiotic prophylaxis during labor and delivery.

6. What is Eisenmenger's syndrome?

A congenital communication between the pulmonary and systemic circulation causing increased pulmonary vascular resistance (PVR) either to the systemic level or greater than the systemic level. Once the PVR becomes greater than the systemic vascular resistance a right-to-left shunt develops along with significant pulmonary hypertension. The most common cause of Eisenmenger's syndrome is a large ventricular septal defect.

7. What are the risks to a pregnant women with Eisenmenger's syndrome?

Women with Eisenmenger's syndrome have a mortality rate of 50%, a fetal mortality rate of 50%, and a preterm delivery rate of 85%. Sudden death can occur at any time; however, the risk is greatest during labor and delivery and the early postpartum period.

Women with Eisenmenger's syndrome have a high PVR. Management during pregnancy revolves around maintaining pulmonary blood flow. Antenatal care centers on limitation of physical activity, oxygen therapy, and possibly pulmonary vasodilators. Delivery should be planned with central hemodynamic monitoring. It is crucial to maintain preload; therefore, these pregnant women should have an assisted second stage. Cesarean section is reserved for obstetric indications. Despite meticulous care, the mortality rate remains significant, approaching 50%.

8. What is the leading cause of mitral stenosis?

Rheumatic fever is the leading cause of this condition. Congenital mitral stenosis (Lutenbacher syndrome) is very rare.

9. What is the pathophysiology of mitral stenosis?

Mitral stenosis impedes the flow of blood from the left atrium to the left ventricle during diastole. These patients normally have a fixed cardiac output. As stenosis worsens, there can be dilation of the left atrium and pulmonary congestion. Normally the mitral valve area is 4–5 cm^2. When the valve area is ≤ 2.5 cm^2, a women experiences symptoms with exertion, and when the valve area is ≤ 1.5 cm^2, a women experiences symptoms at rest.

During pregnancy, the increased blood volume increases venous return. Increased preload in a women with mitral stenosis causes pulmonary congestion instead of increased cardiac output. In addition, tachycardia of pregnancy shortens diastole and decreases left ventricular filling—and, therefore, cardiac output.

10. How are patients with mitral stenosis managed during pregnancy, labor, and delivery?

In the antepartum period, management focuses on maintaining cardiac output while decreasing pulmonary congestion. This balance is achieved with diuretics and beta-blocker therapy. Good pain control is important during labor and delivery to reduce the maternal heart rate and increase diastole. Patients should be given antibiotic prophylaxis for bacterial endocarditis. In addition, most women cannot tolerate the second stage due to a decreased preload with pushing. As a result, an operative vaginal delivery is necessary. Finally, the postpartum auto-transfusion can produce massive pulmonary edema in a woman with mitral stenosis. Immediate and aggressive diuresis postpartum can significantly decrease this complication.

11. Describe the pathophysiology of aortic stenosis.

The majority of aortic stenosis is a combination of congenital lesions and rheumatic fever. The normal aortic valve area is 3–4 cm^2. Aortic stenosis becomes significant when the valve area is ≤ 1 cm^2. As stenosis progresses, the left ventricle initially hypertrophies in response to the increased pressure gradient. Eventually the left ventricle dilates. A patient will present with angina, near-syncope/syncope, and congestive heart failure.

12. How is a patient with aortic stenosis managed during pregnancy, labor, and delivery?

Women with aortic stenosis have a fixed cardiac output. It is essential that their preload be maintained during pregnancy, labor, and delivery. Any hypotension can cause sudden death, and women with a valve gradient > 100 mmHg are at greatest risk. During labor and delivery, women with severe disease may require central hemodynamic monitoring. In addition, regional anesthesia should be used with caution because of the risks for hypotension. These women cannot tolerate the second stage due to a decreased preload with pushing, and an operative vaginal delivery is necessary. Postpartum blood loss can also significantly reduce preload, and volume resuscitation with fluid or blood may be necessary. Finally, patients should be given antibiotic prophylaxis for bacterial endocarditis.

13. What are the management issues for a women with primary pulmonary hypertension?

Women with severe pulmonary hypertension have an obstruction to right ventricular outflow. The major physiologic concern is maintenance of pulmonary blood flow. Anything that decreases preload decreases pulmonary blood flow. Antenatal care revolves around limitation of physical activity, oxygen therapy, and possibly pulmonary vasodilators. Despite meticulous care, the mortality rate remains significant, approaching 50%. *Women with this condition should be strongly advised against pregnancy.*

14. What is Marfan syndrome?

Marfan syndrome is an autosomal dominant genetic disorder with a prevalence of 4–6/10,000. An abnormal fibrillin gene on chromosome 15 causes the disease. Abnormal fibrillin causes connective tissue abnormalities all over the body, the most significant being aortic root dilation, optic lens dislocation, long limbs, scoliosis, and joint laxity. These patients have an increased mortality from aortic dissection or rupture.

15. What is the optimum management for pregnant women with Marfan syndrome?

Women with an aortic root < 4 cm can attempt pregnancy with a modest risk. Women with an aortic root > 5.5 cm should have aortic graft and aortic valve replacement prior to attempting pregnancy.

Women with an aortic root 4.0–5.5 cm have the greatest risk during pregnancy because cardiac surgery is premature. During pregnancy, beta blockade should be used to protect the aortic root from the increased hemodynamic forces of pregnancy. The goal is to maintain a resting pulse of 70 bpm. Follow the aortic root with sequential echocardiograms.

During labor and delivery, women with an aortic root < 4 cm can have a vaginal delivery with prevention of tachycardia. In women with dilated aortic roots, the delivery management is controversial. Some authorities recommend a cesarean delivery to minimize the increased pressures that occur during pregnancy. At the present there is no data to support or refute this delivery plan.

16. What are the diagnostic criteria for peripartum cardiomyopathy?

- Heart failure within the last month of pregnancy or 5 months postpartum
- Absence of prior heart disease
- No determinable cause
- Echocardiographic indication of left ventricular dysfunction: ejection fraction < 45%, fractional shortening < 30%, or left ventricular end-diastolic dimension > 2.7cm/m^2.

17. What is the treatment of peripartum cardiomyopathy?

Women with peripartum cardiomyopathy should be treated with diuretics and afterload reduction. If a patient is pregnant, use hydralazine as the afterload-reducing medication; if the patient is postpartum, an ACE inhibitor is preferred.

18. What is the prognosis for women with peripartum cardiomyopathy?

Women with peripartum cardiomyopathy whose left ventricular (LV) size and function remain abnormal 6 months after delivery have a 5-year mortality of 50–85%. These women should be counseled against subsequent pregnancies.

Women whose LV size and function normalize within 6 months of delivery have a greatly reduced 5-year mortality. However, they also have a 25% recurrence rate during a subsequent pregnancy.

BIBLIOGRAPHY

1. Easterling TR, Otto C: Heart disease. In Gabbe SG, Niebyl JR, Simpson JL (eds): Obstetrics—Normal and Problem Pregnancies, 4th ed. New York, Churchill Livingstone, 2002.
2. Pearson GD, Veille JC, Rahimtoola S, et al: Peripartum Cardiomyopathy. National Heart, Lung, and Blood Institute and Office of Rare Diseases (National Institutes of Health) Workshop Recommendations and Review. JAMA 283:1183–1188, 2000.
3. Shabetai R: Cardiac diseases. In Creasy R, Resnik R (eds): Maternal Fetal Medicine, 4th ed. Philadelphia, W.B. Saunders, 1999.

43. PULMONARY DISEASE IN PREGNANCY

Harish M. Sehdev, M.D.

1. Describe how pregnancy changes pulmonary mechanics.

In normal pregnancy, the shape of the thoracic cage is changed. The diaphragm is displaced superiorly (up to 4 cm); the transverse diameter of the chest increases (up to 2 cm); and the overall chest circumference increases 5–7 cm. As a result of these changes, there is an increase in the subcostal angle.

2. How does pregnancy change lung volumes and pulmonary physiology?

Tidal volume increases 30–40% while expiratory reserve volume decreases about 20%. Vital capacity, inspiratory reserve volume, and respiratory rate remain essentially stable. Overall lung volume is decreased (5%) due to elevation of the diaphragm. Residual capacity is also reduced, approximately 20%. Inspiratory capacity increases slightly. Large airway function is preserved as suggested by stable airflow measurements (forced expiratory volume in 1 second and and forced vital capacity).

3. Describe the pulmonary changes in gas exchange associated with pregnancy.

Pregnancy is associated with an increase in oxygen consumption (up to 30%) and increase in minute ventilation (30–40%). Pregnancy is associated with an increase in arterial oxygen levels and a decrease in arterial carbon dioxide ($PaCO_2$) levels. $PaCO_2$ decreases from 40 mmHg (nonpregnant) to 27–32 mmHg (last half of pregnancy), and this important change aids in the transfer of CO_2 from the fetal to the maternal circulation. Despite the fall in maternal $PaCO_2$, maternal arterial pH is maintained by an increase in renal excretion of bicarbonate, which leads to a lower maternal serum bicarbonate concentration.

4. What is dyspnea of pregnancy?

Most pregnant women (up to 70%) complain of dsypnea. Progesterone levels are increased in pregnancy, and progesterone appears to stimulate the respiratory center. While the exact etiology is unknown, the combination of increased progesterone levels and decreased $PaCO_2$ may play a role in this sensation. Despite this being a common complaint, it is important to evaluate the patient for pathologic causes of dyspnea.

5. Does pregnancy affect asthma?

Asthma, which affects about 1% of all pregnancies, is the most common obstructive disease encountered during pregnancy. Approximately 10% of those with asthma have exacerbations requiring admission. Recent information suggests that during pregnancy up to 70% of patients with asthma show improvement, approximately 20% show no change, and up to 10% experience worsening symptoms. Evidence suggests that in adolescents with asthma, those who become pregnant experience a higher percentage of exacerbations, and over 50% may require systemic steroids. Noncompliance with treatment and respiratory tract infections are factors associated with asthma flares.

6. Does asthma affect pregnancy?

The evidence concerning an increase in adverse perinatal outcome in patients with asthma is conflicting. A recent case-control study revealed that perinatal mortality is *not* affected in well-controlled and actively managed asthmatics.

7. How should the pregnant asthmatic be treated?

The goals of therapy in pregnant asthmatics include adequate oxygenation for both mother and fetus and reduction of attacks (including prevention of status asthmaticus). In general, asthmatic patients should follow their peak flow measurements and seek therapy, or make additions to their therapy, when their peak flow falls below 80% of baseline measures. Over the last few years, the treatment of asthma in pregnancy has changed. There is less reliance on the use of aminophylline. Pregnancy usually requires an increase in the dose of aminophylline, and toxicity is exhibited with nausea, vomiting, and even cardiac arrhythmias.

The main therapy for asthma in pregnancy, as well as in those who are not pregnant, is inhaled **β-agonists** (bronchodilator), either on a scheduled or as-needed basis. Inhaled **steroids** can also be used with β-agonists. **Cromolyn** (prevents mast cell degranulation) can also be used in pregnancy, although it typically is not used alone. If these agents are not adequate, systemic steroids (those with less mineralocorticoid activity, such as prednisone or methylprednisolone), either orally or parentally, may be used. As for safety in pregnancy, these medications do not appear to increase the risk of fetal malformations. Use of systemic steroids rarely causes fetal adrenal suppression, given that only 10–30% of the maternal dose enters the fetal compartment because of degradation by placental hormones. In general, if a patient has taken systemic steroids during the course of the pregnancy, she should receive intravenous steroids during labor and for up to 24 hours after delivery.

Some **prostaglandins** can increase airway resistance. Therefore, they should be used judiciously in a pregnant patient with asthma.

8. How should status asthmaticus be treated in pregnancy?

Status asthmaticus is a severe asthma exacerbation in which oxygenation becomes difficult despite therapy. Patients with this complication require immediate attention, and in general care is the same as in nonpregnant patients with status asthmaticus. Therapy includes humidified oxygen (30–40%), nebulized β-agonists, subcutaneous catecholamines (either epinephrine or terbutaline), and intravenous steroids if the patient does not respond to subcutaneous catecholamines. If the patient does not respond with these measures, and it is difficult to maintain adequate oxygenation, intubation becomes necessary. During treatment, fetal monitoring should be used (if the patient is more than 24 weeks pregnant) as well as assessment of maternal oxygenation to guide effectiveness of therapy.

9. Does pregnancy increase the risk for pulmonary embolism?

Compared to nonpregnant women, the risk of thromboembolism in pregnancy is increased approximately 5 fold. Between 0.5 and 3 of every 1000 pregnancies is complicated by symptomatic venous thrombosis. If untreated, up to 25% develop a pulmonary embolism, of which up to 15% are fatal. Pulmonary embolism remains a leading cause of maternal mortality in the United States and worldwide. Pregnancy increases the risk for thrombosis because of an increase in many clotting factors. Up to 50% of women who develop a thrombosis have an acquired or congenital thrombophilia (5% carry the factor V Leiden mutation, and 2% carry the prothrombin gene mutation G20210A).

10. How is a thromboembolic disease diagnosed?

Patients can present with tachypnea, tachycardia, shortness of breath, and/or chest pain. Physical exam may reveal a pleural rub, and there may be apparent EKG abnormalities. Chest x-ray often is unremarkable, and there usually is a decrease in PO_2 on an arterial blood gas. Studies used to make the diagnosis include impedence plethysmography (positive predictive value 83%), Doppler ultrasound with compression (positive predictive value 93%), and even magnetic resonance imaging. To diagnosis a pulmonary embolism, a ventilation and perfusion (V/Q) scan (radiation dose to the fetus of less than .05 rads) can be used if the chest x-ray is normal. If necessary, selective pulmonary angiography should be performed. In experienced hands and with abdominal shielding, the radiation exposure to the fetus approaches that of a V/Q scan.

11. How should thromboembolic disease in pregnancy be treated?

Anticoagulation is the recommended treatment for thromboembolic disease. As in nonpregnant patients, therapy is initiated with heparin. However, because coumadin crosses the placenta and causes embryo toxicity and malformations, heparin is continued after initial therapeutic anticoagulation. Anticoagulation is continued throughout the pregnancy and for up to 3 months post partum. Heparin is associated with decreased bone mineralization, and therefore patients should be treated with additional calcium supplementation. Furthermore, some patients can experience heparin-induced thrombocytopenia.

Experience is accumulating on the use of low-molecular-weight heparin in pregnancy. It is associated with fewer side effects than heparin and can be used with once or twice a day dosing. However, it is more expensive and should be considered when a patient has a complication with heparin.

12. What organisms are associated with pneumonia in pregnancy?

Streptococcus pneumoniae is the most common organism associated with bacterial pneumonia in pregnancy. Other causative bacterial organisms include *Hemophilus influenzae* and *Klebsiella pneumoniae*. Other causative agents include influenza A, varicella, and mycoplasma. Pregnant women with pneumonia, especially those with other medical comorbidities, are at greater risk for intubation, other maternal complications, and preterm delivery. Pregnant patients with varicella pneumonia have a significantly increased risk of mortality and of adverse perinatal outcome compared to nonpregnant patients with varicella pneumonia.

13. How is tuberculosis diagnosed in pregnancy?

Mycobacterium tuberculosis is an acid-fast bacillus that causes the pulmonary infection tuberculosis. Recently, tuberculosis has been increasing in the U.S., especially in urban areas, due to increased immigration from developing nations. Patients at risk should be screened by skin testing with a purified protein derivative (PPD). Most women with tuberculosis are asymptomatic, and active disease will develop in less than 10% of those with a positive PPD who are not immunocompromised. Patients who have received vaccination with bacillus Calmette-Guérin will have a positive PPD. If the diagnosis is suspected, a chest x-ray with abdominal shielding should be performed. Definitive diagnosis is made by sputum culture for *M. tuberculosis* or specific staining. Culture is extremely important given the increase in resistant strains of *M. tuberculosis*.

14. Describe the treatment of tuberculosis in pregnancy.

Pregnancy does not affect the course of tuberculosis, and adequate treatment does not appear to adversely affect pregnancy outcome. If the diagnosis is confirmed, treatment should be initiated during pregnancy with isoniazid and rifampin. Isoniazid treatment should be given in conjunction with pyridoxine to decrease the risk of peripheral neuropathy. Furthermore, liver function tests should be followed, as liver transaminases will elevate in up to 20% of patients.

Prophylaxis for women with a newly positive PPD during pregnancy is controversial. Treatment may be delayed until the postpartum period. The risk of congenital tuberculosis is small, and perinatal infections can be reduced with treatment of the newborn for the duration of maternal treatment.

15. What is sarcoidosis? Is it a contraindication to pregnancy?

Sarcoidosis is a noncaseating granulomatous disease of unknown etiology. It is diagnosed most commonly in the third and fourth decade of life and can affect the lungs, heart, lymph nodes, skin, central nervous system, liver, and eyes. It is usually diagnosed on routine chest x-ray in asymptomatic patients and requires biopsy to make the diagnosis.

Sarcoidosis occurs in approximately 0.05% of all pregnancies, and it does not appear to adversely affect pregnancy or be affected by pregnancy. Most pregnant women with sarcoidosis experience improvement in their symptoms, but relapses can occur in the postpartum period. When patients with sarcoidosis become pregnant, they should be screened for hepatic and renal involvement. Steroids are used for progression of pulmonary complications related to sarcoidosis.

16. What is cystic fibrosis? Can women with cystic fibrosis consider pregnancy?

Cystic fibrosis is an autosomal recessive disease that affects mucous glands in the respiratory, digestive, and reproductive tracts. Old data concerning pregnancy in women with cystic fibrosis reported a high maternal mortality rate and perinatal mortality rate. However, with careful management by a team including a perinatologist, a pulmonologist, a cardiologist, and a nutritionist, successful pregnancy can be realized in women with cystic fibrosis.

Women with cystic fibrosis are at greater risk for pulmonary infections and must have their pulmonary and cardiac status assessed constantly throughout gestation for evidence of deterioration. Given pancreatic dysfunction and malabsorption in these patients, special attention needs to be given to their nutritional status. There is a greater risk for intrauterine growth restriction.

17. What is an amniotic fluid embolism?

Fortunately, amniotic fluid embolism is a rare complication of pregnancy. It is an unpredictable event with no clear risk factors that cannot be prevented. While it most commonly occurs during labor, it can occur at any time during gestation (including after a second-trimester abortion) and up to 48 hours post partum. Amniotic fluid embolism presents with cardiovascular collapse, and a significant portion of patients have seizures at the time of presentation. Cardiovasular compromise probably arises from pulmonary vasculature obstruction, and with resulting inflammatory reactions, disseminated intravascular coagulation can develop.

18. Describe the treatment of amniotic fluid embolism.

Care is supportive, with initial attention paid to stabilize maternal oxygenation and hemodynamic function. Anemia and coagulation abnormalities are corrected with appropriate transfusion. The fetal status should be assessed, as the timing and manner of fetus delivery could compromise maternal resuscitation. Maternal mortality is approximately 50%. Even if the mother survives, neurologic status may be adversely affected from the initial hypoxia, hypotension, and seizure activity.

Diagnosis can be confirmed at autopsy with the finding of fetal squamous cells in the pulmonary vasculature. However, this finding is neither specific nor sensitive.

BIBLIOGRAPHY

1. Clark SC: New concepts of amniotic fluid embolism: A review. Obstet Gynecol Survey 45:360–368, 1990.
2. Elkus R, Popovich J Jr: Respiratory physiology in pregnancy. Clin Chest Med 13:555–565, 1992.
3. Ginsberg JS: Management of venous thromboembolism. N Engl J Med 335:1816–1828, 1996.
4. Grandone E, Margaglione M, Colaizzo D, et al: Genetic susceptibility in pregnancy-related thromboembolism: Roles of factor V Leiden, prothrombin G20210A, and methylenetetrahydrofolate reductase C577T mutations. Am J Obstet Gynecol 176:1324–1328, 1998.
5. Haake DA, Zakowski PC, Haake DL, Bryson YJ: Early treatment with acyclovir for varicella pneumonia in otherwise healthy adults: A retrospective controlled study and review. Rev Infect Dis 12:788–798, 1990.
6. Haynes de Regt R: Sarcoidosis and pregnancy. Obstet Gynecol 70:369–372, 1987.
7. McColgin SW, Glee L, Brian BA: Pulmonary disorders complicating pregnancy. Obstet Cynecol Clin North Am 19:697–717, 1992.
8. Moore-Gillon J: Asthma in pregnancy. Br J Obstet Gynaecol 101:658–660, 1994.
9. Schatz M, Zeiger RS, Hoffman CP: Perinatal outcomes in the pregnancies of asthmatic women: A prospective controlled analysis. Am J Resp Crit Care Med 151:1170–1174, 1995.
10. Toglia MR, Weg JG: Venous thromboembolism during pregnancy. N Engl J Med 335:108–114, 1996.
11. White RJ, Coutts II, Gibbs CJ, MacIntyre C: A prospective study of asthma in pregnancy and the puerperium. Respir Med 83:103–106, 1989.
12. Working Group on Asthma in Pregnancy: Management of Asthma during Pregnancy. NIH Publication no. 93-3279, September 1993.

44. RENAL DISEASE IN PREGNANCY

Harish M. Sehdev, M.D.

1. What are the normal changes in the anatomy of the urinary system associated with pregnancy?

During normal pregnancy, the kidneys enlarge approximately 1 cm in length, with the right kidney enlarging slightly more than the left kidney. By the second month of pregnancy, the renal pelvis and ureters also begin to increase is size. Again, the right side tends to enlarge greater than the left. The ureters increase in diameter (above the pelvic brim) by as much as 2 cm, while the right and left renal pelvis dilates on average 15 mm and 5 mm, respectively.

The reason for the overall dilation appears to be related to both mechanical obstruction by the growing uterus and smooth muscle relaxation from increasing progesterone levels. Such expansion affects interpretation of urologic studies and increases the incidence of asymptomatic bacteriuria and pyelonephritis.

2. In normal pregnancy, what changes occur in renal hemodynamics?

In pregnancy, dramatic changes occur with respect to both renal plasma flow and glomerular filtration. By the second trimester, renal plasma flow increases approximately 75% above baseline, and then decreases by the end of the third trimester. The glomerular filtration rate is increased almost 50% by the end of the first trimester, and this rate is maintained throughout gestation. Glomerular filtration is clinically assessed by creatinine clearance, and because creatinine is also secreted by the renal tubules, the actual glomerular filtration rate is less than the measured creatinine clearance. The overall effect of the increase in both renal plasma flow and glomerular filtration rate causes a decrease in the filtration fraction until the third trimester, when renal plasma flow falls slightly.

3. What are the effects on serum chemistry measurements resulting from the altered renal hemodynamics?

Both serum creatinine and blood urea nitrogen levels decrease approximately 25% from non-pregnant levels as a result of the increased glomerular filtration rate. By mid pregnancy, serum uric levels are decreased approximately 50%, but increase to normal levels by the third trimester as renal tubular resorption increases.

4. In pregnancy, is glucosuria an abnormal finding?

No. More glucose is excreted through the glomeruli because of the increased glomerular filtration. The reabsorptive capacity of the renal tubules can be exceeded, and therefore it is normal for most pregnant women to excrete up to 10 grams of glucose a day. If glucosuria is detected, the patient should be screened for diabetes if she has risk factors, or if she had no risk factors but has not been previously screened.

While urinary protein loss should not increase, excretion of amino acids, vitamin B_{12}, and folate is increased.

5. How is sodium balance maintained in normal pregnancy?

In normal pregnancy, plasma osmolality is decreased approximately 10 mOsm/kg H_2O due to a decrease in the concentration of sodium. Despite the decreased serum concentration, there is an overall increase of almost 1000 mEq of sodium in the maternal intravascular and interstitial fluids, fetus, and placenta. Sodium loss is increased by the elevated glomerular filtration rate and by progesterone (promotes natriuresis). This is offset by a dramatic increase in renal tubular reabsorption of sodium, which is due to a dramatic increase in levels of the hormones aldosterone, deoxycortisone, and estrogen. Furthermore, angiotensinogen (renin substrate), angiotensin, and renin (the proteolytic enzyme that converts angiotensinogen to angiotensin I) levels jump, as well. The increase in these latter hormones aids in the increased production of aldosterone, which prevents sodium diuresis.

Angiotensin II, a product of angiotensin I, is a potent vasoconstrictor. In normal pregnancy, sensitivity to the vasopressor effect of angiotensin II is reduced. It is believed that increased production of uterine and placental prostaglandins, namely prostacyclin, plays an important role in blunting the normal vasoconstrictor effects of angiotensin II. It is also believed that pregnancies that do not exhibit the normal decreased sensitivity to angiotensin II are at greater risk for developing preeclampsia.

6. Are pregnant women at greater risk for developing pyelonephritis?

Yes. Pyelonephritis occurs in approximately 1–2% of all pregnancies, and it is the most common reason for nonobstetric admission during pregnancy. It is also a risk factor for increased maternal morbidity and adverse perinatal outcome. Pregnant women are at greater risk for developing asymptomatic bacteriuria, most commonly *Escherichia coli*. If untreated, up to 40% of women with asymptomatic bacteriuria will develop symptomatic urinary tract infections (UTIs), cystitis and pyelonephritis.

The etiology for the increase in UTIs includes anatomic changes, increased progesterone levels, and increased glucose and amino acid levels in urine. Screening of all pregnant patients for asymptomatic bacteriuria can reduce the risk of symptomatic infections by approximately 70%, and should be done routinely at the first prenatal visit.

7. Does pregnancy increase the incidence of urolithiasis?

No. Urolithiasis affects less than 1 in 2000 pregnancies, and pregnancy does not appear to increase the incidence. The diagnosis can be made by urine microscopy, by straining urine for the presence of stones, and by ultrasound. If a patient is diagnosed with urolithiasis, consider measuring serum phosphorous and calcium levels to evaluate for hyperparathyroidism.

8. How can chronic renal disease be diagnosed in pregnancy?

In many cases, obstetricians may make the initial diagnosis of chronic renal disease in patients without other medical conditions. In general, renal disease may be silent in early stages. At a patient's first prenatal visit, a urine analysis is performed, and the presence of glucose, protein, or casts should prompt an evaluation. A 24-hour urine collection for creatinine clearance and total protein should be done on patients with greater than trace protein on urine dip-stick analysis (and no UTI). In normal pregnancy, total protein excretion should be less than 0.3 grams per day. Creatinine clearance can decrease by almost 70% before there is an increase in serum blood urea nitrogen or creatinine.

9. What are the effects of pregnancy on chronic renal disease?

In general, the long-term effects of pregnancy on renal disease are unclear. Creatinine clearance will still increase in patients with baseline dysfunction. As pregnancy nears completion, creatinine clearance decreases in those with underlying renal disease, and this fall reverses after delivery. In patients with mild renal disease (serum creatinine < 1.4 mg/dl), pregnancy should not cause a worsening of renal function, but these patients are at greater risk for pyelonephritis. Patients with moderate to severe renal insufficiency (serum creatinine > 1.4 mg/dl and 2.5 mg/dl, respectively) can experience deterioration of renal function that may not improve after delivery.

Comorbid conditions such as hypertension and diabetes can also increase the risk for irreversible renal function with pregnancy. Hypertension should be controlled above levels of 160 mmHg systolic and 110 mmHg diastolic. These patients are at high risk for developing complications from their hypertension—aside from worsening renal disease and superimposed preeclampsia. Worsening proteinuria is common, and this can make the diagnosis of superimposed preeclampsia difficult.

10. What are the effects of chronic renal disease on pregnancy outcome?

In general, patients with renal insufficiency are at greater risk for miscarriage, intrauterine growth restriction, preeclampsia, and preterm delivery (both spontaneous and iatrogenic, due to preeclampsia). Perinatal mortality has decreased as a result of advances in neonatal care, maternal administration of antenatal steroids, and increased antepartum surveillance, but it is still significantly increased in patients with moderate to severe renal dysfunction.

11. In the nondiabetic gravida, what is the most common cause of nephrotic syndrome?

Etiologies for nephrotic syndrome (> 3.5 grams protein/24 hours) include diabetes, systemic lupus erythematosus, minimal change disease, membranous glomerulonephritis, and membranoproliferative glomerulonephritis. Some of these diseases respond to steroids, and therefore when significant proteinuria is documented, it is important to identify the etiology. Pregnancy outcome depends on the etiology of the proteinuria, the presence of other medical conditions such as hypertension, and the gestational age at diagnosis.

The most common etiology for nephrotic-range proteinuria remains preeclampsia, and again, pregnancy outcome depends on gestational age at presentation as well as the presence of other manifestations of severe preeclampsia (pulmonary edema, liver function abnormalities, oliguria, fetal growth restriction, and coagulopathy).

12. Can women requiring dialysis therapy conceive?

Women with chronic renal failure usually have oligomenorrhea, and therefore have significantly decreased fertility. If they do become pregnant, they usually require more frequent and longer dialysis sessions. Hemodialysis can cause significant fluid shifts, and fetal monitoring should be used when fetal viability is attained. Treat anemia with transfusion and erythropoietin. Patients on dialysis have a significantly increased risk of miscarriage, fetal demise, fetal growth restriction, and preterm delivery. There is some evidence that patients on peritoneal dialysis may have better outcomes with fewer complications than those receiving hemodialysis.

13. Should women who have had renal transplantation and become pregnant stop or change their medication regimen?

Many women who experienced oligomenorrhea with chronic renal disease regain fertility as renal function improves after renal transplantation. Immunosuppressive medications (steroids, azathioprine, and cyclosporine) should *not* be stopped after conception. The rate of fetal malformations does not appear to be increased. Azathioprine and cyclosporine can be associated with fetal growth restriction. While there may be some maternal and fetal side effects to these medications, these risks must be weighed against the risk of rejection.

14. What are the risks in pregnancy for women who have had renal transplantation?

The risk for allograft rejection in pregnancy is about 9%, no different than in nonpregnant women. Making the diagnosis of rejection can be difficult in the pregnant patient. Pregnancies in women with renal transplantation are at greater risk for preeclampsia (approximately 30%), fetal growth restriction (approximately 20%), spontaneous abortion, fetal death, and preterm delivery (up to 45%). Because the kidney is denervated, pain may not be experienced when pyelonephritis is present. Women should be screened frequently for urinary tract colonization and infection, and treated appropriately. In late pregnancy, renal function may decrease in up to 15% of patients.

In general, it is recommended that women defer conception for 1 year after receiving a transplant from a living donor and 2 years after a cadaveric transplant.

15. Does pregnancy adversely affect women with adult polycystic kidney disease?

Adult polycystic kidney disease is an autosomal dominant disorder with an incidence of 1 in 400 to 1000 that usually presents in the fourth or fifth decade of life. The disease is associated with hypertension, and pregnancy could worsen the hypertension. In general, pregnancy does not appear to worsen the course of this disease.

BIBLIOGRAPHY

1. Cunningham FG, Cox SG, Harstad TW, et al: Chronic renal disease and pregnancy outcome. Am J Obstet Gynecol 163:453–459, 1990.
2. Davidson J: Changes in renal function and other aspects of homeostasis in early pregnancy. J Obstet Gynaecol Br Commonw 81:1003–1008, 1974.
3. Davison JM: Renal transplantation and pregnancy. Am J Kidney Dis: 374–380, 1987.
4. Gilstrap LC, Leveno KG, Cunningham FG, et al: Renal infection and pregnancy outcome. Am J Obstet Gynecol 141:709–716, 1981.
5. Harris R, Dunnihoo DR: The incidence and significance of urinary calculi in pregnancy. Am J Obstet Gynecol 99:237–241, 1967.
6. Hou S, Orlowski J, Pahl M, et al: Pregnancy in women with end-stage renal disease: Treatment of anemia and premature labor. Am J Kidney Dis 21:16–22, 1993.
7. Imbasciati E, Ponticelli C: Pregnancy and renal disease: Predictors for fetal and maternal outcome. Am J Nephrol 11:353–362, 1991.
8. Lindheimer MD, Katz AI: Pregnancy in the renal transplant patient. Am J Kidney Dis 19:173–176, 1992.
9. Redrow M, Cheron L, Elliot J, et al: Dialysis in the management of pregnany patients with renal insufficiency. Medicine 67:199–208, 1988.
10. Settler RW, Cunningham FG: Natural history of chronic proteinuria complicating pregnancy. Am J Obstet Gynecol 167:1219–1224, 1992.
11. Surian M, Imbasciati E, Banfi G, et al: Glomerular disease and pregnancy. Neprhon 36:101–105, 1984.

45. INFECTIONS DURING PREGNANCY

Thomas J. Bader, M.D.

1. Are pregnant women immunocompromised?

Pregnancy presents a unique immunologic situation in which two individuals with different genetic make-ups coexist with no deleterious immune response. However, this is not accomplished through immunosuppression of the mother. All objective measures of maternal immunocompetence show little or no change with pregnancy. Infections (e.g., pneumonia, pyelonephritis) may be more severe in pregnancy, but this is due to anatomic and physiologic changes associated with pregnancy, not a poorly functioning immune system.

2. Why are infections in pregnancy important?

Infections during pregnancy are important for two reasons. Some infections can cause significant maternal morbidity or even mortality (e.g., pneumococcal pneumonia). This is obviously deleterious to the mother and can indirectly harm the fetus. Other infections may be of little or no clinical significance to the mother but can harm the fetus through fetal or placental infection (e.g., toxoplasmosis).

3. What neonatal conditions are caused by group B streptococcus? How can they be prevented?

Group B strep can lead to two different clinical entities in the neonate: **early-onset infection** (characterized by septicemia) and **late-onset disease** (usually meningitis). Both of these infections occur more commonly in preterm infants, but they can affect term newborns.

A variety of prevention strategies featuring screening cultures and antibiotic regimens have been advocated. Currently there are **two strategies** that have the support of the American College of Obstetricians and Gynecologists, the American Academy of Pediatrics, and the Centers for Disease Control and Prevention:

(1) Screen all pregnant women between 35 and 37 weeks' gestation and to treat those women with positive cultures with ampicillin or penicillin in labor.

(2) The second strategy omits screening cultures and relies instead on identifying women with risk factors for neonatal infection. These risk factors are: preterm (< 37 weeks) delivery, rupture of membranes for more than 18 hours, interpartum fever (≥ 38°C), or a prior child affected with group B strep. In addition, both strategies treat all women with a history of group B strep bacteruria as these women tend to have persistent high colony counts. Both strategies effectively reduce—but do not eliminate—the risk of neonatal disease.

4. Which common genital infections are implicated in preterm birth?

Bacterial vaginosis has been associated with preterm birth, and treatment of bacterial vaginosis in high-risk women has been shown in some studies to reduce the incidence of preterm birth. Other genital infections, such as Trichomonas, gonorrhea and Chlamydia, have been inconsistently associated with preterm premature rupture of membranes and/or preterm delivery.

5. What are examples of infections with minimal maternal effects but the potential for significant fetal compromise?

Parvovirus infection, cytomegalovirus infection and toxoplasmosis.

6. What maternal and fetal effects are caused by parvovirus?

Parvovirus infection, also known as fifth disease, is a relatively common infection which is usually asymptomatic or mildly symptomatic in adults. Most infections of pregnant women occur following exposure to infected children. Although the effect on the mother is insignificant, parvovirus can infect the fetus and lead to anemia with subsequent fetal hydrops and even death. The diagnosis is made by serial maternal serologies. If fetal infection is likely and ultrasound shows fetal hydrops, in utero transfusion may be necessary.

7. How does cytomegalovirus affect the fetus?

Cytomegalovirus is a common pathogen. The majority of adults have detectable antibodies demonstrating prior exposure. Unfortunately, prior infection and the development of antibodies doesn't provide protection from subsequent infections. Given this lack of protection and the ubiquitous nature of the organism, infections during pregnancy are not uncommon. The mother is asymptomatic or mildly symptomatic. The fetus, however, can suffer severe effects involving the nervous system. Fetal growth restriction can also occur as a result of in utero cytomegalovirus infection.

8. Should pregnant women be screened for antibodies to cytomegalovirus?

No. Most women have antibodies, and antibodies detected during screening almost always represent prior disease, which poses no risk to the mother or fetus. Moreover, the presence of antibodies does not provide immunity against future infection. Even in cases of suspected acute maternal infection, antibody titers are of limited value.

9. What is the significance of toxoplasmosis in pregnancy?

Toxoplasma gondii is a parasite that is transmitted by ingestion of infected meat or exposure to infected cat feces. In immunocompetent adults, the infection is inconsequential. If maternal infection occurs during pregnancy, however, fetal infection can occur. The later in pregnancy the maternal infection occurs, the more likely the infection will pass to the fetus. Conversely it is fetal infections that occur early in gestation that are most likely to cause fetal sequelae. There is a wide range of fetal effects from toxoplasmosis, including subclinical disease, growth retardation, and severe effects on multiple systems including the central nervous system (CNS). If the diagnosis is made antenatally, antiparasitic therapy can be initiated to prevent sequelae.

Prior maternal exposure to *T. gondii* provides protection against fetal infection. Simple preventative steps should be emphasized to all pregnant women. These include avoiding cat litter, proper handwashing before handling food, and avoiding poorly prepared meat.

10. Does maternal varicella infection pose risks during pregnancy? What about herpes zoster?

Acute varicella infection (or chicken pox) and herpes zoster (or shingles) are both caused by the varicella-zoster virus. The initial infection with the virus causes varicella usually involving the skin alone. Subsequent re-activation of the dormant virus can lead to zoster usually affecting a single, unilateral dermatome.

Acute maternal varicella infection can be a severe illness for both the mother and the fetus. Adults generally suffer greater morbidity from varicella infection than do children or adolescents. Pneumonia in particular poses a risk to maternal health. Fetal effects can include skeletal deformities, as well as effects on the eyes, CNS, and kidneys. There is risk to the fetus only if maternal infection occurs during one of two time periods: between 13 and 20 weeks, or at the time of delivery. Infection in the second trimester can cause congenital disease; peripartum exposure can lead to neonatal varicella infection.

Zoster outbreaks during pregnancy cause maternal discomfort, but do not pose a risk to the fetus. However, a susceptible woman can develop a varicella outbreak if she is exposed to an individual with active zoster.

11. Can varicella-zoster infection be prevented?

Varicella infection can be prevented through immunization of infected individuals or by the administration of varicella-zoster immunoglobulin (VZIG) to susceptible individuals who are exposed to the virus. The vaccine should not be administered during pregnancy. VZIG can and should be administered in appropriate situations to susceptible pregnant women. Not only will the mother be protected from the effects of the disease, but her fetus will also benefit by avoiding the potential for in utero or neonatal disease.

12. How does infection with the human immunodeficiency virus (HIV) impact pregnancy?

As with all maternal infections during pregnancy, there are maternal and fetal concerns. For the mother, the major health concern is control of the disease. For the fetus, the main concern is the prevention of vertical transmission. Pregnancy does not appear to worsen the disease in the mother. Nor does the presence of maternal infection appear to carry risk to the fetus outside of the risk of neonatal infection.

13. Can anti-retroviral therapy be safely used in pregnancy?

There are obvious concerns about the use of anti-viral agents to treat HIV infection in pregnant mothers. The agents used can be toxic, and there is limited human data regarding their safety in pregnancy. However, the safety concerns need to be balanced against the potential benefit to mother and baby. Depending on the severity of maternal disease, medical therapy may provide significant maternal benefit. For the baby, the benefit is more straightforward. The likelihood of vertical transmission is directly related to maternal viral load, and anti-viral therapy reduces viral load. Pregnant women should be offered medical therapy even if they have a relatively low disease burden (as evidenced by CD-4 counts and viral counts). Current management of HIV infection usually includes multi-drug therapy.

14. What steps can be taken to reduce the risk of vertical transmission?

Prevention of vertical transmission is accomplished through a multi-stage strategy. First, women with significant viral load should receive medical therapy during the antepartum period. Second, if the maternal viral load is greater than 1000 copies per ml, cesarean section should be offered. Third, women with HIV should not breastfeed.

Cesarean section only appears to reduce the rate of transmission in women with higher viral loads. The benefit of cesarean section applies even if the membranes are ruptured.

Together, these approaches should reduce the risk of vertical transmission to < 5%. This compares with a transmission rate of 15–25% in women who receive no treatment and who undergo vaginal delivery.

15. Should pregnant women be routinely screened for HIV infection?

Yes. There is a consensus that all pregnant women should be offered screening for HIV. Targeted testing only of women with risk factors misses too many cases. This testing should be voluntary and accompanied by appropriate counseling.

16. What is the significance of rubella in pregnancy?

Rubella causes german measles, which is a minor maternal illness, but which can cause significant fetal illness leading to severe effects on multiple systems, including the heart and nervous system. Rubella can also lead to growth restriction. Fetal infection is more likely if maternal illness occurs early in pregnancy. Fetal infection in the first trimester is also more likely to lead to serious sequelae.

Fortunately, maternal infection and its sequelae can be largely prevented through immunization of women of child-bearing age. Women should be assessed for immunity, and vaccination should be recommended to susceptible individuals. This should be a part of preconception counseling and is required by many states prior to issuing a marriage license.

17. What are the fetal effects of congenital syphylis?

Fetal infection with *Treponema pallidum* can cause significant sequelae, including hydrops and hepatosplenomegaly. It can also lead to stillbirth. Fetal effects can be prevented by screening pregnant women for syphylis and treating appropriately based on the stage of the illness. Treatment during pregnancy is always with penicillin. Women who are believed to be allergic should be tested and desensitized if necessary.

The prevalence of syphylis in the general population has declined in the last decade. This development, combined with effective screening, should make congenital syphylis very rare.

18. How does herpes simplex virus (HSV) affect pregnancy?

HSV is a relatively common genital infection. This virus causes an initial infection and is then latent. Some infected women only suffer the initial, or primary, outbreak, but many women experience secondary outbreaks as frequently as several times each year. The main concern with maternal HSV infection is transmission to the newborn. Transmission only occurs if the mother is experiencing an outbreak around the time of delivery. Neonatal disease ranges from asymptomatic infection to disseminated disease and death.

19. How is transmission of HSV to the fetus/newborn prevented?

If at the time of labor she is symptomatic (with a viral prodrome) or has a visible genital herpes lesion, then cesarean section is recommended. The risk to the newborn is much more significant if the mother is experiencing an initial outbreak as opposed to a recurrence. In recurrent or secondary outbreaks, maternal antibodies likely provide some passive immunity to the newborn. Although the risk is much lower with secondary outbreaks, cesarean section is still routinely recommended.

The frequency of secondary herpes outbreaks can be reduced with daily medication with antivirals (acyclovir and others). If a woman has frequent outbreaks before or during pregnancy, many providers use daily prophylaxis beginning at 36 weeks to reduce the likelihood of a peripartum outbreak and to avoid the need for a cesarean section.

20. For which infections should pregnant women be screened?

Currently, universal screening is only conducted for a limited number of diseases: HIV, syphylis, and group B streptococcus. Pregnant women are also screened for immunity to rubella, but this screening is done to identify susceptible individuals for post-partum immunization, not for disease identification.

There are advocates for screening for several other diseases (e.g., toxoplasmosis, bacterial vaginosis). When considering use of a screening test, make your decison based on its accuracy (as defined by sensitivity and specificity), the prevalence of the disease, the severity of the disease, the ability to improve outcome through early identification, and the costs (of screening, confirmation, and treatment). The availability of a screening test doesn't necessarily warrant its universal application.

BIBLIOGRAPHY

1. Alger LS, Lovchik JC, Hebel JR, et al: The association of *Chlamydia trachomatis, Neisseria gonorrhoeae*, and group B streptococci with preterm rupture of the membranes and pregnancy outcome. Am J Obstet Gynecol 1988;159:397–404.
2. American College of Obstetricians and Gynecologists: Perinatal viral and parasitic infections. Practice Bulletin No. 20, 2000.
3. American Academy of Pediatrics and the American College of Obstetricians and Gynecologists: Joint Statement on Human Immunodeficiency Virus Screening. Policy Statement. May, 1999.
4. American College of Obstetricians and Gynecologists. Management of herpes in pregnancy. Practice Bulletin No. 8, 1999.
5. American College of Obstetricians and Gynecologists: Prevention of early-onset group B streptococcal disease in newborns. Committee Opinion No. 173, 1996.
6. American College of Obstetricians and Gynecologists: Scheduled cesarean delivery and the prevention of vertical transmission of HIV infection. Committee Opinion No. 234, 2000.
7. Centers for Disease Control and Prevention: 1998 guidelines for treatment of sexually transmitted diseases. MMWR 1998;47:1–111.
8. Cunningham FG, Gant NF, Leveno KJ (eds): Williams Obstetrics, 21st ed. New York, McGraw Hill, 2001.

9. Enders G, Miller E, Cradock-Watson J, et al: Consequences of varicella and herpes zoster in pregnancy: Prospective study of 1739 cases. Lancet 1994;343:1548–1551.

10. Hauth JC, Goldenberg RL, Andrews WW, et al: Reduced incidence of preterm delivery with metronidazole and erythromycin in women with bacterial vaginosis. N Engl J Med 1995;333:1732–1736.

11. McGregor JA, French JI, Parker R, et al: Prevention of premature birth by screening and treatment for common genital tract infections: Results of a prospective controlled evaluation. Am J Obstet Gynecol 1995;173:157–167.

12. Mercer BM, Arheart KL: Antimicrombial therapy in expectant management of preterm premature rupture of the membranes. Lancet 1995;346:1271–1279.

13. Pastuszak Al, Levy M, Schick B, et al: Outcome after maternal varicella infetion in the first 20 weeks of pregnancy. N Engl J Med 1994;330:901–905.

14. Randolph AG, Washington AE, Prober CG: Cesarean delivery for women presenting with genital herpes lseions. Efficacy, risks, and costs. JAMA 1993;270:77–82.

15. Scott LL, Sanchez PJ, Jackson GL, et al: Acyclovir supression to prevent cesarean section after first-episode genital herpes. Obstet Gynecol 1996;87:69–73.

16. Watts DH: Management of human immunodeficiency virus infection in pregnancy. New Eng J Med 2002;346:1879–1891.

46. AUTOIMMUNE DISEASE IN PREGNANCY

Mohammed Elkousy, M.D.

1. What is autoimmunity? What are the autoimmune diseases?

In normal individuals, the immune system allows a host to distinguish between self and non-self tissue and to defend itself against foreign pathogens. A disturbance in this balance results in autoantibody production and autoimmune disease. Autoantibodies may be organ and non-organ specific. Examples of organ-specific antibodies include antithyroid and antismooth-muscle antibodies. Non-organ-specific antibodies are the antiphospholipid antibodies (ACA, LA), antinuclear antibodies, and antihistone antibodies (see table).

Autoimmune diseases include the antiphospholipid syndrome, systemic lupus erythematosus (SLE), rheumatoid arthritis, myasthenia gravis, and idiopathic thrombocytopenic purpura (also known as autoimmune thrombocytopenia). Thyroid disease and diabetes are discussed elsewhere.

AUTOIMMUNE DISEASE	ASSOCIATED AUTOANTIBODIES
Antiphospholipid syndrome	ACA, LA
Systemic lupus erythematosus	ANA, Anti-DNA, Anti-SSA, Anti-SSB, ACA Anti-SM
Myasthenia gravis	Anti-acetylcholine receptor antibodies
Rheumatoid arthritis	Rheumatoid factor
Idiopathic thrombocytopenic purpura	Antibody to antigens on platelet glycoproteins (IIb-IIIa or Ib-IX)

ACA = anticardiolipin antibody, LA = lupus anticoagulant, ANA = antinuclear antibody, SSA = skin-sensitizing antibody

2. What are lupus anticoagulant, anticardiolipin antibody, and anti-beta 2 glycoprotein antibody?

Lupus anticoagulant and *anticardiolipin* are **antiphospholipid antibodies** (non-organ-specific autoantibodies) that bind to the negatively charged phospholipids found in all cell membranes. Both LA and ACA have been associated with thrombosis and adverse pregnancy outcomes. *Beta-2 glycoprotein I* is an abundant **plasma glycoprotein** that enhances the binding of antiphospholipid antibodies to phospholipid. Although it has been reported that the presence of anti-beta-2 glycoprotein antibodies may be more specific markers for the medical complications of the antiphospholipid syndrome, their use in this regard is still investigational. The role of treating pregnant women with isolated elevations of anti-beta-2 glycoprotein is unknown.

3. What are the implications of antiphospholipid antibodies in pregnancy?

Antiphospholipid antibodies have been associated with arterial and venous thrombosis, recurrent pregnancy loss, thrombocytopenia, fetal growth restriction, preterm birth, and preeclampsia. The presence of these autoantibodies when there is no other underlying disease is suggestive of a primary antiphospholipid syndrome (APS). When the antibodies are present with other diseases such as the collagen vascular or rheumatic diseases (e.g., SLE), a secondary APS is suggested. The diagnosis of APS is made after specific clinical *and* laboratory criteria are met.

4. How is lupus anticoagulant detected in plasma?

LA is detected by using a phospholipid-dependent clotting assay (e.g., activated partial thromboplastin time, kaolin clotting time, or dilute Russell viper venom time). In all of these assays, phospholipid is used as a template for the cofactors and enzymes of the clotting cascade.

If LA is present, it binds to the phospholipid, interferes with the clotting cascade, and prolongs the time for clot formation. Other factors can result in prolonged clotting times, including medications and clotting factor deficiencies.

If the presence of LA in plasma is suspected, a mixing study should be performed for confirmation. In this test, the suspected plasma is mixed with normal plasma. If the prolonged clotting time is due to the absence of a factor, the clotting time will be normal; if it remains prolonged, then LA is present. The addition of excess phospholipid to the plasma should correct or shorten the clotting time in the presence of LA.

5. How is anticardiolipin antibody detected?

Use a standardized, enzyme-linked, immunosorbent assay that detects the anionic phospholipid cardiolipin for the detection of ACA. The antibody levels are reported in a standard nomenclature: GPL = immunoglobulin G, MPL = immunoglobulin M, APL = immunoglobulin A. All values are reported as negative, low, medium, or high positive. Only the medium- to high-positive GPL and MPL are used for the diagnosis of APS.

6. How is the diagnosis of antiphospholipid syndrome made?

In 1998, an international conference of experts convened and proposed criteria for the classification of APS. One of the primary goals of the conference was to standardize the classification to facilitate studies of treatment and causation. Diagnosis of APS is confirmed if at least one of the clinical and one of the laboratory criteria are met.

Clinical Criteria

1. *Vascular thrombosis*: One or more clinical episodes of arterial, venous or small vessel thrombosis, in any tissue or organ. Thrombosis must be confirmed by imaging or Doppler studies, or by histopathology, with the exception of superficial venous thrombosis. For histopathologic confirmation, thrombosis should be present without significant evidence of inflammation in the vessel wall.

2. *Pregnancy morbidity*:
   (a) One or more unexplained fetal deaths of a morphologically normal fetus at or beyond the 10th week of gestation, with normal fetal morphology documented by ultrasound or by direct examination of the fetus, *or*
   (b) One or more premature births of a morphologically normal neonate at or before the 34th week of gestation because of severe preeclampsia or eclampsia, or severe placental insufficiency, *or*
   (c) Three or more unexplained consecutive spontaneous abortions before the 10th week of gestation, with maternal anatomic or hormonal abnormalities and paternal and maternal chromosomal causes excluded.

Laboratory Criteria

1. *Anticardiolipin antibody of IgG and/or IgM isotype* in blood, present in medium or high titer, on two or more occasions, at least 6 weeks apart, measured by a standardized enzyme-linked immunosorbent assay for beta-2 glycoprotein I-dependent anticardiolipin antibodies

2. *Lupus anticoagulant* present in plasma, on two or more occasions at least 6 weeks apart, detected according to the guidelines of the International Society of Thrombosis and Hemostasis, in the following steps:
   (a) Prolonged phospholipid-dependent coagulation demonstrated on a screening test (e.g., activated partial thromboplastin time, kaolin clotting time, dilute Russell viper venom time, dilute prothrombin time, Textarin time)
   (b) Failure to correct the prolonged coagulation time on the screening test by mixing with normal platelet-poor plasma
   (c) Shortening or correction of the prolonged coagulation time on the screening test by the addition of excess phospholipid
   (d) Exclusion of other coagulopathies.

7. What are the indications for testing for antiphospholipid antibodies (APA)?

The American College of Obstetricians and Gynecologists has adopted a list of indications for testing for APA. **Obstetric indications include**: otherwise unexplained fetal death or still-birth; recurrent pregnancy loss (three or more spontaneous abortions with no more than one live birth, or unexplained second- or third-trimester fetal death); severe pregnancy-induced hyperten-sion at less than 34 weeks of gestation; and severe fetal growth restriction or other evidence of uteroplacental insufficiency in the second or early third trimester.

Medical indications include: nontraumatic thrombosis or venous or arterial thromboem-bolism; stroke in an individual less than 50–55 years of age; autoimmune thrombocytopenia; transient ischemic attacks or amaurosis fugax in individuals less than 50–55 years of age; livedo reticularis; hemolytic anemia; SLE; or a false positive serologic test for syphilis.

8. How is APS treated during pregnancy?

Patients who are diagnosed with APS using the previously mentioned strict clinical and lab-oratory criteria are candidates for treatment. *Traditional regimens* have included prednisone, pro-phylactic or therapeutic heparin, and low-dose aspirin. *Current recommendations* include prophylactic heparin in divided subcutaneous doses with low-dose aspirin daily in those who have had a prior fetal death or recurrent pregnancy loss. Women who have experienced a prior thrombosis or stroke may be candidates for therapeutic heparin dosing. In women who have APS without a prior history of pregnancy loss or thrombosis, the best management is uncertain. All patients receiving heparin therapy should be counseled on the adverse effects, including bruising, bleeding complications, osteoporosis, and heparin-induced thrombocytopenia.

Recently, the use of **low-molecular-weight heparin** (LMWH) has been more common, al-though experience is limited during pregnancy. LMWH is produced through an enzymatic break-down of unfractionated heparin. It has no effect on aPTT; therefore measurement of anti factor Xa levels may be necessary. LMWH has a longer half-life than unfractionated heparin, resulting in questions surrounding its use with epidural anesthesia.

9. How is systemic lupus erythematosus diagnosed?

SLE is a multisystemic disease in which tissues and cells are damaged by autoantibodies and immune complexes. Several drugs can cause a syndrome that resembles SLE, including pro-cainamide, hydralazine, and methyldopa. After excluding drug-induced SLE, the diagnosis is made when 4 of 11 criteria are present at any time during the course of disease. The 11 criteria are:
- Malar rash
- Discoid rash
- Photosensitivity
- Oral ulcers
- Arthritis
- Serositis
- Renal manifestations (proteinuria)
- Neurologic manifestations (seizures, psychosis)
- Hematologic disorder (e.g., hemolytic anemia, leukopenia, lymphopenia, thrombocytopenia)
- Immunologic manifestation (positive LE cell preparation, anti-ds-DNA or anti-SM anti-bodies, or false positive VDRL [test for syphilis])
- Antinuclear antibodies (abnormal titers of ANA)

10. Describe the course of SLE during pregnancy.

Ninety percent of SLE occurs in women of childbearing age; therefore, its occurrence during pregnancy is common. Pregnancy is not thought to affect the long-term prognosis of lupus. However, flares may increase during pregnancy and the puerperium. The effect of SLE on preg-nancy is dependent on the disease activity. Mild disease generally has a good prognosis, but active disease—especially active renal disease and maternal hypertension—have been associated with fetal loss, premature birth, and intrauterine growth restriction.

It is generally recommended that prior to planning a pregnancy, a woman with lupus should be without a flare for at least 6 months. Patients who do become pregnant will have their disease activity monitored by measuring levels of total serum complement. In addition, these patients should have ultrasounds to follow fetal growth, and antenatal testing should be initiated between 28 and 32 weeks.

11. What is neonatal lupus?

Neonatal lupus is defined by two criteria: the presence of maternal antibodies to the 52-kD SSA/Ro, 60-kD SSA/Ro, or 48-kD SSB/La ribonucleoproteins; and the presence of heart block or a transient skin rash. Neonatal lupus may also be associated with hepatic and hematologic abnormalities. Only the development of heart block is permanent and results in significant morbidity and mortality. Available treatment includes oral corticosteroids, which may slow the progression of the heart block, and postnatal pacemaker placement.

12. What is rheumatoid arthritis (RA)? What is its course during pregnancy?

RA is a chronic, multisystem disease characterized by a persistent inflammatory synovitis involving the peripheral joints in a symmetric distribution. The synovial inflammation can cause cartilage destruction and bone erosions that result in joint deformities. Women are affected more frequently than men, and the prevalence increases with age.

RA generally improves during pregnancy, probably due to the elevated cortisol levels that are present. In those patients who require treatment, steroids and analgesics may be used. Other drugs include paracetamol, aspirin, gold, chloroquine, sulfasalazine, penicillamine, and immunosuppressants such as azathioprine.

13. What is myasthenia gravis? What is its course during pregnancy?

Myasthenia gravis is characterized by a reduced number of acetylcholine receptors at the neuromuscular junction. This results in weakness and fatigability of the muscles. Muscle weakness generally starts with the cranial muscles. Diplopia and ptosis are common complaints, as is facial weakness. Speech and swallowing may be affected, and the muscle weakness can generalize to the limb muscles.

During pregnancy and the puerperium, relapses and remissions are variable. Management during pregnancy should be the same as in patients who are not pregnant. Treatment includes the use of anticholinesterase medications, immunosuppressive agents (e.g., glucocorticoids, azathioprine), thymectomy, and plasmapheresis. Intrapartum issues that must be addressed include the use of regional anesthesia over general anesthesia and the avoidance of muscle relaxants. Do not use magnesium sulfate, because it may precipitate a myasthenic crisis. Some patients may require assistance during the second stage of labor to have a successful vaginal delivery.

14. What is neonatal myasthenia?

Neonatal myasthenia is a transient disorder and occurs in about 10-15% of infants born to myasthenic mothers. The infant may show signs of a weak cry, respiratory difficulties, and weak movements. The symptoms generally become apparent within the first 72 hours after birth. Infants can be treated with anticholinesterase drugs.

15. What is idiopathic thrombocytopenic purpura (ITP)?

ITP (autoimmune thrombocytopenia) is an autoimmune disorder in which IgG antibodies are directed to platelet antigens. These immune complexes are then sequestered and destroyed in the reticuloendothelial system, especially the spleen. During pregnancy, the disorder places the mother at risk for hemorrhage postpartum, and because IgG antibodies can cross the placental barrier, the fetus is at risk for thrombocytopenia.

16. How is the diagnosis of ITP determined?

The diagnosis of ITP is one of exclusion, and the differential diagnosis of thrombocytopenia should include laboratory error, SLE, antiphospholipid syndrome, HIV infection, drug-induced thrombocytopenia, thrombotic thrombocytopenic purpura, and diffuse intravascular coagulation. During pregnancy, other possible causes of thrombocytopenia include preeclampsia and gestational thrombocytopenia. Most women with ITP have a history of easy bruising and menorrhagia. Currently, the use of assays that measure antiplatelet antibodies are not recommended for the routine evaluation of possible ITP, and a bone marrow biopsy may be required to diagnose the disorder.

Confusion can occur during pregnancy because gestational thrombocytopenia, which occurs in 5% of pregnancies, may lead to platelet counts as low as 80,000/μL. Gestational thrombocytopenia is a benign condition that has no maternal or fetal affects.

17. What are the maternal management issues of ITP during pregnancy?

Management during pregnancy should take into consideration both the mother and fetus. The goal for maternal therapy is to minimize the risk of hemorrhage. Generally, maternal platelet counts above 50,000/μL are not treated. As platelet counts fall below 50,000/μL in the second trimester, **prednisone** may be started. In those cases refractory to prednisone, intravenous **immunoglobulin** (IG) can be used. Platelet transfusions are a temporary measure to control hemorrhage. Transfused platelets have a shortened lifespan because of the presence of antiplatelet antibodies.

Splenectomy results in remission in 80% of cases. It can be performed during pregnancy and is generally reserved for women who have not responded to steroids or intravenous IG.

18. What are the fetal considerations in the management of ITP?

The main fetal risk is that of intracranial hemorrhage (ICH). IgG antiplatelet antibodies cause maternal thrombocytopenia and cross the placental barrier, resulting in fetal thrombocytopenia. There is no correlation between maternal and fetal platelet counts. Although there is only a 1% risk of fetal ICH due to ITP, this low risk has led to concern and controversy about the mode of delivery. Many have recommended cesarean section for women who have ITP. Others have recommended that fetal platelet counts be determined prior to allowing vaginal delivery. If the fetal platelet count is > 50,000/μL, then vaginal delivery may be allowed.

Suggested methods of assessing fetal platelet counts have included fetal scalp sampling and cordocentesis. Fetal scalp sampling often incorrectly diagnoses low fetal platelets, and cordocentesis may have a complication rate up to 5%. A recent decision analysis suggests that cordocentesis is preferable to fetal scalp sampling. Currently, the optimal intrapartum management remains controversial.

BIBLIOGRAPHY

 1. American College of Obstetricians and Gynecologists: ACOG Educational Bulletin—Antiphospholipid Syndrome. Number 244, February 1998, pp 302–311.
 2. Aminoff MJ: Neurologic disorders. In Creasy RK, Resnick R (eds): Maternal-Fetal Medicine, 4th ed. Philadelphia, WB Saunders, 1999, pp 1091–1119.
 3. Cowchock S: Treatment of antiphospholipid syndrome in pregnancy. Lupus 7(suppl 2):S95–S97, 1998.
 4. Coulam CB, Gleicher N: Autoimmunity. In Gleicher (ed): Principles and Practice of Medical Therapy in Pregnancy, 3rd ed. Stamford, Appleton and Lange, 1998, pp 521–529.
 5. De Swiet M: Rheumatologic and connective tissue disorders. In Creasy RK, Resnick R (eds): Maternal-Fetal Medicine, 4th ed. Philadelphia, WB Saunders, 1999, pp 1082–1090.
 6. Dulitzki M, Pauzner R, Langevitz P, et al: Low-molecular-weight heparin during pregnancy and delivery: Preliminary experience with 41 pregnancies. Obstet Gynecol 87(3), 1996.
 7. Greaves M: Antiphospholipid antibodies and thrombosis. Lancet 353:1348–1353, 1999.
 8. Lee RM, Emlen W, Scott JR, et al: Anti-beta-2 glycoprotein I antibodies in women with recurrent spontaneous abortion, unexplained fetal death, and antiphospholipid syndrome. Am J Obstet Gynecol 181(3):642–648, 1999.
 9. Meng C, Lockshin M: Pregnancy in lupus. Curr Opin Rheumatol 11:348–351, 1999.
10. Silver RM, Branch DW: Immunologic disorders. In Creasy RK, Resnick R (eds): Maternal-Fetal Medicine, 4th ed. Philadelphia, WB Saunders, 1999, pp 465–483.
11. Stamilio DM, Macones GA: Selection of delivery method in pregnancies complicated by autoimmune thrombocytopenia: A decision analysis. Obstet Gynecol 94(1):41–47, 1999.
12. Wilson WA, Gharavi AE, Koike T, et al: International Consensus Statement on Preliminary Classification Criteria for Definite Antiphospholipid Syndrome. Report of an international workshop. Arth Rheum 42(7):1309–1311, 1999.

47. ALCOHOL AND DRUG ABUSE DURING PREGNANCY

Serdar H. *Ural,* M.D.

ALCOHOL

1. Why is alcohol use during pregnancy of clinical importance?
Maternal alcohol consumption during pregnancy is one of the most common preventable causes of birth defects and childhood disabilities. Varying levels of fetal abnormalities can occur from fetal alcohol exposure. These appear in a spectrum of alcohol-related disabling conditions, ranging from cognitive and behavioral problems to fetal alcohol syndrome (FAS). According to the latest available data from the U.S. Centers for Disease Control, the FAS rate has dramatically risen. Alcohol is the most commonly abused substance during pregnancy.

2. What are the features of fetal alcohol syndrome?
Growth deficiency before and after birth
Mental retardation
Abnormalities of the head and face
Congenital heart defects
Behavioral disturbances
Central nervous system anomalies

3. Is there a "safe" limit of alcohol consumption?
No safe level of alcohol consumption in pregnancy has been identified. The safest thing to do is not to drink alcohol at all. An advisory not to drink alcohol both for women who are pregnant and women attempting conception was issued by the U.S. Surgeon General in 1981 and by the Secretary of Health and Human Services in 1990.

4. Is there a dose/response relationship between alcohol consumption and pregnancy outcome?
No. Among offspring of women who consume 5 ounces of alcohol daily, about one-third of the infants have FAS, one-third show some prenatal toxic effects, and the remaining one-third appear to be normal. When 1–2 ounces of alcohol are consumed daily, approximately 10% of offspring may exhibit characteristics of FAS. Even smaller amounts of alcohol have been associated with FAS! Alcohol consumption within the social drinking range has been associated with persistent effects on IQ and learning problems in young children who have no apparent anatomic abnormalities.

5. How much does a woman have to be drinking to consume 5 ounces of alcohol per day?
Beer is generally 5% alcohol; one 12-oz can contains 0.6 oz of absolute alcohol. Wine contains approximately 0.5 oz per glass, as does a shot of liquor. Four to five ounces of alcohol may be reached through various combinations of the above, such as a couple of "mixed" drinks before and after dinner with four glasses of wine at dinner, or a six-pack of beer plus four glasses of wine.

6. Does alcohol cross the placenta?
Ethyl alcohol does cross the placenta. Fetal blood alcohol levels approximate those of the mother.

7. Should an alcoholic pregnant woman stop drinking on her own?

A pregnant woman who is physically dependent on alcohol requires medically supervised detoxification. The risk of preterm labor is significantly increased with alcohol withdrawal.

8. When do the signs and symptoms of alcohol withdrawal appear during pregnancy?

Withdrawal symptoms begin when blood alcohol concentrations decline sharply after cessation or reduction, usually within 4–12 hours. However, it is possible for withdrawal symptoms to develop even a few days after abstinence. Untreated withdrawal symptoms reach their peak intensity at 48 hours and may persist for up to 3–6 months at lower levels of intensity. Signs and symptoms of alcohol withdrawal include tremulousness, anxiety, increased heart rate, increased blood pressure, sweating, nausea, hyperreflexia, and insomnia, depending on the severity of previous alcohol dependence and the general condition of the patient.

9. Once a pregnancy is recognized, does decreasing alcohol intake affect the rate of fetal abnormalities produced?

Ethanol or ethyl alcohol crosses the placenta and the fetal blood-brain barrier freely. It is thought that the effects are caused by the direct toxicity of alcohol and its metabolites. Stopping or slowing down consumption of alcohol once pregnancy is diagnosed may lead to a decrease in anomaly rates. However, there is always a possibility that this may not be the case. Therefore, further studies are needed to evaluate this accurately.

COCAINE

10. True or false: Cocaine use in pregnancy is increasing.

True. There has been a rise in the use of cocaine in the pregnant population, corresponding to the rise in the general population. The availability of inexpensive crack cocaine is a major reason for this.

11. How does cocaine affect the pregnant patient?

Cocaine prevents reuptake of norepinephrine and dopamine. The increase in norepinephrine causes vasoconstriction, tachycardia, and rapid rise in maternal and fetal arterial pressure. Uterine and placental blood flow decreases, with resultant fetal tachycardia and increased fetal oxygen consumption. Uterine contractility also increases.

12. What risks are associated with cocaine use during pregnancy?

Pregnancy risks associated with cocaine use include irregularities in placental blood flow, abruptio placentae, and premature labor and delivery. Use of cocaine in the third trimester increases the risk of abruption. Abruption and stillbirth have been documented in 8% of cocaine abusers. Cocaine use in the first trimester results in a spontaneous abortion rate of 40%. In terms of fetal development, reported risks include low birth weight, congenital anomalies, urogenital anomalies, mild neurodysfunction, transient electroencephalographic abnormalities, intrauterine growth restriction, increased risk of intrauterine fetal demise, certain congenital anomalies, and cerebral infarction and seizures. Hypertonicity, spasticity and convulsions, hyperreflexia, and irritability have been observed in children exposed to cocaine in utero.

13. How long do cocaine metabolites remain in the urine?

Cocaine use can be detected in a urine sample for up to 3 days after last use.

HEROIN

14. What is the prevalence of opiate abuse or dependence during pregnancy?

The true extent of opiate abuse and dependence by women is unknown. Overall, women account for about 25% of all opiate-dependent individuals, and most of the estimated 300,000 women are untreated for their addiction.

15. What risks are incurred by opiate dependence during pregnancy?

Heroin does not seem to cause an increase in congenital anomaly rates. However, prematurity, intrauterine growth restriction, stillbirth, perinatal death, and multiple neonatal problems have been reported.

16. What is the best treatment for opiate dependence during pregnancy?

Methadone maintenance confers several treatment benefits for the pregnant opiate-dependent woman. It eliminates the need for illicit behavior to support a drug habit, prevents fluctuations in maternal heroin levels, and removes the patient from a drug-seeking environment.

17. Should a woman on methadone be weaned during pregnancy?

No. Although it is desirable to use the lowest possible dose, reduction below 20 mg/day may precipitate in utero withdrawal. Whatever dose is required to prevent symptoms in the mother is also best for the fetus, and no attempt should be made to taper and discontinue methadone until after delivery.

18. Does methadone prevent withdrawal in the newborn period?

No. About 80% of infants exposed to methadone require treatment for neonatal withdrawal in contrast to 100% of infants exposed to heroin. The incidence of withdrawal is reduced in infants of mothers on the lowest methadone doses.

19. What are the symptoms of neonatal withdrawal from heroin or methadone?

The classic symptom complex of neonatal abstinence syndrome (NAS) includes central nervous system hyperirritability, gastrointestinal dysfunction, respiratory distress, tremors, high-pitched cry, poor feeding, and electrolyte imbalance.

20. Is methadone harmful?

Methadone is not known to cause an increase in congenital anomalies. However, it has been reported to be associated with low birthweights.

21. Should patients who abuse drugs breastfeed?

Breastfeeding is not recommended. Alcohol, cocaine, and opiates cross into breast milk to some extent. Breastfeeding is *contraindicated* for cocaine users, because cocaine may cause significant cardiovascular changes in neonates.

22. List the signs of substance abuse.

Agitation
Sedation
Disorientation
Tachycardia
Hallucinations
Hypertension
Unusual skin infections

23. How should I manage substance abuse in pregnancy?

Hospitalization may be necessary for detoxification purposes. Referral to treatment centers, social services, and counseling is important.

TOBACCO

24. What are some of the potential complications that have been associated with tobacco use?

Pregnant mothers who smoke are at increased risk for spontaneous abortion, placental abruption, preterm delivery, premature rupture of membranes, and low-birth-weight infants. An increase in congenital anomalies has not been reported thus far. There is no known "safe" amount of cigarette smoking. From experience with other toxic substances, it is assumed that the more a mother smokes, the greater the associated risk. Patients should be counseled that the safest approach is not to smoke at all.

25. What are the effective cessation techniques for smoking?

Twenty-five percent of reproductive-age women are smokers. Effective techniques in controlling tobacco addiction include counseling, continued reassurance, periodic and frequent contact with a health provider, and medication. Medical treatment consists of nicotine replacement, which is available either as a chewing gum or as a skin patch. If used appropriately along with continued support and counseling, both medications are effective.

MARIJUANA

26. What are the risks of marijuana use during pregnancy?

Marijuana is the most commonly used illicit substance among pregnant women. There is no evidence that marijuana is associated with congenital anomalies in humans. However, maternal marijuana use may be associated with increased perinatal mortality, preterm delivery, infants of lower birth weight, and premature rupture of membranes. It is not clear if marijuana itself is the cause, or if the associated use of other illicit drugs leads to these complications.

27. When should a woman stop smoking marijuana during pregnancy?

It is unclear if there is a particular gestational age when marijuana use carries the greatest risk. Nor is there clear data to suggest that stopping marijuana at a certain gestational age improves outcomes. Therefore the safest recommendation is to avoid marijuana use throughout pregnancy.

BIBLIOGRAPHY

1. Centers for Disease Control. Update: Trends in fetal alcohol syndrome—United States, 1979–1993. MMWR 44:249–253, 1995.
2. Chasnoff IJ, Griffith DR, Freier C, Murray J: Cocaine/polydrug use in pregnancy: Two-year follow-up. Pediatrics 89:284–289, 1992.
3. Cyr MG, Moulton AW: Substance abuse in women. Obstet Gynecol Clin North Am 17:905–925, 1990.
4. Dombrowski M, Wolfe H, Welch R, Evans M: Cocaine abuse is associated with abruptio placentae and decreased birth weight, but not shorter labor. Obstet Gynecol 77:139, 1991.
5. Finnegan LP, Kandall SR: Maternal and neonatal effects of alcohol and drugs. In Lowinsin JH, Ruiz P, Millman RB, Langrod JG (eds): Substance abuse: A Comprehensive Textbook, 2nd ed. Baltimore, Williams and Wilkins, 1992, pp 628–656.
6. Mastrogiannis D, Decavalas G, Verma U, Tejani N: Perinatal outcome after recent cocaine usage. Obstet Gynecol 76:8, 1990.
7. Streissguth AP, Barr HM, Sampson PD: Moderate alcohol exposure: Effects on child IQ and learning problems at 7 1/2 years. Alcohol Clin Exp Res 14:662–669, 1990.
8. Wiemann CM, Berenson AB, San Miguel VV: Tobacco, alcohol, and illicit drug use among pregnant women. J Reprod Med 39:769–776, 1994.
9. American College of Obstetricians and Gynecologists: Substance abuse in pregnancy. ACOG Tech Bull195, 1994.
10. Creasy RK, Resnik R: Maternal Fetal Medicine, 4th ed. Philadelphia, W.B. Saunders, 1999, pp 145–164.

48. PSYCHIATRIC ISSUES DURING PREGNANCY

Dominic Marchiano, M.D., and Sharon Zwillinger, M.D.

1. Describe the normal reactions and psychological adjustments to a normal pregnancy.

For women, adjustment to pregnancy involves a developmental crisis, with reworking of old relationships (especially with her mother and father), revisiting issues of attachment and separation, gaining a sense of mastery, and coming to terms with her own femaleness. Normal reactions can also include anxiety, fear, ambivalence, and mixed anticipation. Social, cultural, economic, and emotional factors in the environment mediate many of the responses.

For men, adjustment to pregnancy often involves satisfaction of the desires to reproduce, identify with their offspring, and promulgate the family line. It can also be a time of reworking old relationships and gaining a new sense of purposefulness and seriousness. However, normal pregnancy can also stimulate concerns about personal health, finances, job security, and personal freedom. Men may feel left out and resentful of the new mother-child dyad. Once again, social, cultural, economic, and emotional issues mediate these adjustments.

2. What psychiatric symptoms and emotional reactions are associated with problem pregnancies or pregnancy losses?

Patients and couples who have to deal with these situations are faced with many different feelings and reactions. Determinants of response include premorbid adjustment, personality traits, and coping styles. However, many persons share the following cluster of symptoms:

- Sadness, grief, depression, helplessness, and somatic symptoms
- Shock, denial, and acceptance
- Anxiety, guilt, isolation, withdrawal, anger, and shame
- Narcissistic vulnerability, including difficulties with self-esteem and sense of self
- Problems with attachment and separation
- Loss of libido and impaired sexual functioning
- Symptoms similar to those of chronic illness or disability
- Symptoms of post-traumatic stress disorder
- Sense of injustice, envy, and resentment of the healthy
- Severe stress in the marital/couple relationship
- Disruption of normal family and social relationships
- Loss of hope for the future and loss of faith.

Even realistic expectations in such situations can be overwhelming. However, when the reactions and symptoms listed above persist and begin to impact on social functioning, and if vegetative symptoms last for more than a few weeks or a month, psychiatric evaluation and treatment may be necessary.

3. How can caregivers help?

Caregivers can help by allowing the woman or couple to mourn or cope in their own individual ways, while keeping watch for serious psychiatric sequelae. Caregivers should be careful not to impose their own values and judgments, and should offer supportive assistance and appropriate referral to counseling and/or psychiatric services. Caring, involvement, and nonabandonment are extremely important.

4. How do existing psychiatric disorders influence pregnancy?

Whether psychiatric *illness* directly influences pregnancy outcome remains controversial. However, *medications* used to treat these illnesses certainly may have adverse effects (see Question 8). Also, severely ill patients may neglect their health or well-being, which can adversely

227

affect pregnancy outcome. Specifically, depressive symptoms can be associated with harmful behaviors such as substance abuse, noncompliance with prenatal care, poor weight gain, and even suicidal thinking. Likewise, eating-disordered pregnancies are at risk for fetal growth disturbances. The adverse influence of harmful behaviors can be seen with virtually any psychiatric illness, including bipolar disorder, schizophrenia, and anxiety disorders.

Some authors report a marginal increase in the incidence of congenital anomalies in schizophrenic patients. Major depression has been associated with preterm birth and low birth weight. However, these findings are inconsistent, and interpretation must include consideration of the confounding effects of socioeconomic status, substance abuse, smoking status, and psychotropic medication use.

5. How does pregnancy influence the course of psychiatric illness?

The physical and emotional stress of pregnancy can lead to a first diagnosis of psychiatric illness or cause greater manifestation of previously diagnosed illness. Reluctance to administer appropriate doses of psychopharmacologic medications can also result in disease exacerbation. Psychiatric illness must be closely monitored throughout pregnancy to detect and effectively address disease exacerbation.

6. What psychiatric illnesses are encountered during pregnancy?

Any psychiatric illness can be encountered in pregnancy. Some more common illnesses include antepartum depression, bipolar disorder, schizophrenia, anxiety disorders, and eating disorders. These illnesses are important to think about in evaluating pregnant women because: (1) they are common, (2) they may be undiagnosed or kept secret, (3) they may worsen during the course of the pregnancy or the puerperium, and (4) if they are not treated, psychiatric and other sequelae may occur.

7. List some general principles to guide treatment of psychiatric illness in pregnancy.

Psychiatric disorders can and should be treated during pregnancy because of significant risks to both the mother and developing fetus. A depressed or overly anxious woman may be unable to adjust to pregnancy and her new role as a mother, and she may be unable to mobilize needed support when the baby arrives. More seriously, she may not be able to maintain an adequate weight gain or good physical health during her pregnancy.

Depending on the severity of illness, *nonpharmacologic treatments* are often used initially, including individual supportive or insight-oriented psychotherapy, couples or family therapy, and/or cognitive behavioral interventions. *Psychopharmacologic treatments* are required when responses to other interventions are inadequate and the severity of the illness poses a greater risk to the mother and fetus than the risk of medication exposure to the developing fetus. Such cases require a complicated risk/benefit assessment, considering the severity of the psychiatric illness, the risk of the untreated psychiatric illness in causing increased morbidity to the mother and fetus, and the risk of medication exposure to the fetus. First-trimester exposure should be avoided whenever possible, and patients should be monitored closely on the lowest possible doses.

Although it is not often used, electroconvulsive therapy (ECT) may be the treatment of choice for severe depression with suicidality or severe bipolar disorder. ECT is considered safe in pregnancy.

8. What are the fetal and neonatal risks associated with prenatal exposure to psychopharmacologic medications?

Tricyclic antidepressants: TCAs are considered relatively safe during all trimesters and are not associated with increased risk of congenital malformations or developmental delay. Less anticholinergic preparations, such as nortriptyline (Pamelor) and desipramine (Norpramin), should be considered first.

Serotonin reuptake inhibitors: Fluoxetine (Prozac) appears relatively safe during pregnancy and has not been associated with an increased risk of congenital anomalies. However, fewer data are available regarding sertraline (Zoloft) and paroxetine (Paxil), and even less is known about the newer agents. There are no studies regarding behavioral development and these medications. Because these medications are new, caution is advised—especially in the first trimester.

Mood stabilizers: Lithium has been associated with an increased risk of cardiac malformations—most notably Ebstein's anomaly, with a reported 20 times greater risk (1/1000 vs. 1/20,000) with first-trimester exposure. Newer data, however, may reveal a lower risk. Hypotonia and cyanosis or "floppy baby" syndrome may occur in newborns exposed near term. Valproic acid (Depakote) and carbamazepine (Tegretol) are associated with neural tube defects, craniofacial defects, and possibly growth retardation. Behavioral difficulties have not been described.

Benzodiazepines: Diazepam (Valium) is the best studied benzodiazepine. Based on studies mainly involving epilepsy, it is designated a class D medication in pregnancy, meaning that its use should be avoided. First-trimester exposure has been linked to craniofacial malformations such as cleft lip and palate. Second-trimester exposure has been linked with hemangiomas and cardiovascular defects. Third-trimester exposure does not seem to have any teratogenic effects, but has been linked to a specific syndrome of neonatal benzodiazepine withdrawl. Although other benzodiazepines have not been extensively studied, they are commonly assigned a similar risk profile. Substitute other medications whenever possible, especially in the first trimester.

Antipsychotics: Higher-potency neuroleptics such as haloperidol (Haldol) are recommended over low-potency drugs like thioridazine (Thorazine). However, each of these is fairly safe to use during pregnancy. Few data are available about newer antipsychotic agents such as risperidone (Risperdal), Olanzipine (Zyprexa), and clozapine (Clozaril).

9. What are the main psychiatric disorders during the postpartum period? How are they treated?

Postpartum or maternity "blues" is very common, occurring in 50–80% of all new mothers. Symptoms include emotional lability, sleep disturbance, and difficulty in concentrating. Symptoms may begin shortly after delivery and usually resolve spontaneously by 2 weeks postpartum. Helpful interventions include education, supportive therapy, and reassurance. If symptoms persist beyond 2 weeks, consider other disorders.

Postpartum depression is a more serious and clinically significant disorder, with a prevalence rate of 8–15%. Symptoms may begin early, immediately following delivery or the "blues" or anytime during the first year postpartum, peaking at 2–4 months. The hallmarks are depression longer than 2 weeks and neurovegetative signs such as depressed mood, changes in appetite, sleep disturbance, guilt, fatigue, concentration difficulties, and suicidal ideation. Intrusive thoughts about harming the baby may or may not be present. The patient may be unable to care for her infant adequately, and antidepressants are often required. Hospitalization is sometimes necessary.

Postpartum psychosis: The most serious of the postpartum disorders occurs in 1–2 per 1000 deliveries and may develop within hours or days postpartum. Symptoms often include severe anxiety, agitation, restlessness, insomnia, and, at times, disorganization and confusion. Delusions about the baby and hallucinations about harming one's self or the baby may also be present. This situation can be dangerous because of the risk of suicide and/or infanticide. Psychiatric hospitalization is nearly always required, as is treatment with antipsychotic or other psychopharmacologic medications.

Postpartum anxiety disorders, including obsessive-compulsive disorders, are now being described. They may be variants of postpartum depression or they may be independent disorders. The incidence rate is still unknown.

10. What risk factors identify women who may be vulnerable to postpartum depression and psychosis?

Risk factors for *postpartum depression* include:
- A history of previous antepartum or postpartum depression
- Depression during pregnancy

  • A family history of depression
  • Lack of adequate social supports
  • Negative life events late in pregnancy.
Additional risk factors for *postpartum psychosis* include:
  • A history of bipolar disorder or psychotic disorder
  • A family history of bipolar disorder or psychosis
  • Previous postpartum psychosis
  • Primiparity.

11. Does postpartum depression recur?
Yes. Women with a history of postpartum depression have a 50% recurrence rate with the next pregnancy and even higher recurrence rates after multiple affected pregnancies.

12. Can postpartum depression be prevented?
Recurrences may be significantly decreased with initiation of peripartum psychopharmacologic medication. Women with bipolar disorder, who are at significant risk for developing postpartum psychosis (50%), are less likely to suffer this serious complication if treated either during the pregnancy or just prior to delivery with mood-stabilizing medications.

13. What is known and recommended about the use of psychopharmacologic medication during lactation?
  Facts
  • All psychopharmacologic medications are secreted into breast milk.
  • Lithium is the one drug that most experts agree is *absolutely contraindicated* in breastfeeding women.
  • True risks to the infant with respect to short- or long-term sequelae are not well-documented or understood.
  • Serum levels of psychopharmacologic agents in infants are often inaccurate.
  • Premature infants may be at more risk from medication exposure because of immature development of their kidneys and liver.
  Recommendations
Decisions about use of psychopharmacologic medication during breastfeeding involve a complicated risk/benefit analysis. The assessment should include the risk to the mother and infant when the psychiatric condition is treated and not treated and an exploration of alternative treatment methods and supports.

The pediatrician, obstetrician, internist, and psychiatrist should be involved in the decision-making process for optimal care.

If medication is used, care should include (1) careful monitoring of mother and infant, (2) use of lowest possible doses of medication, (3) use of medications with short half-lives and few or no active metabolites, and (4) possible adjustments of feeding schedule relative to peak and trough levels of medications.

BIBLIOGRAPHY

1. Aminoff MJ: Neurologic disorders. In Creasy RK and Resnick R (eds): Maternal-Fetal Medicine, 4th ed. Philadelphia, W.B. Saunders Company, 1999, pp 1115–1116.
2. Bennedsen BE, et al: Congenital malformations, stillbirths, and infant deaths among children of women with schizophrenia. Arch Gen Psychiatry 58(7):674–679, 2001.
3. Briggs GG, Freeman RK, Yaffe SJ: Drugs in Pregnancy and Lactation, 5th ed. Philadelphia, Lipincott, Williams, and Wilkins, 1998.
4. Cohen LS, Rosenbaum JF: Psychotropic drug use during pregnancy. J Clin Psychol 59 (Suppl 2):18–28, 1998.
5. Depression in women. ACOG Educational Bulletin 182. Washington DC, American College of Obstetricians and Gynecologists, 1993.

6. Kuller JA, et al: Pharmacologic treatment of psychiatric disease in pregnancy and lactation: Fetal and neonatal effects. Obstet Gynecol 87(5 Pt 1):789–794, 2000.
7. Marcus SM, et al: Treatment guidelines for depression in pregnancy. Int J Gynecol Obstet 72:61–70, 2001.
8. Nonacs R, Cohen LS: Postpartum mood disorders: Diagnosis and treatment guidelines. J Clin Psychol 59(Supp. 2):34–40, 1998.
9. Wisner KL, et al: Pharmacologic treatment of depression during pregnancy. JAMA 282(13):1264–1269, 1999.

49. SURGICAL DISEASE IN PREGNANCY

Martha E. Rode, M.D.

1. What is the most common non-obstetric cause of acute abdominal pain leading to exploratory laparotomy?

Acute appendicitis. The incidence of proven appendicitis is close to one in 1500 deliveries.

2. Is appendicitis more common in pregnant than non-pregnant women?

No.

3. Is the diagnosis of appendicitis more difficult in pregnancy?

Yes, and more so as pregnancy progresses. One study notes no delay of diagnosis in the first trimester, while delays occurred in 18% in the second trimester and 75% in the third trimester. The gravid uterus displaces the anterior peritoneum, and this can lead to vague symptoms and generalized pain (though generally believed to be displaced upward and laterally, the appendix is found near its usual location in pregnancy). The frequency of rupture (55%) is higher than that reported outside pregnancy.

4. What signs and symptoms associated with pregnancy can confuse the diagnosis of appendicitis?

Nausea, anorexia, mild leukocytosis.

5. What gynecologic pathology can be confused with appendicitis?

Degenerating myomata and adnexal torsion.

6. Does the management of biliary tract disease differ in pregnancy?

No. Initial preoperative management includes IV fluids and stopping all oral intake. Antibiotic therapy should be initiated for acute cholecystitis, choledocholithiasis, or a poor response to conservative medical management. Patients who fail to respond to the above or have recurrent symptoms after successful initial treatment are then candidates for surgical management.

7. Which surgical procedures may be performed laparoscopically during pregnancy?

Appendectomy and cholecystectomy. The laparoscopic approach is likely not an option by mid-gestation, as the expanding fundus limits accessibility.

8. Is laparoscopic surgery advisable during pregnancy?

Pregnancy was once believed to be a contraindication to laparoscopic surgery. It is now frequently reported without an associated negative impact on fetal or maternal outcome. Benefits of this approach are decreased hospitalization time, decreased use of narcotics, and a faster return to a regular diet. Some believe the decreased uterine manipulation may lead to a lower risk of preterm labor.

9. What pathophysiologic changes associated with pregnancy should be considered during induction of general anesthesia in a pregnant patient?

Delayed gastric emptying and **increased residual gastric volume** significantly increase the risk of aspiration of gastric contents during intubation. The use of Bicitra preoperatively neutralizes gastric contents (and will decrease the severity of an associated pneumonitis should aspiration occur). Employ awake intubation (with preservation of airway reflexes) or rapid sequence induction with cricoid pressure to prevent passive reflux.

Hyperemia can cause sufficient narrowing of the upper airways and increase risk for upper airway trauma or failed intubation. Small endotracheal tubes (6–7 mm) may be required.

Decreased functional residual capacity may lower oxygen reserve enough that a short period of apnea may significantly lower the PO_2. Therefore, administer 100% oxygen prior to an attempt at intubation. If not successful after 30 seconds, stop and ventilate (bag and mask) with 100% oxygen again before a repeat attempt.

Uterine compression of the inferior vena cava and associated **maternal and fetal hypotension**. Left uterine displacement (lateral tilt of at least 15 degrees) is advisable after the first trimester.

Hypercoagulability with associated risk of **thromboembolic events**. Use perioperative prophylactic heparin or pneumatic compression stockings to reduce the risk of thrombosis.

10. Should radiologic studies be avoided in pregnancy?

Yes and no. Any imaging that is required for the diagnosis and treatment of the patient should certainly be obtained. If possible, radiation exposure should be limited (by the number of views/films and shielding of the abdomen).

11. What are the associated risks of diagnostic radiologic procedures during pregnancy?

Serious risk to the fetus does not occur until the absorbed dose is 10 rad or more. Large doses of maternal radiation used in radiation therapy are associated with microcephaly and mental retardation in offspring exposed *in utero* (see table).

Estimated Ovarian Radiation Exposure From Common Radiologic Procedures (mrad)

Chest x-ray	8
Choleycystography	300
Upper GI series	558
Intravenous pyelography	407
Barium enema	805
Abdominal x-ray	289
Lumbar x-ray	275
Pelvic x-ray	41

12. What conditions specific to pregnancy may present as right upper quadrant pain?

- Severe preeclampsia—nausea, vomiting, and right upper quadrant pain may all be present.
- Hepatic capsule rupture—a dramatic complication of severe preeclampsia/HELLP syndrome, marked by sudden onset of upper abdominal pain, nausea, vomiting, and fever. Rupture may be heralded by shock and hypotension; the diagnosis is rarely made prior to emergent laparotomy. Maternal mortality has historically exceeded 60%, but is thought to be decreasing secondary to advances in imaging techniques and heightened awareness.
- Acute fatty liver of pregnancy—newly associated with a heterozygous deficiency of long-chain 3-hydroxyacyl-CoA dehydrogenase and the patient carrying an affected (homozygous) fetus. In this rare condition (approximately one in 1000 deliveries), the patient presents with acute liver failure, renal failure, hypoglycemia which may lead to coma, bleeding diatheses, and metabolic acidosis. The maternal and fetal mortality is approximately 25%.

13. Which surgical conditions are more likely to occur during periods of rapid change in uterine size (second trimester and postpartum)?

- Adnexal torsion—the presence of an adnexal mass increases this risk. Laparotomy and unilateral salpingo-oophorectomy is often necessary.
- Intestinal obstruction—adhesions (usually related to prior surgical procedures) may incarcerate loops of bowel as the intra-abdominal contents shift with growth of the uterus.

14. What is the cause of hemorrhoids in pregnancy? How are they treated?

Approximately one-third of pregnant patients suffer from hemorrhoids. The increased incidence in pregnancy is thought to be secondary to straining with constipation, increased rectal venous pressure, and increased intra-abdominal pressure. Mild hemorrhoids usually respond to increased dietary fiber, over-the-counter medications, and hemorrhoidal suppositories. Severe hemorrhoids can be treated with banding. When the complications of thrombosis or severe pain occur, hemorrhoidectomy is indicated.

15. How is fetal well-being established intraoperatively?

Some advocate intermittent intraoperative monitoring of the heart rates of viable fetuses, if possible. Others recommend obtaining fetal heart tones before and after the procedure. Women whose pregnancies are of a periviable or greater gestational age are likely to be better served if they are transported to a labor and delivery unit for postoperative recovery and monitoring.

16. Does surgery itself cause labor?

Probably not. Most researchers feel that it is the condition requiring surgery (e.g., infection, inflammation, dehydration) that leads to the increased risk of preterm labor following surgery. Unless contraindications exist, tocolysis is indicated for patients with preterm gestations experiencing labor following surgery.

17. What two rare conditions that present with left upper quadrant pain occur more frequently during pregnancy?

- Splenic rupture—the hypervolemia and relative anemia associated with pregnancy contribute to hypersplenism and the increased risk for spontaneous rupture.
- Splenic artery aneurysm rupture—25% of cases of this rare but catastrophic event occur in pregnant women. Diseased vessels are further compromised by the moderate displacement of the spleen by the gravid uterus and pregnancy-induced hypersplenism. Immediate laparotomy is warranted; despite prompt treatment, mortality is high.

BIBLIOGRAPHY

1. Firstenberg MS, Malangioni MA: Gastrointestinal surgery during pregnancy. Gastro Clin North Am 27(1):73–88, 1998.
2. Jones KL: Effects of therapeutic, diagnostic, and environmental agents. In Creasy RK, Resnick R (eds): Maternal-Fetal Medicine, 4th ed. Philadelphia, W.B. Saunders, 1999, pp 132–144.
3. Tracey M, Fletcher HS: Appendicitis in pregnancy. Am Surg 66(6):555–559, 2000.
4. Van Hook JW: Ventilator therapy and airway management. In Clark SL, Cotton DB, Hankins GDV, Phelan JP (eds): Critical Care Obstetrics, 3rd ed. Malden, Blackwell Science, 1997, pp 143–171.

50. TRAUMA IN PREGNANCY

Martha E. Rode, M.D.

1. What is the frequency of trauma in pregnancy? Why is it significant?

Trauma, either accidental or intentional (e.g., suicide, homicide, or domestic violence), is a leading cause of death in women of reproductive age. It is estimated that physical trauma complicates approximately one in every 12 pregnancies. Trauma is the leading cause of non-obstetrical maternal death.

2. What are the three most frequent causes of trauma complicating pregnancies in industrialized nations?

Motor vehicle accidents (MVAs), falls, and direct assaults to the abdomen. Two-thirds of all trauma in pregnancy are secondary to MVAs. Domestic abuse is known to escalate during pregnancy.

3. What is the risk of fetal loss with significant maternal trauma? With minor injuries?

Life-threatening trauma (e.g., shock, head injury with coma, emergent laparotomy for maternal indications) is associated with a 40–50% fetal loss rate. For minor injuries, the rate is 1–5%. As minor trauma is much more common, it is responsible for a higher number of pregnancy losses.

4. How is the risk to the fetus different with blunt trauma versus penetrating trauma?

- Blunt trauma—the fetus is at risk due to abruptio placentae or other placental injury, direct fetal injury, uterine rupture, maternal shock or death, or some combination thereof.
- Penetrating trauma—fetal loss usually occurs through direct fetal injury or damage to the umbilical cord or placenta.

Overall, maternal loss of life is the most frequent cause of fetal death.

5. How does gestational age affect the above?

In pregnancies < 13 weeks, fetal or uterine injury is rare because of the protection afforded by the pelvic bones. Therefore, trauma rarely is a cause of pregnancy loss in the first trimester. With further enlargement of the uterus, fetal injury becomes more likely. A gestational age consistent with extrauterine survival may significantly impact management decisions if there is evidence of fetal compromise.

6. Is it advantageous for a victim of abdominal penetrating trauma to be pregnant?

In some situations, yes. Maternal outcome is overall improved, as the maternal viscera are shielded by the uterus and its contents, which absorb most of the projectile energy (in the case of gunshot wounds) or prevent penetrating wounds from reaching vital organs. However, as a result of cephalad displacement of the bowel by the uterus, upper abdominal stab wounds may result in more complex bowel injury than in the non-pregnant woman.

7. If a trauma patient is pregnant, should the initial evaluation be altered?

No. The standard protocol for assessment and stabilization should be followed (airway, breathing, circulation). When attention is drawn to the fetus before the mother is stabilized, serious or life-threatening maternal injuries may be overlooked. Following stabilization, a more detailed secondary survey of the patient, including fetal evaluation, should be performed.

8. Is radiologic imaging prudent in the assessment of the extent of trauma in a pregnant patient?

Yes. Any imaging necessary for optimal treatment of the mother should be performed, with shielding of the fetus whenever possible.

9. What is the role of diagnostic peritoneal lavage (DPL) in the diagnosis of intraperitoneal hemorrhage during pregnancy?

Peritoneal lavage is unnecessary if clinically obvious intraperitoneal bleeding is present. Although controversial, most trauma surgeons respect the 98% accuracy of DPL and consider it useful in the gravid patient as long as an open (usually periumbilical) technique is employed to avoid injury of the uterus. The following are some of the indications for DPL following trauma during pregnancy:
- Abdominal signs or symptoms suggestive of intraperitoneal bleeding
- Altered sensorium
- Unexplained shock
- Major thoracic injuries
- Multiple major orthopedic injuries

Alternatively, if the patient is relatively stable, a **CT scan** is another option. This is less invasive, provides injury-specific data, and is superior for the evaluation of retroperitoneal injuries. However, its sensitivity is likely lower than DPL and, in contrast to most x-ray imaging, abdomino-pelvic CT employs a radiation dose (3.5 rads) near the threshold of fetal effect (5 rads). **Ultrasound** is increasingly being used in the trauma setting, and is attractive because of its lack of associated radiation exposure.

10. What physiologic changes that occur in pregnancy may confuse the diagnosis of serious injury or influence the pathophysiologic response the mother manifests to trauma?

PARAMETER	ADAPTATION	IMPACT ON TRAUMA PATIENT
Plasma volume	50% increase	Relative resistance to limited blood loss
Red cell mass	30% increase	Dilutional anemia
Cardiac output	30–50% increase	Relative resistance to limited blood loss
Heart rate	10–15 beats	May be interpreted as hypovolemia
Blood pressure	Fall in second trimester only	May be interpreted as hypovolemia
Coagulation factors	Increased (I, VII, VIII, IX, X)	Increased risk of deep vein thrombosis
Uteroplacetal blood flow	20–30% shunt	Uterine injury may predispose to increased blood loss
Uterine size	Dramatic increase	Compression of vena cava/aorta (supine hypotension); shifting of abdominal contents
Minute ventilation	25% increase	Decreased $PaCO_2$; decreased buffering capacity
Functional residual capacity	Decreased	Increased propensity for atelectasis and hypoxemia
Gastric emptying	Slowed	Increased risk of aspiration

11. In addition to the standard work-up, what additional facts must be established for a pregnant trauma patient?
- Estimated gestational age: based upon estimated date of conception, history, last menstruation period, clinical exam, ultrasound
- Fetal status: ultrasound with fetal heart rate, external fetal monitoring
- Assessment for labor, rupture of membranes, possible abruption

12. What additional laboratory studies should be obtained from a gravid trauma patient?

Blood type and Kleihauer-Betke (K-B). The K-B screens for fetal cells in the maternal circulation (evidence of a fetal-maternal hemorrhage). There is no evidence that this testing can predict immediate adverse sequelae (severe fetal anemia, cardiac arrhythmias, and death) due to hemorrhage. If hemorrhage occurs, the mean estimated blood volume of injected fetal blood usually is < 15 ml, and more than 90% of fetal-maternal hemorrhages are fetal blood volume < 30 ml. Therefore, administration of 300 micrograms (one ampule) of D immune globulin protects nearly all D-negative women from D alloimmunization. The K-B is used to determine which D-negative unsensitized women have a > 30 ml transfusion. Additional D immune globulin should be administered to these patients. This appears to effectively prevent alloimmunization when administered within 72 hours post trauma.

13. How long does a pregnant patient have to be monitored to rule out abruption?
    This is controversial. Because abruption usually becomes apparent shortly after injury, monitoring should be initiated as soon as the woman is stabilized. The recommended minimum time of post-trauma monitoring is 2–6 hours. No large prospective study has validated this recommendation. Monitoring should be continued and further evaluation carried out if uterine contractions, non-reassuring fetal testing, vaginal bleeding, uterine tenderness, serious maternal injury, or amniotic rupture is present.

14. In hypovolemic shock, is the fetus preferentially perfused?
    No. The fetus is treated as an expendable peripheral organ. Blood is preferentially shunted to the maternal brain and heart.

15. What maneuvers are performed to attempt to maximize uteroplacental (and therefore fetal) perfusion during evaluation and treatment of the pregnant patient?
    • Left uterine displacement: poor fetal perfusion occurs secondary to maternal hypotension stemming from uterine compression of the inferior vena cava (IVC) when the mother is in the supine position. Displacement of the uterus, either by tilting the patient or manual displacement (if the patient must remain supine) can alleviate this.
    • Administration of oxygen to the mother
    • IV hydration: expansion of the intravascular volume (a standard therapy in any trauma protocol) may increase uteroplacental perfusion.

16. Should military anti-shock trousers (MAST) be used to treat shock in the pregnant trauma patient?
    The lower extremity portion may be useful, especially in splinting fractures. The abdominal portion should not be inflated, as this may cause further compression of the IVC or aorta.

17. Are the indications for laparotomy after blunt trauma different for pregnant patients?
    No, but additional indications do exist. Standard reasons include overt peritonitis, massive hemoperitoneum, positive DPL, and significant injury on imaging study (hollow viscus or major solid organ). Pregnancy-specific indications include uterine rupture, placental abruption, and fetal distress (viable fetus).

18. Does pregnancy change the management of stab wounds?
    This is controversial. The standard management protocol limits laparotomy to patients with violation of the peritoneum and positive DPL. In pregnant trauma patients, some advocate further restriction if the injury overlies the uterus, as all but the bladder is protected. If fetal testing is reassuring and cystoscopy normal, observation may be appropriate.

19. In what circumstances is cesarean section indicated during laparotomy?
    • Damage to uterine vessels or lacerations/rupture of uterus that may threaten the health of fetus/mother if left unrepaired; cesarean hysterectomy may be necessary in this situation.
    • Mechanical obstruction by gravid uterus, preventing exposure for surgical repair
    • The risk of potential injury to fetus from continuing the pregnancy is felt to exceed risks of prematurity.

• Unstable thoracolumbar spinal injury with mature fetus
• Evidence of worsening disseminated intravascular coagulation
• Persistent maternal shock/imminent maternal death

Cesarean section adds to the total blood loss, both from the surgery and from placental separation, by about 500 ml.

20. Is intrauterine fetal demise an indication for cesarean delivery?

No! It is *not* an indication for cesarean delivery. This approach incurs increased risk to the mother and may lead to complications which could otherwise have been avoided (e.g., coagulopathy, injury from surgery, infection).

21. Is vaginal delivery possible in patients with pelvic fractures?

Yes. Pelvic fracture is not a definite contraindication to vaginal delivery. However, a severe, dislocated, or unstable fracture or a large healing callus may preclude an attempt at vaginal delivery.

22. Will labor cause dehiscence of a relatively recent abdominal incision?

No. Labor and vaginal delivery is well tolerated even in the early postoperative period.

23. When is it necessary to perform a hysterectomy?

This should be a very rare requirement. Uterine repair is faster and preserves fertility, while hysterectomy can be time-consuming and bloody. Hysterectomy should only be performed when access to other injuries remains obstructed by an empty uterus; there is severe uterine or broad ligament bleeding despite multiple maneuvers (hypogastric, uterine, or ovarian artery ligation); or uterine injury is such that repair is impossible.

24. What are the indications for perimortem cesarean delivery?

There are no clear guidelines. Neurologically intact fetal survival is highly unlikely if more than 15–20 minutes have elapsed since the loss of maternal vital signs. Based on isolated case reports, cesarean delivery should be considered for maternal benefit 4 minutes after cardiopulmonary arrest in the late second or third trimester.

25. When and how should pregnant women wear seatbelts?

Seat belts should *always* be worn. The pregnant woman positions the lap belt low under the abdomen and over both anterior superior iliac spines and the pubic symphysis. The shoulder harness should be positioned diagonally, between the breasts. Placement of the lap belt over the dome of the uterus has been associated with significant uterine and fetal injury.

26. How does pregnancy affect the outcome of gravidas who are burn victims?

Pregnancy does not appear to have an impact on maternal outcome. Fetal prognosis is related to the extent of the burns and the development of maternal complications. Burns affecting less than one-third of the body surface area have little effect on the outcome of pregnancy. Burns of more than two-thirds of the surface area are associated with an extremely high maternal mortality rate. Fetal survival is strongly influenced by the development of maternal complications such as hypoxia, hypotension, and sepsis. It has been suggested by some that delivery should be performed for fetuses of a viable gestation prior to the development of such complications.

27. What is the fetal risk following maternal electrical injuries?

The uterus and amniotic fluid offer low resistance to the passage of electricity. The risk of fetal mortality is approximately 50%. If the fetus survives, there is a risk of intrauterine growth retardation, oligohydramnios, and late intrauterine death.

28. Are suicide attempts less frequent in pregnancy?

No. Attempted suicide is at least as common among gravidas as among non-pregnant women of comparable age, but rarely successful. Attempts occur most frequently at the time of pregnancy diagnosis and early in the third trimester. They are most common among teenagers, primigravidas, and unmarried women with limited social supports. Early involvement of psychiatry is essential; patients are again at increased risk in the pueriperium.

BIBLIOGRAPHY

1. American College of Obstetrics and Gynecology: Obstetric aspects of trauma management. ACOG Technical Bulletin No. 251, 1998.
2. Hankins GDV, Van Hook JW: Trauma and envenomation. In Clark SL, Cotton DD, Hankins GDV, Phelan JP (eds): Critical Care Obstetrics, 3rd ed. Malden, MA, Blackwell Science, 1997, pp 597–628.
3. Henderson SO, Mallon WK: Trauma in pregnancy. Emerg Med Clin North Am 16(1):209–228, 1998.
4. Mighty H: Trauma in pregnancy. Crit Care Clin 10(3):623–634, 1994.
5. Stone IK: Trauma in the obstetric patient. Obstet Gynecol Clin North Am 26(3):459–467, 1999.
6. Vaizey CJ, Jacobson MJ, Cross FW: Trauma in pregnancy. Br J Surg 81(10):1406–1415, 1994.

51. TWIN PREGNANCY

Nina M. Boe, M.D., and John G. McFee, M.D.

1. How often do twins occur?

Twins occur in 1 of 100 pregnancies among white women, 1 of 80 pregnancies in black women, and in only 1 of 155 pregnancies in Asian women. Monozygotic twins occur in 1 in 250 births and are independent of race, heredity, age, and parity. Dizygotic (DZ) twinning, however, is affected by each of these factors and also by fertility drugs. A woman who is a DZ twin is twice as likely to give birth to DZ twins.

Assisted reproductive technologies also increase the rate of multiple gestations: the rate is 16–40% with gonadotropin induction of ovulation, 25–30% with superovulation, and 7–13% with clomiphene (Clomid) therapy. Additionally, women undergoing in vitro fertilization often have multiple embryos placed into the uterus; of such pregnancies that reach viability, 22% are multiple. Among women using assisted reproductive technologies, twins occur in 25–30%, triplets in 5%, and higher-order multiple gestation in 0.5–1.0%.

2. What are the mechanisms that lead to identical twins?

Identical or monozygotic (MZ) twins arise from division of one fertilized ovum into two separate embryos. The timing of this division has important implications.

Division within the first 72 hours after conception results in a **diamniotic, dichorionic (di/di)** monozygotic twin pregnancy. As neither the inner cell mass nor the outer layer of blastocyst (destined to become chorion) has formed, each embryo will have a separate amnion and chorion. This occurs in about 30% of MZ twins and has the lowest mortality rate—about 9%.

Division 4–8 days after fertilization results in a **diamniotic, monochorionic (di/mono)** twin pregnancy. As the amnion is not yet differentiated, separate amniotic sacs but shared chorion will result. This is the most frequent type of monozygotic twinning (68%), and in some series the mortality rate is as high as 25% due to complications of vascular anastomoses within the placentas.

Division 8–13 days after fertilization results in **monoamniotic, monochorionic (mono/mono)** twins. These MZ twins occur least often (2% or less) but have the highest mortality rate—up to 50%.

Division at 2 weeks after fertilization, after the amniotic sac and embryonic disk are formed but division of the embryonic disk is incomplete, results in **conjoined** twins. The frequency of conjoined twins is not well established, but is on the order of 1 in 60,000 births.

3. What mechanisms lead to fraternal twins?

Fraternal or dizygotic twins arise from the fertilization of two separate ova. **Superfecundation** refers to fertilization of different ova in the same menstrual cycle, at two separate episodes of intercourse. **Superfetation** occurs when two ova are fertilized during separate menstrual cycles, i.e., the second ovulation occurred after the first pregnancy was established; this is rare.

4. How does examination of the placenta help to establish zygosity?

Twins of the opposite sex (barring genetic abnormalities) are always dizygotic; placental examination reveals zygosity in cases of like-sex twins. Determination is based on the chorion/amnion status (see Question 2). **Histologic evaluation of the membranes** as they join the body of the placenta at the so-called "T-section" (transverse section) may be needed to establish the presence of one or two chorions. Demonstration of **vascular anastomoses** by injection of milk or dye through the vessels may reveal communications between the placentas and also indicates MZ twinning. In indeterminate situations, zygosity can be established by blood types and chromosomal or DNA polymorphisms.

5. How does ultrasound help to establish zygosity?

If fetal gender can be identified on ultrasound, twins of opposite sex are almost always dizygotic. If the separating membrane between the twins measures > 2 mm in thickness, the pregnancy is probably dichorionic. If two separate placentas are scanned, the pregnancy is dizygotic.

6. What characteristics of multiple gestations distinguish them from singleton pregnancies?

Preterm delivery: close to 50% are premature (born before 37 weeks). Prematurity is the most common cause of neonatal morbidity and mortality in multiple gestations. Overall, twins account for about 10% of all premature infants. The mean length of gestation in twins is 35 weeks, in triplets 33 weeks, and in quadruplets 31 weeks.

Intrauterine growth restriction (IUGR): occurs in up to two-thirds of twins. Although twin growth is similar to singleton gestations up to 28–30 weeks, after that point, a falloff in the growth rate can be expected. Growth restriction may occur in one or both fetuses. Asymmetric or discordant growth is identified in 10–25% of twin pregnancies and carries a higher perinatal mortality. IUGR in multiple gestations may be caused by placental insufficiency, velamentous cord insertion, and twin-twin transfusion as well as all intrinsic fetal conditions affecting a singleton pregnancy. IUGR is more common in MZ twins. Growth discordance is defined as a greater than 20% difference in the estimated fetal weights (EFW) of the twins (based on the EFW of the larger twin). If the EFW is < the 10th percentile for gestational age, IUGR is diagnosed. These twins are followed with antepartum testing, serial ultrasound evaluations for interval growth, amniotic fluid volume assessment, and Doppler velocimetry of the umbilical artery.

Perinatal mortality: averaging five times higher than singletons. The risk is higher for MZ twins and twins displaying discordant growth. The largest single cause of perinatal death, however, is prematurity. Twins are responsible for 25% of preterm perinatal deaths and 10% of all perinatal mortality. In addition to prematurity, etiologies include congenital malformations, twin-twin transfusion syndrome, uteroplacental insufficiency, and birth trauma or hypoxia.

Spontaneous abortion: at least twice as often as singleton pregnancies. With increasing use of ultrasound, early abortion or resorption of one twin—the "vanishing twin syndrome"—has been observed to occur in 21–63% of spontaneous twin gestations. It is estimated that only 50% of twins diagnosed by ultrasound in the early first trimester continue as such until delivery.

Congenital malformations: twice as frequent; increased risk is confined to MZ sets.

Pregnancy-induced hypertension: 3–5 times more often in multiple gestations, and increasing frequency correlates with higher-order gestations (e.g., triplets); apt to occur earlier in pregnancy and to be more severe as compared with singleton pregnancies. It occurs with equal frequency in MZ and DZ twin pregnancies.

Anemia: due to iron deficiency because of increased fetal requirements. Rarely, megaloblastic anemia from folic acid deficiency occurs. Additionally, physiologic dilution from plasma volume expansion contributes.

Polyhydramnios: in one or both sacs, to a greater or lesser degree in 5–8% of twin pregnancies overall. It tends to be more common in MZ sets, usually from the twin-twin transfusion syndrome.

Fetal malpresentation at birth: one of the main factors leading to more frequent cesarean delivery of twins.

Abruptio placentae: may occur with the sudden decompression of the uterus immediately after delivery of the first twin.

Placenta previa: the placenta occupies a much larger area of the uterine cavity than in singleton pregnancies, and therefore is more likely to cover the internal os of the cervix.

7. What are the risks from placental vascular anastomoses in a monochorionic placenta?

The *twin-twin transfusion syndrome* occurs when one placenta is fed by an artery from the first twin and drained by a vein that leads to the second twin. This syndrome develops in 15% of MZ sets and varies in severity. In its full-blown picture, the donor twin is hypoperfused, anemic, undergrown, and hypotensive, and oligohydramnios develops. The oligohydramnios may be so severe that the donor twin appears "stuck." The hyperperfused twin is polycythemic; has hypertension, cardiac hypertrophy, and edema; and polyhydramnios develops.

Moderate and severe twin-twin transfusion syndrome usually manifests before 28 weeks' gestation. The hallmark is a rapidly expanding uterus with polyhydramnios and discordant fetal growth. Perinatal mortality is high—only 20–45% survive if diagnosed before 28 weeks. If one fetus dies, significant problems may occur in the remaining twin, such as multicystic encephalomalacia and renal cortical necrosis. Current theory holds that such defects result from significant hypotension, as the living twin loses blood to the dead twin through placental vascular anastomoses, rather than embolic events.

The placentas in twin-twin transfusion syndrome often reflect the difference in perfusion. The recipient placenta has a more plethoric appearance and is larger, whereas the donor placenta appears pale and is somewhat smaller.

8. How are twin-twin transfusion syndromes managed?

Management begins with **ultrasound documentation** of discordant fetal growth (> 20% of the larger fetus's weight) and amniotic fluid volumes in monochorionic twins. In the third trimester, pregnancies are followed by **serial ultrasounds and nonstress tests** for fetal well-being. The patient should keep **daily fetal movement charts**, which may reveal decreased fetal movement in the donor twin due to the oligohydramnios. If fetal hydrops develops, consider delivery by **cesarean section**. Gestational age and the effect of the syndrome on the other twin influence the timing of delivery.

Polyhydramnios in the recipient twin may cause preterm labor due to distention of the uterus. **Therapeutic amniocentesis** (amnioreduction) to remove excessive amniotic fluid may help and often must be repeated at frequent intervals as the fluid rapidly reaccumulates. It is important to remove excessive fluid slowly, because rapid decompression may increase the risk of abruption. The use of this technique results in a 60% survival rate.

Fetoscopic laser coagulation of the communicating placental vessels is a promising new technique to treat twin-twin transfusion syndrome. It is available only in a few centers, but may result in a higher survival rate and perhaps a lower risk of neurologic disability. **Selective feto-cide** of the smaller infant with umbilical cord occlusion is also under study.

9. What are the principles of prenatal care for twin pregnancies?
  • Early diagnosis is associated with an improved perinatal outcome.
  • Frequent antenatal visits, at least every 2 weeks from 20–36 weeks
  • Diet: additional calories (+300 kcal/day) and protein (to 80 g/day); 60–100 mg/day of iron supplementation; folic acid, 1 mg/day; weight gain 35–45 pounds
  • Extra bedrest
  • Educate the patient about the signs and symptoms of preterm labor. Inquire about these at every prenatal visit.
  • Prevent, recognize, and aggressively treat preterm labor.
  • Follow fetal growth by serial ultrasound examinations to detect discordant growth and IUGR; manage accordingly.
  • Watch for and treat pregnancy-induced hypertension and preeclampsia.
  • Watch for and manage less common complications: polyhydramnios, twin-twin transfusion syndrome, intrauterine death.
  • Institute antepartum testing if IUGR, significant growth discordance (> 20% difference in EFW), oligohydramnios or polyhydramnios, preeclampsia, fetal anomalies, or monoamniotic monochorionic twins are present. (Many physicians institute antepartum testing at 32–34 weeks for twins in general, since they have a significantly increased perinatal morbidity and mortality.)
  • Have parents make plans for two babies at home.

10. How can preterm delivery be prevented?

There is a higher incidence of preterm labor with twins due to increased uterine distention, and prematurity in multiple gestation is associated with substantial morbidity and mortality.

Therefore, a major effort must be devoted to preventing preterm labor. The overall objective, in the absence of other problems, is to achieve **34 weeks' gestation**, beyond which poor outcomes owing to prematurity are unusual. The critical period for these efforts is 24–32 weeks.

Bed rest, hospitalization, prophylactic oral tocolytic drugs (beta-mimetics), routine weekly cervical examination, and prophylactic cerclage have been promoted as measures to prolong twin gestation. None of these is consistently effective in reducing the rate of preterm delivery in twins.

Results of programs for early detection of preterm labor through frequent contact with healthcare providers and education of the patient have been mixed. The use of home uterine activity monitoring to identify uterine contractions has not been found to be effective. Oral tocolytic agents were not effective in preventing preterm labor or preterm delivery in twin gestations.

11. How is the management of preterm labor different for multiple gestations?

Intervention is similar to a singleton pregnancy, with additional consideration of the altered maternal physiologic characteristics of multiple pregnancy. Plasma volume with twins exceeds that of normal pregnancy (as much as 50–60% of the nonpregnant state vs. 45%), and cardiac output (heart rate and stroke volume) is increased over that of a singleton gestation. Such changes pose a special risk with intravenous fluids and beta-mimetic tocolytics. Pulmonary edema and other cardiac problems are seen more often with tocolysis of twin gestation, which dictates that tocolytic agents be used with caution. Magnesium sulfate may be the best initial tocolytic drug. Strict monitoring of patient fluid volume is mandatory. The use of nifedipine or indomethacin in patients who fail magnesium sulfate may be successful. Administer a single course of steroid therapy (betamethasone) to accelerate fetal lung maturity in patients with documented preterm labor between 24–34 weeks' gestation.

12. How should parents of multiple gestations plan for the future?

The diagnosis of twins usually comes as a shock to most parents, especially the mother. Increasing physical discomfort causes difficulty in performing the usual household chores, caring for other children in the family, and continuing with employment. At home following delivery, the reality of caring for two babies at once, especially if they are premature and/or have other medical problems, is a real challenge. Parents may feel exhausted and overwhelmed. Prospective parents of multiple gestations should plan ahead, and arrange for additional help from family and friends in the home after delivery. Many communities have twin parent support groups. Information about such groups should be made available to the parents early in the pregnancy.

13. What happens if one twin dies in utero?

- If death occurs *in the first trimester*, the dead fetus may be completely resorbed or may persist as a fetus papyraceous (small, flattened, dried-out fetus). If the patient did not have an ultrasound during this time, the twin gestation may not be identified.
- If death occurs *in the second or third trimester* (incidence 0.5–6.8%), the surviving fetus may face significant morbidity and mortality. Prognostic factors include the etiology of the demise, type of zygosity and placentation, gestational age at the time of demise, and length of time between death of the first twin and delivery of the surviving twin. Monozygotic twins with monoamniotic/monochorionic or diamniotic/monochorionic placentation are at highest risk of complications.

14. Describe morbidity in the surviving twin. Are there any risks to the mother?

Neonatal morbidity in the surviving MZ twin involves structural defects of the central nervous system, skin, and kidneys. Cerebral palsy, microcephaly, multicystic encephalomalacia, renal cortical necrosis, and aplasia cutis have been reported. Thromboplastin from the dead twin was thought to cross via placental anastomoses to the living twin and to cause infarction of various organs. Current theory holds that such defects result from significant, prolonged hypotension as the living twin loses blood to the dead twin through placental vascular anastomoses. Maternal morbidity from disseminated intravascular coagulation is rare and usually does not occur until 4 or more weeks after fetal death.

Early delivery does not prevent or decrease the risk of such complications, which are likely to have occurred at the time of demise. Delivery should be done for the usual obstetric indications. Vaginal delivery is appropriate unless there is an obstetric indication for cesarean section.

15. Do twins differ from singletons in developing pulmonary maturity? How should pulmonary maturity be assessed?

Overall, twins appear to develop pulmonary maturity 3–4 weeks earlier than singletons, and many achieve maturity by 32 weeks. Lecithin/sphingomyelin (L/S) ratios and the risk of hyaline membrane disease after birth are usually similar for both babies, but occasionally, differences are marked. Pulmonary function is frequently more mature in the smaller, growth-restricted twin of a discordant set and in the presenting twin during preterm labor.

When assessment of pulmonary maturity is necessary, amniocentesis from one twin for an L/S ratio is adequate in most cases. In cases of discordant growth, the sac of the larger twin should be tapped. In preterm labor, the sac of the nonpresenting twin should be sampled.

16. How are twins managed in labor and delivery?

Anticipate and recognize the increased potential for complications of labor and delivery in twins. Delivery should take place in the operating room with equipment for either vaginal or cesarean delivery. Continuous electronic fetal monitoring of both twins, intravenous fluid access, surveillance of patient and fetuses by a trained obstetric nurse, presence of an obstetrician, and immediate availability of anesthesia are *mandatory*. In addition, pediatricians and/or other nursery personnel are needed for neonatal resuscitation. Complications to be anticipated include uterine dysfunction, pregnancy-induced hypertension, fetal malpresentations, prolapse of the umbilical cord, abruptio placentae, fetal distress necessitating emergent delivery, and postpartum hemorrhage.

17. What are the most common presentations of twins at labor and delivery?

Vertex-vertex	42%	Vertex-transverse	18%
Vertex-breech	27%	Others	8%
Breech-breech	5%		

18. What are locked twins?

Although rare (1 in 817 twins), the phenomenon of locked twins occurs when the first fetus is breech and the second is vertex. The chin of the first (breech) fetus locks in the neck and chin of the second (vertex) fetus. This situation may occur in both single- and double-sac twins. Unless they spontaneously disengage, delivery must be accomplished by cesarean section.

19. How does fetal presentation affect labor and delivery of twins?

On admission, the presentation of both twins is established by ultrasound examination. Generally, vertex-vertex twins are delivered vaginally, and sets in which twin A is nonvertex are delivered by cesarean section. The management of vertex-nonvertex twins is controversial.

20. How is delivery of vertex-vertex twins managed?

After delivery of the first twin, the cord is left clamped and no blood is taken; placental anastomoses may compromise the blood supply to the second twin. Until the second twin's head is well engaged, its amniotic sac is left intact if possible. Unless electronic fetal monitoring is non-reassuring or bleeding suggests an abruption, the uterus is allowed to resume labor for delivery of the second twin. Oxytocin may be needed to restart uterine contractions. Generally, the second twin delivers within 15–30 minutes of the first twin. With continuous electronic fetal monitoring, this interval may be prolonged as long as the fetal heart rate tracing remains reassuring. Delivery, as with twin A, may be expedited by vacuum extraction or low forceps, if indicated.

21. What are the delivery options if the presentation is vertex-breech?

Breech extraction of the second twin is successful in 83–96% of attempts. The prerequisites for breech extraction are the same as for singleton breech deliveries—i.e., adequate pelvis, estimated fetal weight of 2000–3800 g, flexed or military head, a physician experienced in performing breech extraction, and the *immediate* availability of general anesthesia. Adequate anesthesia is mandatory for managing soft-tissue dystocia, nuchal arms, and other problems with delivery of the aftercoming head, which is the cause of most morbidity in vaginal breech delivery. Many practitioners do not attempt this form of delivery if the estimated fetal weight of twin B is significantly greater than that of twin A.

External cephalic version of the second (breech) twin to a vertex presentation under ultrasound guidance is another option. Versions are successful in 46–73% of attempts, depending on gestational age and maternal habitus. Delivery then proceeds as in a singleton vertex delivery. The disadvantages are fetal distress secondary to the version or other factors and unsuccessful version. In such cases, the woman must undergo immediate cesarean section or breech extraction for delivery of the second twin. For these reasons, this approach is used much less frequently.

In light of the potential problems associated with either external cephalic version or breech extraction, it seems reasonable to offer **cesarean section** as an option to patients with a vertex-breech presentation, if the physician involved is not adequately trained in breech extraction or external cephalic version.

22. What are the postpartum risks for twin pregnancies?

Because the uterus of a multiple gestation is overdistended, it frequently contracts inadequately after delivery. Postpartum hemorrhage from uterine atony must be anticipated and steps taken for its prevention.

23. What is the role of selective reduction in multiple gestations?

With assisted reproductive technologies, higher-order gestations occur more frequently. Both maternal and neonatal outcomes from pregnancies complicated by quadruplets or greater are believed to be significantly improved by reducing the pregnancy to a lower gestational number early in gestation. Usually performed at 10–13 weeks, selective reduction is generally undertaken by intracardiac/intrafetal injection of potassium chloride.

For pregnancies with triplets, studies have been varied with regard to the overall benefits of selective reduction to twins. Although many report comparable perinatal outcomes in selectively reduced triplets (to twins) compared with triplets managed with close surveillance, some studies suggest selective reduction of triplet pregnancies to twins leads to reduced perinatal morbidity and mortality. The risk of loss of the entire pregnancy after multi-fetal reduction is 8–12% in the centers with the most experience in reducing triplets to twins.

BIBLIOGRAPHY

1. American College of Obstetricians and Gynecologists. Special Problems of Multiple Gestation. ACOG Educational Bulletin No. 253. Washington DC, American College of Obstetricians and Gynecologists, 1998.
2. Benirschke K: Multiple gestation: Incidence, etiology, and inheritance. In Creasy RK, Resnik R (eds): Maternal-Fetal Medicine: Principles and Practice, 4th ed. Philadelphia, W.B. Saunders, 1999, pp 585–597.
3. Boggess KA, Chisholm CA: Delivery of the nonvertex second twin: A review of the literature. Obstet Gynecol Surv 52 (12):728–735, 1997.
4. Chitkara U, Berkowitz RL: Multiple gestations. In Gabbe SG, Niebyl JR, Simpson JL (eds): Obstetrics: Normal and Problem Pregnancies, 4th ed. New York, Churchill Livingstone, 2002, pp 827–867.
5. Cunningham FG, Gant NF, Levens KJ, et al (eds): Williams Obstetrics, 21st ed. New York, McGraw-Hill, 2001, pp 765–810.
6. Malone FD, D'Alton ME: Multiple gestation: Clinical characteristics and management. In Creasy RK, Resnik R (eds): Maternal-Fetal Medicine: Principles and Practice, 4th ed. Philadelphia, W.B. Saunders, 1999, pp 598–615.

52. ISOIMMUNIZATION IN PREGNANCY

Mohammed Elkousy, M.D.

1. What is red cell isoimmunization?

Red blood cells (RBCs) have numerous cell surface antigens that are involved in maintaining membrane stability and assist in transmembrane exchange. One group of antigens on RBCs is part of the Rh system and is composed of D, C, c, E, and e antigens. Other antigens include those from other blood group systems such as Kell, Kidd, Duffy, and Lewis. Red cell isoimmunization occurs when women who lack a particular red cell antigen are exposed to that antigen and produce antibodies.

Fetal hemolytic disease occurs when these antibodies pass through the placenta to the fetus that is carrying that antigen. The antibodies form a complex with the RBC, and fetal RBC destruction occurs. This sequence of events is possible with many of the RBC antigens to varying degrees, but the most commonly studied has been the Rh blood group system.

2. How can women become exposed to foreign red cell antigens?

A mother can become exposed to foreign red cell antigens if she is carrying a fetus that is carrying the antigen that she lacks. In Rh disease, an Rh-negative mother would be exposed to the RBC of an Rh-positive fetus. Fetal RBCs are known to cross into the maternal circulation, exposing the mother's immune system to the foreign antigen.

Another mode of exposure is through blood transfusion. Blood is routinely tested for Rh-D and ABO compatibility. This is not the case for the irregular antigens.

3. Why is Kell isoimmunization different?

Although isoimmunization by Kell antigen results in fetal anemia through red cell destruction, it is believed that Kell also causes anemia through erythroid suppression. This makes management more complicated than for Rh isoimmunization.

4. What is the significance of the Lewis antibodies Le(a) and Le(b)?

These antibodies do not cause fetal anemia because they are IgM antibodies, and their structure does not allow them to cross the placenta. In addition, these antigens are poorly expressed on fetal RBC.

5. What is the current preventive strategy for Rh disease?

Currently, prevention of Rh disease is by testing women at their first prenatal visit with a blood type and antibody screen. In those women who are Rh negative with a negative antibody screen, 300-ug (one vial) of anti-D globulin (IgG) is given at 28 weeks of gestation if the antibody screen has remained negative. At the time of delivery, if the newborn is Rh positive, the anti-D globulin is readministered. Administration of anti-D globulin will cause maternal serum antibody titers to be positive to no greater than a titer of 1:4 for several weeks after administration.

6. Providing anti-D globulin will protect against what quantity of fetal blood in the maternal circulation?

One vial will protect against 30 cc of fetal whole blood or 15 cc of fetal packed red blood cells.

7. If you suspect a fetal-maternal hemorrhage that exposes the mother to more than 30 cc of fetal whole blood, what test should you order?

The Kleihauer-Betke (KB) test will tell you the percentage of fetal cells in the maternal circulation. Generally we assume that the maternal blood volume is 5 liters during pregnancy.

Multiplying your KB result by 5000 cc will give you the amount of fetal blood in the maternal circulation. For example, a KB of 0.2% should be calculated as .002 × 5000 = 10 cc of fetal blood. If more than 30 cc of fetal blood has passed into the maternal circulation, then more than one vial of anti-D globulin is required.

8. What is the next step in management of a mother who has a positive antibody screen for an antibody that is known to cause fetal hemolytic disease?

Determine paternity and then evaluate the paternal antigen status. If the father's antigen status is negative, then no further evaluation is required. In the case of D-antigen status, a person may be either heterozygous or homozygous at the D gene locus. Charts are available to assist in determining the most likely zygosity based on the presence or absence of the other antigens in the Rh system, and the paternal race.

9. What is the critical titer?

The critical titer is the antibody level in the maternal serum that signifies that more invasive testing is needed to manage an isoimmunized pregnancy. Antibody titers are measured using an indirect Coombs' test (the amount of antibody in the maternal serum that is not bound to red cells). A critical titer is considered to be 1:16. An exception to this rule is for anti-Kell, for which the critical titer used to initiate invasive testing is 1:8.

10. What is the Du antigen?

The Du antigen is a cell surface marker that is part of the D antigen. There have been reports of Du-positive women becoming sensitized to the D antigen. Anti-D globulin may be given to Du-positive women.

11. Which invasive tests can be used to assess the fetal condition?

Amniocentesis or cordocentesis can both be used. Amniotic fluid contains bilirubin, which is an indirect marker of fetal hemolytic disease. Amniocentesis can be performed every 1–3 weeks to obtain delta OD450 measurements. Cordocentesis is a direct sampling through the fetal umbilical cord to determine fetal hemoglobin and hematocrit levels. Although the data for delta OD450 measurements mainly comes from RH disease (anti-D), it is still applied to other irregular antibodies. Its utility is limited for anti-Kell because the mechanism for this antibody is also thought to include erythroid suppression. Recently, a noninvasive method utilizing Doppler ultrasound measurements for the peak systolic velocity of the fetal middle cerebral artery has been more useful for managing anti-Kell pregnancies.

12. What is the Liley graph?

The Liley graph is a plot on semi-logarithmic paper between the change in optical density at 450 nm (delta OD450) of the amniotic fluid bilirubin plotted against gestational age between 27 and 41 weeks. The graph is divided into three zones. Zone 1 indicates an unaffected fetus, Zone 2 is an affected fetus, and Zone 3 indicates a fetus that is at risk for intrauterine death. Prior to 27 weeks, data have been published for the extrapolation of the curve.

13. What is the management of a fetus that falls into Zone 2?

Management of fetuses in Zone 2 is essentially continuing with amniocentesis every 2–3 weeks. After the first amniocentesis, the second is usually performed 2 weeks later, and if the trend of the delta OD450 appears to be decreasing, the amniocentesis can be performed at greater intervals. Remember, every time an amniocentesis is performed, you run the risk of increasing the maternal antibody response.

14. What is the management of a fetus that falls into Zone 3?

Cordocentesis with intrauterine blood transfusion.

15. What are the sonographic findings in a fetus that is moderately to severely affected?

Cardiomegaly, pericardial effusions, ascites, hepatosplenomegaly, umbilical vein dilation, subcutaneous edema, increased placental size, and polyhydramnios.

16. Describe middle cerebral artery Doppler ultrasound.

Recently, it was discovered that the peak velocity of systolic blood flow in the middle cerebral artery is increased in fetuses with anemia. These measurements are now being used as a noninvasive method to detect fetuses with moderate or severe anemia.

BIBLIOGRAPHY

1. American College of Obstetricians and Gynecologists: ACOG Educational Bulletin—Management of Isoimmunization in Pregnancy. Number 227, August 1996, pp 581–587.
2. Berry SM: Red cell isoimmunization and fetal hemolytic disease. In Gleicher (ed): Principles and Practice of Medical Therapy in Pregnancy, 3rd ed. Stamford, Appleton and Lange, 1998, pp 213–222.
3. Mari G: Noninvasive diagnosis by Doppler ultrasonography of fetal anemia due to maternal red-cell alloimmunization. New Engl J Med 342(1), 2000.
4. Mckenna DS, Nagaraja HN, O'Shaughnessy R: Management of pregnancies complicated by anti-Kell isoimmunization. Obstet Gynecol 93(5; part 1):667–673, 1999.
5. Nicolaides KH, Rodeck CH, Mibashan RS, Kemp JR: Have Liley charts outlived their usefulness? Am J Obstet Gynecol 155(1):90–94, 1986.
6. Queenan JT: Diagnosis and treatment of Rh-erythroblastosis fetalis. Contemp OB/GYN 48–52, 61–62, July, 1994.
7. Queenan JT, Tomai TP, Ural SH, King JC: Deviation in amniotic fluid optical density at a wavelength of 450 nm in Rh-immunized pregnancies from 14 to 40 weeks' gestation: A proposal for clinical management. Am J Obstet Gynecol 168(5):1370–1376, 1993.

VI. The Fetus and Placenta

53. PRENATAL DIAGNOSIS

Serdar H. *Ural*, M.D.

1. Who should be offered prenatal diagnosis?
Mothers at risk for having a fetus with any of the following:
　Chromosome abnormality
　Genetic disease
　Neural tube defect
　Congenital malformations
Mothers with:
　Teratogen exposure
　Abnormal maternal serum screening tests
　Abnormal ultrasound exam
　Family history of chromosomal/congenital abnormalities
　Exposure to infections

2. What are other indications for prenatal diagnosis?
- History of prior neonatal death
- Hemoglobinopathies
- Tay-Sachs disease
- Cystic fibrosis
- Fragile X syndrome

3. List the risk factors for having an infant with a chromosomal abnormality.
- Maternal age of 35 years or older
- Previous child with a chromosomal abnormality
- Chromosome abnormality in either parent, including balanced translocation, aneuploidy, or mosaicism
- Chromosome abnormality in a close family member
- Abnormal fetus on ultrasound exam
- Abnormal maternal serum screening tests/abnormal triple screen (alpha-fetoprotein (AFP), estriol (uE3), beta-hcG)
- Prior child with neural tube defect

4. Why are women over age 35 at risk for having infants with chromosomal abnormalities?
Increased maternal age poses increased risk for a fetus with nondisjunction of a chromosome. *Nondisjunction* is an error in meiosis that results in a gamete with one chromosome too few or too many. Fertilization of the gamete with one extra chromosome results in a conception with 47 chromosomes. **Aneuploidy** occurs when the chromosome number is not an exact multiple of 23. The most common aneuploidies are trisomy 21 (Down syndrome), trisomy 13 (Patau syndrome), and trisomy 18 (Edwards syndrome). Nondisjunction may involve the sex chromosomes; therefore, abnormalities such as 47,XXY, 47,XYY, and 47,XXX also increase with increasing maternal age.

5. If a parent is a translocation carrier, what is the risk of an unbalanced offspring?

An unbalanced offspring has an abnormal amount of chromosomal material. All people have two copies of chromosomes except for the sex chromosomes. The offspring of a translocation carrier may have three copies of one chromosome and only one copy of another. Translocation may involve whole chromosomes or portions of chromosomes. The specific risk of having an abnormal child varies according to the type of translocation.

6. How should a couple with a previous child with spina bifida be screened?

If the couple appears to have a child with an isolated neural tube defect (NTD), the risk for recurrence with that couple is around 3% for each pregnancy. Because serum screening may miss a proportion of abnormalities, an ultrasonographic assessment of fetal anatomy—including an evaluation of the neural tube/spinal column—is necessary. Amniocentesis for amniotic fluid alpha-fetoprotein (AFP) and possibly acetylcholinesterase may be necessary. Review the couple's family and medical histories, and examine the medical records of the previous child to see if a specific diagnosis was made. Sometimes an NTD is part of a syndrome, or it may be due to a chromosomal abnormality. In some cases the recurrence risk may be increased.

7. If a family history identifies a couple at risk for a specific inherited disease, how should they be counseled?

Obtain medical records of the affected family members to determine the specific diagnosis. Then investigate the specific inherited disease to see if prenatal diagnosis is available. The couple can be counseled according to what tests are available. For example, carrier testing for Tay-Sachs disease is available, and if both members of the couple are carriers, prenatal diagnosis is indicated since it is autosomal recessive. The metabolic defect (hexosaminidase A enzyme deficiency) can be determined from cultured amniocytes and chorionic villi. In this case, amniocentesis or chorionic villus sampling can be offered.

8. What DNA techniques are used in prenatal diagnosis?

If the specific, most common mutations are known for a disease, mutations can be looked for in fetal cells such as amniocytes or chorionic villus. When multiple different mutations in a known gene are responsible for a specific disease, such as Duchenne muscular dystrophy, or if the gene has not been identified, linkage to DNA markers can be used. DNA markers are located near the gene on the chromosome. Polymerase chain reaction (PCR) is a commonly used technique today.

9. Which techniques are used most often to make prenatal diagnosis?
- Maternal serum screening/multiple marker screen
- Ultrasound
- Chorionic villus sampling
- Amniocentesis
- Magnetic resonance imaging
- Percutaneous umbilical blood sampling
- Ultrasound-guided tissue biopsy

10. What is genetic amniocentesis?

Amniocentesis is a technique in which amniotic fluid is removed from around the fetus. The fluid or the cells suspended in the fluid can be used for specific metabolic tests, recombinant DNA technique, or obtaining a karyotype (chromosomes). Traditionally, amniocentesis is done between 16 and 18 weeks of pregnancy. The risk of procedure-related loss is stated to be 1/200–300. Amniotic fluid AFP can be assessed to screen for neural tube defects.

Early amniocentesis is done before 16 weeks. Present data does not support safety equal to traditional amniocentesis.

11. What is chorionic villus sampling (CVS)?

CVS is a procedure in which placental tissue is removed between 10 and 12 weeks. The tissue can be obtained by either a transabdominal or transcervical approach and can be used for recombinant DNA techniques, PCR, enzyme assays, or cytogenetic testing. The *advantage* of the procedure is earlier diagnosis, which may result in decreased medical risks associated with earlier termination. The *disadvantages* include a fetal loss rate of about 1/100. Limb reduction defects have also been reported. An amniotic fluid AFP cannot be done simultaneously. As a result, maternal serum AFP and a fetal anatomic ultrasound survey are recommended at around 16 weeks and at 18–20 weeks, respectively.

12. What concern has been raised about birth defects among infants exposed to CVS?

Initial studies suggested a markedly higher rate of limb reduction abnormalities in infants exposed to CVS. Similar anomalies have been noted in animals secondary to ischemic damage as a result of vasoconstriction/vascular trauma. General recommendations include preprocedural counseling about limb reduction defects.

13. What is the function of the triple test and the multiple marker screen?

These tests use biochemical markers in the maternal serum to calculate the risk for a birth defect and chromosomal anomaly. The most common abnormalities for which risk can be calculated are neural tube defect, trisomy 21, trisomy 18, and trisomy 13.

14. What markers are used in the triple test?

- Alpha-fetoprotein
- Human chorionic gonadotropin (hCG)
- Unconjugated estriol (uE3)

15. How are the markers in the triple test interpreted?

AFP was the first fetal biochemical analog found to have altered serum concentration in the mother of a fetus with Down syndrome. AFP is produced by the yolk sac first, then fetal gastrointestinal tract and fetal liver. The AFP level and maternal age can be used to calculate a risk for Down syndrome. About 25% of fetuses with Down syndrome can be detected with AFP alone, and about 60% using the multiple marker screen; amniocentesis and chromosome studies are needed in 3–5% of screened pregnancies. The AFP is about 20% lower in the serum of mothers of a fetus with Down syndrome. **hCG** is produced by the placenta and is about twice as high in the serum of women with a fetus with Down syndrome. **uE3** is 25% lower than normal. It is produced by the fetal adrenal gland, fetal liver, and placenta. The three values are combined, and a specific risk for an individual pregnancy is given.

16. What other information is included in the calculation of the triple test?

- Maternal age
- Gestational age
- Race
- Diabetes mellitus
- Maternal weight

17. What are the advantages and disadvantages of percutaneous umbilical blood sampling for prenatal diagnosis?

Ultrasound-guided aspiration of a fetal blood sample can be obtained generally from 18 weeks' gestation onward. Sampling can be done from the umbilical cord and fetal intrahepatic vein. The fetus may need to be immobilized via medication.

Advantages include access to the entire spectrum of diagnostic studies afforded by a peripheral blood sample, including karyotype in 48 hours and hematologic, infectious, immunologic, and acid/base assessment, and treatment for such conditions as fetal arrythmia. *Disadvantages* include a 3–5/100 fetal loss rate, depending on circumstances.

18. What are some of the ultrasound findings for trisomy 21?
- Small-for-dates fetus
- Short femur
- Echogenic bowel
- Heart malformations
- Thickened nuchal fold

19. What new prenatal diagnostic options are on the horizon?

Preimplantation diagnosis. Early in human gestation, when the vast majority of cells are destined for trophoblastic development, a single cell at the 8-cell stage or a dozen cells at the blastocyst stage can be removed without subsequent damage to the fetus. These cells provide sufficient DNA for PCR-directed molecular analyses of inherited diseases or fluorescent in situ hybridization for aneuploidy. Preimplantation biopsy for prenatal diagnosis involves participation in an in vitro fertilization program and is currently available for a limited number of genetic conditions.

Fetal cells in maternal circulation. Acquisition of fetal DNA without invasive studies has been an area of research for several decades. Attempts are underway to identify the most efficient means of isolating the few fetal cells from the overwhelming number of maternal cells. Once isolated, fetal cells provide information about the fetus through PCR and molecular studies as well as fluorescent in situ hybridization for aneuploidy.

BIBLIOGRAPHY

1. American College of Obstetricians and Gynecologists: Genetic Technologies. ACOG Tech Bull 208, 1995.
2. American College of Obstetricians and Gynecologists: Maternal serum screening. ACOG Educ Bull 228, 1996.
3. Burton BK: Outcome of pregnancies with unexplained elevated or low levels of maternal serum alpha fetoprotein. Obstet Gynecol 72:709, 1988.
4. Campbell TL: Maternal serum alpha fetoprotein screening: Benefits, risks and costs. J Fam Pract 25:461, 1987.
5. Crandall BF: Risks associated with an elevated maternal serum alpha fetoprotein level. Am J Obstet Gynecol 165:581, 1991.
6. Creasy RK, Resnick R: Maternal Fetal Medicine, 4th ed. Philadelphia, W.B. Saunders, 1999, pp 1–62, 341–364.
7. Haddow JE, Palomaki GE, Knight GJ, et al: Prenatal screening for Down's syndrome with use of maternal serum markers. N Engl J Med 327:588, 1992.
8. Hook EB, Cross PK, Schreinmachers DM: Chromosome abnormality rate at amniocentesis and in live-born infants. JAMA 249:2034–2038, 1983.
9. Stoll C, Tenconi R, Clementi M: Detection of congenital anomalies by fetal ultrasonographic examination across Europe. Community Genet 4(4):233–238, 2001.

54. GENETICS IN PREGNANCY

Deborah A. Driscoll, M.D.

GENETIC COUNSELING AND SCREENING

1. When should genetic counseling occur?

Ideally, counseling should be offered prior to conception or early in pregnancy to assess a couple's or individual's risk of having a child with a chromosomal abnormality, genetic disorder, or congenital malformation. The risk depends on the family history, medical history, prior history of stillbirths or miscarriages, ethnicity, medication, and exposures (Table 1).

At the counseling session, a three-generation pedigree is obtained, risk is determined, and prenatal testing and reproductive options are discussed. The benefits, risks, and limitations of testing are reviewed.

Table 1. *Common Indications for Genetic Counseling*

Advanced maternal age (≥ 35)
Previous child or parent with chromosomal abnormality
Previous child or relative with mental retardation
Previous child, parent, or relative with congenital malformation
Previous child, parent, or relative with a single-gene disorder
Recurrent miscarriages or stillbirth
Teratogen exposure
Consanguinity (e.g., first cousins)

2. What screening tests should be offered to determine if an individual is a carrier of a single-gene disorder?

Specific screening tests for single-gene disorders are offered to individuals based on their ethnicity and/or family history. The incidence and carrier risk for some genetic disorders is increased among certain ethnic groups and has led to the current recommendations for carrier screening (Table 2). Individuals of Jewish ancestry may also consider carrier testing for Gaucher disease, Niemann-Pick disease, Fanconi pancytopenia syndrome, and cystic fibrosis (CF). These are DNA-based tests, which screen for the common mutations that have been identified in this specific population.

For many genetic diseases such as CF and Duchenne muscular dystrophy, the gene and disease-causing mutations have been characterized, and carrier testing is available for individuals with a known family history. In 2001, the American College of Obstetrics and Gynecology recommended that CF carrier screening be offered to all pregnant women and women contemplating pregnancy.

Table 2. *Recommendations for Carrier Screening*

ETHNICITY	GENETIC DISEASE	CARRIER RISK	SCREENING TEST
African-American	Sickle cell	1/10	Hemoglobin electrophoresis
Asian	α-Thalassemia	1/25	Mean corpuscular volume (MCV)
Mediterranean	β-Thalassemia	1/30	Mean corpuscular volume (MCV)
Ashkenazi Jewish	Tay-Sachs	1/30	Hexosaminidase A or DNA mutation testing
	Canavan	1/40	DNA mutation testing

3. What percentage of children are born with birth defects? What causes them?

Two to three percent of liveborns have a major malformation; 5% have a minor malformation. The etiology is heterogeneous and includes chromosomal abnormalities, single-gene disorders, teratogenic exposures, maternal diseases (e.g., insulin-dependent diabetes, phenylketonuria), and infections (e.g., cytomegalovirus, rubella). The majority of isolated malformations are presumed to be multifactorial.

4. Can fetal malformations be prevented?

Folic acid has been shown to reduce the risk of neural tube defects (NTDs). All reproductive-age women should consume 0.4 mg of folate daily. Women who have had an NTD in a previous pregnancy should take 4 mg of folate per day beginning 3 months prior to conception and through the first trimester.

The risk for fetal malformations such as cardiac and NTDs in women with insulin-dependent diabetes is reduced with optimal glucose control prior to pregnancy. Women with phenylketonuria can reduce their risk for fetal malformations (e.g., cardiac defects, microcephaly) and mental retardation by adherence to a phenylalanine-restricted diet prior to and throughout pregnancy.

5. What screening tests are recommended during pregnancy to determine whether the fetus has a congenital malformation?

Standard obstetrical practice is to offer **maternal serum alpha-fetoprotein (MSAFP) testing** at 15–18 weeks' gestation as a screening test for NTDs. Amniotic fluid AFP levels are elevated when the fetus has an NTD. MSAFP screening identifies approximately 80% of fetuses with open spina bifida and 90% with anencephaly. Other conditions associated with an elevated MSAFP include multiple gestation, gastroschisis, omphalocele, fetal demise, and incorrect dating of the pregnancy.

Ultrasonography at 18–22 weeks' gestation is a useful tool to detect major congenital malformations, although some studies have questioned the efficacy of routine ultrasound screening for anatomical defects. For pregnancies at risk of a malformation or a genetic disorder based on family history, results of MSAFP screening, exposure to teratogens or infections, or maternal condition, ultrasonography is indicated.

Fetal **echocardiography** to determine if the fetus has a congenital heart defect is indicated when a first-degree relative (sibling or parent) has a cardiac defect; the fetus has a chromosomal abnormality, malformation, or suspected cardiac defect detected by ultrasonography; the fetus is at risk for a genetic disorder associated with a cardiac defect; the mother has insulin-dependent diabetes; or the mother uses a medication associated with a cardiac defect (e.g., Accutane).

6. Can a parental history of infertility affect the fetus?

Some causes of infertility can increase the risk of having a fetus with a chromosomal abnormality or a genetic disease such as CF. Severe oligospermia and azospermia are associated with balanced translocations (3–5%), Klinefelter's syndrome (47,XXY), and abnormalities and microdeletions of the Y chromosome. Individuals with sex chromosome abnormalities associated with subfertility—including XYY males, XXX females, and females with Turner syndrome mosaicism—have an increased risk for offspring with chromosomal abnormalities. Approximately two-thirds of males with congenital bilateral absence of the vas deferens (CBAVD) have at least one CF mutation.

Partners of males with CBAVD and a CF mutation should be offered CF screening to determine if they are carriers, too. Since affected men are candidates for testicular aspiration and biopsy with intracytoplasmic sperm injection, prior knowledge of one's risk for having a child with CF may influence choice of reproductive options.

CHROMOSOMAL DISORDERS

7. How often do chromosomal abnormalities occur in newborns? Stillbirths? Spontaneous abortions?

The incidence of chromosomal abnormalities increases with advancing maternal age, due to non-disjunction. The incidence of chromosomal abnormalities in livebirths is 0.5%, stillbirths

5%, and spontaneous abortions 50%. In livebirths, the most common autosomal disorder is trisomy 21 (1 in 800); trisomy 18 and 13 are less frequent (Table 3). Trisomy 16 is the most common autosomal disorder in first-trimester spontaneous abortions. Trisomy 18 is most common in stillbirths.

At 35 years of age, women are routinely offered genetic counseling and prenatal diagnostic testing for chromosomal abnormalities by either amniocentesis at 15–17 weeks or chorionic villus sampling at 10–12 weeks' gestation. Testing is offered at any age for individuals with a chromosome abnormality (e.g., balanced translocation). Individuals with a previous trisomy have a 1% recurrence risk in each subsequent pregnancy and, hence, are offered testing.

Table 3. Autosomal Chromosomal Disorders

CHROMOSOME ABNORMALITY	PREVALENCE AT BIRTH	CLINICAL FEATURES
Trisomy 21	1/800	Cardiac defects, duodenal atresia, characteristic facies, mental retardation
Trisomy 18	1/6000	Cardiac defects, omphalocele, IUGR, clenched fists with overlapping fingers, severe mental retardation, < 10% survive to 1 year
Trisomy 13	1/10,000	Oral-facial clefts, ocular and CNS malformations, scalp defects, severe mental retardation, < 10% survive to 1 year

IUGR = intrauterine growth restriction, CNS = central nervous system

8. Are sex chromosome abnormalities associated with advanced maternal age?

All with the exception of Turner syndrome (45,X) which can result from loss of the paternal chromosome, mosaicism (45,X/46,XX or 45,X/46,XY), or structural abnormalities of one of the X chromosomes (e.g., deletions, isochromosomes). The recurrence risk for Turner syndrome is negligible.

9. Do sex chromosome abnormalities cause congenital malformations and/or mental retardation?

Congenital anomalies are *not* common in newborns with sex chromosome abnormalities (Table 4). If not diagnosed prenatally, they may not be detected until puberty. Sex chromosome aneuploidy does *not* cause mental retardation, although learning disabilities have been observed in males with 47,XXY and 47,XYY.

Table 4. Sex Chromosome Abnormalities

CHROMOSOME ABNORMALITY	PREVALENCE AT BIRTH	CLINICAL FEATURES
45,X Turner syndrome	1/2500	Coarctation of aorta, renal anomalies, webbed neck, shield chest, lymphedema hands and feet, short stature, streak gonads, primary amenorrhea, usually infertile
47,XXY Klinefelter syndrome	1/500	Taller than average, gynecomastia, most infertile, IQ 10–15 points below siblings, predisposition learning disabilities
47,XYY	1/1000	Taller than average, IQ 10–15 points lower than siblings, ADHD, learning disabilities
47,XXX	1/1000	Menstrual irregularities, some infertile

ADHD = attention deficit-hyperactivity disorder

10. What is a Robertsonian translocation? A reciprocal translocation?

A *Robertsonian translocation* is a fusion between two acrocentric chromosomes (13, 14, 15, 21, 22) at their centromeres, creating a composite chromosome. The carrier of this new chromosome is genetically balanced, but at risk for unbalanced offspring and spontaneous abortion. Robertsonian translocations with chromosome 21 can result in Down syndrome; the risk is 10–15% if the mother carries the translocation, 1–2% if the father is the carrier.

A *reciprocal translocation* is one in which breakage and exchange between segments of two different chromosomes occur. The balanced carrier has the correct number of chromosomes (46), but the rearrangement increases the risk for having unbalanced offspring with deletions and duplications of chromosomal material resulting in an abnormal phenotype.

11. What are microdeletion syndromes?

Microdeletion syndromes (Table 5) are well-recognized disorders associated with submicroscopic deletions of chromosomes that in most cases can only be detected using molecular techniques such as FISH (fluorescence *in situ* hybridization; see Question 13). Testing for these deletions is recommended when a parent is a carrier of the deletion and when a previous child has the deletion. Testing for the 22q11.2 deletion is also recommended when a conotruncal heart defect (e.g., tetralogy of Fallot) is detected by prenatal ultrasonography or echocardiography.

Table 5. *Microdeletion Syndromes*

MICRODELETION SYNDROME	CHROMOSOME DELETION	CLINICAL FEATURES
Angelman	15q11-13	Severe mental retardation, seizures, ataxic gait
DiGeorge/velocardiofacial	22q11.2	Cardiac defects, hypocalcemia, immune deficiency, cleft palate, learning difficulties
Miller-Dieker	17p13.3	Lissencephaly, characteristic facies
Prader-Willi	15q11-13	Mental retardation, short, hypotonia, obesity, characteristic facies, small feet
Williams	7q11.23	Supervalvular aortic stenosis, hypercalcemia, characteristic facies, mental retardation

12. What are the indications for chromosome testing during pregnancy?

Advanced maternal age (> 35 years)
Previous child with aneuploidy
Parent with balanced translocation or other chromosomal abnormality
Parent with mosaicism for a chromosomal abnormality
Fetal malformation
Abnormal serum screening for aneuploidy
Relative with mental retardation or malformations
Prior stillbirth
Recurrent pregnancy loss

13. What is fluorescence *in situ* hybridization? What are the indications for FISH?

FISH is used as an adjunct to routine cytogenetic analysis for the detection of submicroscopic chromosome deletions and duplications that are too small to be detected by conventional cytogenetics. It is also used to assist with the identification of subtle translocations and marker chromosomes. FISH can be performed on metaphase chromosome preparations from cultured lymphocytes, amniocytes, and chorionic villi, and on interphase nuclei from blood, tissue, chorionic villi, and amniotic fluid.

The use of interphase cells is advantageous because neither time nor tissue viability is needed for cell culture. FISH of interphase nuclei is used prenatally when a fetal malformation is detected, for the rapid detection of common aneuploidies such as trisomy 21. The results may influence a couple's reproductive options or obstetrical management.

FISH has also been used for preimplantation genetic diagnosis for carriers of balanced translocations or deletions. FISH only provides information about the specific chromosome(s) studied and does not provide a complete karyotype.

SINGLE-GENE DISORDERS

14. How many single-gene traits have been identified?

Over 11,000 single-gene disorders have been described, and many of these genes have been mapped to specific chromosomes and identified.

15. What are autosomal dominant disorders?

Autosomal dominant disorders occur in approximately 1 in 200 individuals. The disease is usually seen in multiple generations and transmitted from an affected parent to child. The recurrence risk is 50% in each pregnancy. Examples include Huntington disease, Marfan syndrome, neurofibromatosis, achondroplasia, and familial polyposis.

16. Why do autosomal dominant disorders often appear in a newborn with "normal" parents?

New mutation: Increased paternal age has been associated with autosomal dominant disorders such as achondroplasia, neurofibromatosis, and Apert syndrome. The recurrence risk for subsequent children is low.

Variable expression: The severity of the disease can be variable, and a parent may have unrecognized mild or subclinical manifestations.

Reduced penetrance: A parent may have the gene but not exhibit the clinical features.

Non-paternity: The estimated rate of non-paternity is 15%.

17. Can two siblings have an autosomal dominant disorder when there is no family history?

Yes, presumably due to germline mosaicism. The mutation may have only occurred in a population of cells in the gonads, so the parent appears unaffected yet can transmit the mutation to multiple offspring.

18. What are autosomal recessive disorders?

Autosomal recessive disorders are seen in multiple siblings; the parents are both carriers, and the recurrence risk is 25% in each pregnancy. Parents are often unaware that they are carriers until the birth of an affected child. Examples include sickle cell disease, cystic fibrosis, phenylketonuria, Tay-Sachs disease, and Canavan disease.

19. Why do autosomal recessive disorders often have an increased frequency among specific populations?

Some autosomal recessive disorders are more common in a specific population; for example, sickle cell disease among African-Americans and thalassemia among individuals of Asian and Mediterranean ancestry. Tay-Sachs, Canavan, Gaucher, and Niemann-Pick are more common among Ashkenazi Jews.

Gene flow within reproductively isolated populations forms the basis for the differences now seen between various racial and ethnic groups. As each group continues to segregate genes among themselves, mutations are passed silently through carriers, and when expressed in a double dose, a recessive disorder is produced. The normal phenotype of the unsuspecting recessive carrier serves to mask the supply of mutant genes.

20. What are X-linked disorders?

X-linked recessive diseases are transmitted from mother to son. Examples include Duchenne muscular dystrophy and hemophilia. Since females have two copies of the X chromosome they usually appear unaffected; female carriers have a 50% risk of having affected males. X-linked dominant disorders are transmitted from affected mothers to 50% of their sons and daughters. Affected fathers transmit the disease to all of their daughters and none of their sons. Examples include vitamin D–resistant rickets and hereditary hematuria.

21. Can single-gene defects be identified antenatally in the fetus?

The genes for many genetic disorders have been identified. Therefore, if the mutations are known and the parents are carriers, it is possible to determine if the fetus is affected. Molecular diagnostic testing is widely available for a number of single-gene disorders including muscular dystrophies, hemophilia, CF, sickle cell, Tay-Sachs, Canavan, Huntington disease, and fragile X syndrome (see Question 23).

In some cases, a specific molecular diagnostic test may be performed based on sonographic findings; for example, CF for echogenic bowel, FGFR2 (fibroblast growth factor receptor 2) for Apert's syndrome (craniosynostosis), and FGFR3 for thanatophoric dysplasia and achondroplasia.

22. What is a trinucleotide repeat expansion?

Some genes contain a region of triplet repeats (e.g., CGG). This region is unstable and can increase with successive generations—a phenomenon called "anticipation." The number of repeats determines whether an individual is affected. Trinucleotide repeat expansions are the cause of a number of genetic diseases such as fragile X syndrome, myotonic dystrophy, and Huntington disease.

23. What is fragile X syndrome? What are the indications for testing?

Fragile X syndrome is the most common cause of familial mental retardation. Affected males have large ears, prominent jaw, large testes, autistic behavior, and mild to severe mental retardation. Females are less severely affected due to X-inactivation. The gene for fragile X syndrome is on the X chromosome and contains a trinucleotide repeat (CGG). Normal individuals have 6–50 repeats; unaffected female carriers have a premutation of 50–200 repeats, which can expand during female meiosis to a full mutation of greater than 200 repeats. When there is a full mutation, the gene is inactivated by methylation and the fetus is affected. The severity is variable due to random X-inactivation in females, the degree of methylation, and mosaicism for the size of the repeat.

Female carriers of a premutation have a 50% risk of transmitting the gene with the expansion. Males with a premutation are normal, but all of their daughters will be carriers of the premutation; the number of repeats remains stable when transmitted by a male. Fragile X testing to determine the number of repeats and the methylation status is available (Table 6).

Table 6.   *Indications for Fragile X Testing*

Individual with mental retardation, developmental delay, autism
Individual with features of fragile X syndrome
Individuals with family history of fragile X syndrome
Individuals with family history of undiagnosed mental retardation
Fetus of mother who is known carrier

24. What is imprinting?

Imprinting is a process in which the activation of a gene preferentially occurs on either the maternal or paternal chromosome, but not both. Normal development will occur only when both the maternal and paternal copies of the imprinted gene are present. The imprinted gene is the inactive gene; therefore, if the active gene is lost (e.g., deleted) or has a mutation, then the fetus will be affected. Only a portion of genes are imprinted.

25. Name two conditions in which imprinting is important.

Angelman syndrome
Complete hydatidiform molar pregnancies

26. Describe the significance of imprinting in the two conditions named in Question 25.

- **Angelman syndrome (AS):** This disorder is characterized by severe mental retardation, ataxic gait, distinct facies, and paroxysms of laughter and seizures. The AS gene is active only on the maternally inherited chromosome; thus, when there is a deletion on the maternal chromosome 15 or when the maternal copy of the gene has a mutation, the protein product is not made, and the child is affected. AS also can occur when both copies of chromosome 15 are inherited from the father (no maternal copy of chromosome 15). This is called uniparental disomy (UPD). UPD usually occurs through either loss of a chromosome from a trisomic conceptus or gain of a chromosome in a fetus who is monosomic for the chromosome. Each of the two chromosomes can be genetically dissimilar (heterodisomy) or identical (isodisomy), depending on whether the event occurs during the first or second meiotic divisions, respectively.

- **Complete hydatidiform moles**: These pregnancies are typically diploid (46,XX or XY), but are entirely of paternal origin with no maternally derived chromosomes; the fetus fails to develop. Complete moles can coexist with a normal twin, but are at increased risk for maternal complications, including hyperthyroidism, preeclampsia, and preterm birth. In contrast, partial moles are generally triploid (69,XXX, 69,XYY), with an additional set of chromosomes of paternal origin. Triploidy as a result of an additional set of maternal chromosomes is associated with intrauterine growth restriction, congenital malformations, and a small placenta.

27. What is mitochondrial inheritance?

Mitochondria in the cytoplasm of the ovum (not the sperm) are transmitted from mother to offspring. The mitochondria have their own DNA. There are several genetic diseases caused by mutations in mitochondrial DNA, including Leber hereditary optic neuropathy, Leigh's disease, and myoclonic epilepsy with ragged red fibers. Expression of these diseases is variable.

MOLECULAR DIAGNOSTIC TESTING

28. What are the various approaches for molecular diagnosis of genetic disorders in a fetus?

Direct mutation analysis is the most straightforward and accurate method. When a gene has been identified and the disease-causing mutations are characterized, then it is possible to directly test for the absence or presence of the mutation in the parent and the fetus. The polymerase chain reaction (PCR) is used to amplify a region of DNA containing the mutation. Mutations such as deletions, insertions, and duplications that change the size of the expected PCR product may be detected on agarose-gel electrophoresis as an altered DNA fragment or, in the case of a deletion, an absent fragment. This type of testing is frequently used to detect deletions in Duchenne muscular dystrophy.

Allele specific oligonucleotide analysis is frequently used to detect point mutations due to base substitutions. The PCR product is placed on a filter and hybridized with oligonucleotide probes for the normal sequence and the mutation. When the mutation is present, it will bind with the mutant oligonucleotide probe and give a positive signal.

Restriction fragment length polymorphism analysis can be used when a mutation creates or destroys a restriction enzyme recognition site. The PCR product is incubated with the restriction enzyme and analyzed on an agarose gel. The DNA fragments resulting after specific enzyme cleavage are altered in size and gel mobility if a mutation is present.

Linkage analysis is used when the location of a gene is known, but the gene and mutations have not been characterized. DNA markers close to or within the gene are used to track the transmission of the disease gene within a family and can predict the likelihood that a fetus inherited the disease gene.

29. What are the practical considerations of molecular diagnostic testing?

The accuracy of DNA-based testing depends on an accurate diagnosis and knowledge of the specific mutation. When a family member of an affected individual or an at-risk fetus is tested, care should be taken that the mutation within the family is known. For many genetic diseases the detection rate is less than 100%—even when hundreds of mutations have been reported. Many mutations are only present in a single family. Hence, failure to detect a mutation does not always exclude the possibility that an individual is a carrier. Some genetic diseases are caused by mutations in two or more different genes (e.g., tuberous sclerosis) and, conversely, different mutations within a single gene can cause several types of disorders (e.g., FGFR3 mutations cause achondroplasia and craniosynostosis). Additionally, DNA testing assumes correct paternity.

MULTIFACTORIAL INHERITANCE

30. What are characteristics of multifactorial inheritance?

Traits with an increased familial aggregation and recurrence without a Mendelian pattern of gene transmission. The malformation often involves a single organ and has an increased propensity for one sex. Common examples include neural tube defects, cleft lip with or without cleft palate, and cardiac defects.

31. What is the risk of recurrence for multifactorial traits?

In general, if one first-degree relative (sibling or parent) is affected, the recurrence risk is 2–3%. If two first-degree relatives are affected, the risk is 4–6%. Unaffected siblings have a 1–2% risk of having an affected offspring. For traits that are more common in one of the sexes, an affected offspring of the less commonly affected sex carries a higher recurrence risk.

32. Why is a careful examination necessary to exclude other minor malformations when a presumed multifactorial disorder has been identified?

Anomalies commonly inherited in a multifactorial fashion can also be components of genetic syndromes with different prognoses and recurrence rates. For example, neural tube defects can occur in association with polycystic kidneys and polydactyly consistent with Meckel syndrome, an autosomal recessive disorder with a 25% recurrence risk.

BIBLIOGRAPHY

1. American College of Obstetricians and Gynecologists: Maternal serum screening. ACOG Educational Bulletin 228. The 2001 Compendium of Selected Publications. Washington, DC, 2001.
2. Caskey CT: Medical genetics. JAMA 277(23):1869–1870, 1997.
3. Engel EM, DeLozier-Blanchet D: Uniparental disomy, isodisomy and imprinting: Probable effects in man and strategies for their detection. Am J Med Genet 40:432–439, 1991.
4. Jameson JL: Principles of Molecular Medicine. Totowa, NJ, Humana Press, 1998.
5. Jourde LB, Carey JC, Bamshad MJ, White RL: Medical Genetics, 2nd ed. Philadelphia, Mosby, Inc., 2000.
6. Korf BR: Molecular Diagnosis. New Engl J Med 332:1218–1220, 1499–1502, 1995.
7. Simpson JL, Golbus MS: Genetics and Obstetrics and Gynecology, 2nd ed. Philadelphia, W.B. Saunders, 1992.
8. Wilkins-Haug L: Medical genetics. In Ryan KJ, Berkowitz RS, Berbieri RL (eds): Kistner's Gynecology, 6th ed. St. Louis, Mosby, 1995.

55. OBSTETRIC ULTRASOUND

Anthony O. Odibo, M.D., MRCOG

1. Describe the equipment used for obstetric ultrasound.

Ultrasound (US) equipment uses sound waves delivered at a high frequency, usually > 20,000 cycles per second (Hz). Most diagnostic applications of US operate at frequencies of 2–10 million cycles per second (2–10 MHz). The best resolution is obtained with the highest-frequency US, although depth of visualization is compromised. Abdominal US transducers have a linear array with a rectangular image; sector scanners with a pie-shaped image; or curvilinear scanners that combine both principles. These transducers operate at 3.5–5 MHz. Vaginal scanners operate at 5–10 MHz.

2. What are the advantages of transvaginal scanning over abdominal transducers?

The closer proximity of the transducer in vaginal scanning leads to improved resolution of images obtained. In early pregnancy this results in earlier differentiation of intrauterine and ectopic gestations. There is no requirement for a full bladder with transvaginal scanning, and some indices—such as cervical length and placental location—can be more accurately delineated with transvaginal US.

3. Is obstetric ultrasound examination safe?

Theoretically, US can cause biological heating. With the intensity of US used by most laboratories, there have been no confirmed adverse biologic effects on patients, fetuses, or instrument operators.

4. Should all pregnant patients have an ultrasound exam?

Routine performance of obstetric US remains controversial in the United States, although it is performed throughout Europe. Opponents of routine US cite the failure of randomized clinical trials to demonstrate a clear benefit; the deleterious effects of false-positive or false-negative diagnoses; the lack of adequately trained personnel to perform the procedures; and cost. The benefits of routine US screening include detection of unsuspected anomalies, accurate determination of fetal age, and earlier diagnosis of placenta previa or multiple gestation.

5. What should be demonstrated and documented in a first-trimester ultrasound exam?

- Location of the gestational sac
- Identification of the embryo
- Measurement of the crown-rump length
- Presence or absence of fetal cardiac activity
- Fetal number
- Condition of uterus, cervix, and maternal adnexae
- Presence, size, and shape of the yolk sac.

6. What is first trimester nuchal transluceny?

Nuchal translucency (NT) is a translucent area detected behind the fetal neck in first-trimester US. An enlarged NT has been associated with fetal aneuploidy. Attempts are underway to develop NT as a screening test for chromosomal anomalies in the first trimester.

7. What should be demonstrated and documented in a second- or third-trimester exam?

- Presence of fetal cardiac activity
- Fetal number

• Fetal presentation
• Assessment of amniotic fluid volume
• Appearance of the placenta and its location, especially with reference to the cervical os (i.e., presence or absence of placenta previa)
• Gestational age
• Condition of maternal uterus and adnexae

Fetal anatomic examination should include, but is not limited to, evaluation of the cerebral ventricles, four-chamber view of the heart, spine, stomach, bladder, cord insertion, and kidneys. Most third-trimester exams are for evaluating fetal growth.

8. List the helpful landmarks of a normal early pregnancy.

When the mean sac diameter measures > 25 mm by transabdominal US, a living embryo should be identified in a viable pregnancy. This generally occurs by 7–8 weeks of gestation. By transvaginal US, fetal cardiac activity should be documented by 6.5 weeks, or when the mean sac diameter measures 18 mm. A normal gestational sac can be seen transvaginally when the level of human chorionic gonadotropin reaches 1000 mIU/ml.

9. What is a blighted ovum?

A blighted ovum is a fertilized ovum in which development has stopped. The absence of a fetal pole in a gestational sac with a diameter of 3 cm or more is consistent with the diagnosis of blighted ovum.

10. What is the chance of spontaneous abortion in a patient with documented fetal cardiac activity in the first trimester?

In patients with documented fetal cardiac activity in the first trimester, < 5% will subsequently experience a fetal loss. This rate depends somewhat on maternal age and is slightly higher for women over the age of 35. It is also higher for patients already presenting with a threatened abortion.

11. Which measurements are used for gestational dating?

In the first trimester, the fetal crown-rump length is used to assess gestational age. In the second and third trimesters, the biparietal diameter and femur length are the measurements used for pregnancy dating. The head and abdominal circumferences could also be used in the second trimester. It is preferable to use a combination of parameters for dating.

12. What is a quick assessment of fetal age based on crown-rump length (CRL) if tables are not handy?

$$\frac{\text{CRL (in mm)}}{7} + 5.5 \text{ weeks} = \text{weeks of gestation}$$

13. How accurate is ultrasound dating of pregnancy?

US dating of pregnancy becomes less accurate as pregnancy progresses. CRL in the first trimester is accurate within 3–5 days, whereas measurements in the second trimester are approximate within 2 weeks and in the third trimester within 3 weeks.

14. What structural landmarks indicate the appropriate level to measure the biparietal diameter (BPD)?

The BPD is measured in a transverse axial plane at the level of the falx cerebri, the thalamic nuclei, and the cavum septum pellucidi.

15. What cardiac views should be demonstrated on a routine second-trimester US?

The "four chamber" was the only view traditionally obtained. Recent studies have shown that demonstrating the cardiac septa and outflow tracts leads to improved detection of congenital heart defects.

16. Which structures identify the appropriate level to measure the abdominal circumference?

The abdominal circumference is measured in a transverse axial plane at a level including the left portal vein deep in the liver, and the fetal stomach.

17. If you are limited to only one ultrasound exam during pregnancy, when is the best time to perform it?

At 18–20 weeks, you can judge placental position, estimate amniotic fluid volume, recognize early shortening of the cervix, and detect numerous fetal anomalies. Despite the somewhat improved accuracy of dating in the first trimester, these advantages make 18–20 weeks of gestation the ideal time to schedule a single US exam.

18. How accurate is fetal weight calculated by a third-trimester ultrasound exam?

When based on two or more fetal parameters using published regression formulas, an estimated fetal weight by US is predictive with 95% confidence that the true fetal weight is within a range of 15–20% above and below the estimated weight. The later in gestation the exam is performed, the greater the standard deviation.

19. What is the amniotic fluid index?

The amniotic fluid index (AFI) is a quantitative technique to assess amniotic fluid volume. The maternal abdomen is divided into quadrants, using the umbilicus and linea nigra as reference points. The transducer head is maintained perpendicular to the floor, and the largest vertical pocket in each quadrant is measured. The sum of the four measurements (in cm) is the AFI. This is only reliable for singleton gestations. With multiple pregnancies, the single largest pocket is used.

20. Define the terms oligohydramnios and polyhydramnios.

The usual ways of determining amniotic fluid volume are by subjective assessment, measurement of the deepest vertical pocket, or using the AFI. Oligohydramnios is usually defined as a single vertical pocket of < 1–2 cm, or an AFI < 5 cm. Polyhydramnios is usually considered a single vertical pocket > 8 cm, or an AFI ≥ 25 cm.

21. What are the components of a biophysical profile?

The biophysical profile is a sonographic assessment of multiple fetal biophysical activities or components, including fetal body movements, fetal breathing movements, fetal tone, and amniotic fluid volume. The nonstress test is also included as part of the profile. Each component is scored as 0 when abnormal or 2 when normal; thus a normal score is 8 or 10, depending on whether the nonstress test is included.

22. What is M-mode echocardiography?

M-mode echocardiography provides details about structural motion in the heart and accurate measurements of the dimensions of walls and cavities. It is used to document the presence of cardiac activity in early pregnancy, to evaluate ventricular cavity dimension and wall thickness as well as valve and wall motion, and to assess cardiac arrhythmias.

23. Describe the uses of Doppler ultrasound in pregnancy.

Doppler *ultrasonography* demonstrates the direction and characteristics of blood flow and is used in evaluation of the fetal heart and great vessels as well as the uteroplacental and fetoplacental circulation. Doppler *velocimetry* can be used for further assessment of pregnancy complications such as intrauterine growth retardation, fetal hypoxemia or asphyxia, fetal cardiac anomalies, and cord malformations. Recent studies have shown Doppler velocimetry to be useful in predicting fetal anemia, especially that associated with rhesus isoimmunization.

24. Can ultrasound detect Down syndrome or other chromosomal abnormalities?

US can detect many of the malformations associated with chromosomal abnormalities. Fetuses with trisomy 13 and 18 tend to have major malformations, most of which can be detected sonographically. In Down syndrome, many fetuses have either no major malformations or malformations that tend to be detected late in pregnancy, such as duodenal atresia. Thus **only 30%** of Down syndrome fetuses are detected by routine US. Subtle biometric or morphologic abnormalities, such as shortened femurs, thickened nuchal folds, and renal pyelectasis, can be used to screen for and detect some cases of fetal Down syndrome.

25. What causes of an abnormal alpha-fetoprotein screen can be detected by ultrasound?

Maternal serum alpha-fetoprotein (MSAFP) was first noted to be elevated with open fetal neural tube defects. Elevated MSAFP also occurs with underestimation of gestational age, multiple gestation, fetal demise, cystic hygroma and other conditions associated with fetal edema, anterior abdominal wall defects, and other fetal anomalies associated with fetal skin defects. A low AFP can be associated with fetal chromosome abnormalities (e.g., Down syndrome, trisomy 18), dating errors, molar pregnancy, or fetal demise.

26. What ultrasound markers can be used to differentiate chorionicity in twin pregnancy?

Evaluation of chorionicity is an important component of the sonographic assessment of twins. Evidence of dichorionicity includes:
- Separate sacs in the first trimester
- Separate placentas
- Different genders
- Thick intertwin septa
- Presence of a chorionic peak.

A *chorionic peak* is a projecting zone of tissue extending from the chorionic surface of the placenta and tapering within the intertwin membrane.

27. What degree of discrepancy in estimated weight between twins implies a risk of morbidity?

A weight estimate discordance of 20% raises concern of significant birthweight disparity and risk of increased morbidity. Patients beyond viability with this degree of discordance should be monitored for fetal well-being. This may be an indication of possible **twin-twin transfusion syndrome**.

28. Describe the cranial signs suggestive of neural tube defects.

The "banana" and "lemon" signs are two sonographic signs of the Arnold-Chiari malformation seen in spina bifida. The frontal bones of the skull are scalloped, giving a lemonlike configuration. The cerebellum is flattened and centrally curved, obliterating the posterior fossa and giving the cerebellum a bananalike appearance. Ventriculomegaly can also be seen.

29. When does the normal physiologic herniation of the midgut resolve?

Before 12 weeks' gestation, the embryonic bowel is extra-abdominal within the umbilical cord and should not be diagnosed as an abdominal wall defect. After this time, the bowel assumes its normal intra-abdominal location.

30. What are the differences between gastroschisis and omphalocele?

Gastroschisis and omphalocele are both anterior abdominal wall defects. *Gastroschisis* is a right paraumbilical defect through which small bowel (and occasionally other intra-abdominal organs) eviscerates. The loops of bowel are not covered by a membrane. *Omphalocele* is an extrusion of the abdominal contents into the base of the umbilical cord. Thus, in omphalocele, the herniated mass is covered with parietal peritoneum, amnion, and Wharton's jelly.

Gastroschisis is usually an isolated anomaly, whereas omphalocele is commonly associated with other malformations and/or chromosome abnormalities.

31. What are the ultrasound features of hydrops fetalis?

Hydrops fetalis is a condition of excessive fluid accumulation within the fetus. It is characterized by varying degrees of ascites, pleural effusions, pericardial effusions, skin edema, placental edema, and polyhydramnios.

BIBLIOGRAPHY

1. American College of Obstetrics and Gynecology: Ultrasonography in Pregnancy. Washington DC, ACOG Tech Bull 187, 1993.
2. American Institute of Ultrasound in Medicine Bioeffects Committee: Bioeffects considerations for the safety of diagnostic ultrasound. J Ultrasound Med 7(Suppl 9):S1–38, 1988.
3. Callen PW: Ultrasonography in Obstetrics and Gynecology, 4th ed. Philadelphia, W.B. Saunders, 2000.
4. Gabbe SG, Niebyl JR, Simpson JL: Obstetrics: Normal and Problem Pregnancies, 4th ed. New York, Churchill Livingstone, 2002.
5. Simpson JL, Mills JL, Holmes LB, et al: Low fetal loss rates after ultrasound-proven viability in early pregnancy. JAMA 258:2555, 1987.

56. DISORDERS OF FETAL GROWTH

Martha E. Rode, M.D.

INTRAUTERINE GROWTH RESTRICTION

1. What is the definition of intrauterine growth restriction (IUGR)?

Most authors define IUGR (formerly referred to as intrauterine growth *retardation*) as an estimated fetal weight below the tenth percentile for gestational age. As the term IUGR includes normal fetuses at the lower end of the growth curve as well as those who are later found to have been unable to reach their inherent growth potential secondary to various maternal clinical conditions, this definition is not always clinically relevant. Studies suggest that adverse perinatal outcome is generally confined to those infants with weights below the fifth or perhaps even the third percentile for gestational age.

2. What is the difference between "small for gestational age" (SGA) and IUGR?

These terms have often been used as if they are interchangeable. SGA describes an *infant* with a birth weight at the lower extreme of the normal distribution (below the tenth percentile for gestational age). IUGR applies to a *fetus* who meets this criterion.

3. What is the differential diagnosis for IUGR?

The etiologic factors for IUGR can be divided into several broad categories: constitutional, maternal medical conditions, structural anomalies, exposure to drugs and toxins, primary placental disease, multiple gestation, infections, and genetic disorders including aneuploidy. In addition, low socioeconomic status and extremes of maternal age are associated with IUGR.

4. Which maternal medical conditions place the fetus at risk for IUGR?

Those which affect the microcirculation, leading to fetal hypoxemia or a reduction in fetal perfusion. These include elevated blood pressure, pregestational diabetes with end-organ damage, systemic lupus erythematosis, sickle cell disease, antiphospholipid syndrome, and others.

5. How does the placenta play a possible role in the development of IUGR?

Impaired placental perfusion is the most common cause of SGA in otherwise normal infants, as seen in severe early-onset pre-eclampsia. It can also be the primary cause of IUGR (placental mosaicism, chorioangioma). IUGR is also associated with other placental anomalies such as chronic partial abruption, infarcts, placenta previa, and hematoma.

6. Maternal use of which drugs is associated with abnormal fetal growth?

- Alcohol: dose-related, unknown if threshold exists
- Tobacco: 3.5 times risk of SGA infant compared to women who don't smoke; quitting at any point in pregnancy increases birth weight
- Heroin and cocaine: difficult to isolate the risks imposed by frequent concurrent behaviors

7. What is the effect of maternal weight gain on birth weight?

Although low pre-pregnancy weight and low maternal weight gain have been positively correlated with an increased risk of IUGR, there has been no study proving that interventions to increase maternal weight gain lead to increased birth weight. A woman would likely have to limit her daily intake to < 1500 kcal/day to have a negative impact on her infant's birth weight.

8. Why is growth restriction more common in multi-fetal gestations?

It is thought that growth restriction is more common in multi-fetal gestations due to inadequate placental reserve to sustain normal growth of more than one fetus. IUGR is more common in higher-order gestations than twins, and more common and severe in monozygotic twins than dizygotic.

9. Are viral infections a common cause of IUGR?

No. Viral infections are estimated to be the etiology in less than 5% of cases of IUGR. However, the incidence of IUGR is high in documented cases of fetal infection. This association is proven for rubella and cytomegalovirus; postulated for varicella zoster and HIV.

10. Are genetic disorders a common cause of IUGR?

Yes. Many structural anomalies are also associated with an increased risk of abnormal fetal growth.

11. Is perinatal morbidity and mortality increased in fetuses with IUGR?

Yes, especially for those with weights below the third percentile for gestational age. These risks are modified by gestational age at delivery, primary etiology, and whether there has been progression of associated maternal etiologic factors.

12. Why do IUGR fetuses have an increased risk of intrapartum complications?

Increased risk of intrapartum complications is most likely related to the presumed decrease in "placental reserve." Oligohydramnios is a common associated finding (around 80%) and may leave the umbilical cord susceptible to compression with associated variable decelerations. Up to 50% of these fetuses exhibit abnormal heart rate patterns in labor, and there is an increased risk of cesarean delivery. The incidence of low Apgar scores and cord blood acidemia is also elevated in SGA infants.

13. Which complications are seen more frequently among SGA neonates?

Polycythemia
Hypoglycemia
Hyperbilirubinemia
Hypothermia
Apneic spells
Need for intubation in the delivery room
Seizures
Sepsis
Low Apgar scores
Umbilical artery pH < 7
Neonatal death

14. How is the diagnosis of IUGR made?

The more accurate the estimated delivery date (EDD), the easier it is to diagnose IUGR with certainty. In a pregnancy with unsure dates (one with late or no prenatal care) the diagnosis can be difficult. IUGR is suspected when the fundal height on clinical examination lags behind that expected by the EDD, especially in a woman with known risk factors. The diagnosis is confirmed when the sonographic assessment of fetal size is less than the tenth percentile for gestational age. Serial ultrasounds (every 2–4 weeks) are valuable in monitoring fetal growth and confirming the diagnosis when IUGR is suspected.

15. What evaluation should be performed following the diagnosis?

- Obtain maternal history—weight gain in pregnancy, tobacco use, illicit or therapeutic drugs, family history of low birth weights

- Physical examination—maternal body mass index, blood pressure
- Laboratory evaluation—cytomegalovirus and rubella serologies, possible antiphospholipid antibody/anticardiolipin antibodies
- Fetal assessment—thorough anatomic survey for anomalies, evaluation of the placenta, Doppler studies, karyotype, and nonstress test (NST) or biophysical profile (BPP) if gestational age is appropriate
- Placental pathology—following delivery, may help determine etiology for counseling regarding future pregnancies

16. What is the role of Doppler velocimetry of the umbilical artery in evaluating fetuses with suspected IUGR?

Although not useful as a screening technique, Doppler studies are useful once the diagnosis has been made. Doppler velocimetry has been shown to reduce interventions and improve outcome in IUGR pregnancies.

17. What interventions improve pregnancy outcome once IUGR is diagnosed?

Avoidance of smoking. Other proposed interventions (bed rest, early delivery with abnormal Doppler studies, nutrient supplementation, plasma volume expansion, maternal oxygen therapy, heparin, and low-dose aspirin) have been insufficiently studied to arrive at a conclusion regarding efficacy. These fetuses should undergo serial antenatal testing (BPP or NST) and ultrasounds with Doppler studies to predict which are at risk for intrauterine fetal demise and may benefit from early delivery.

18. When should a growth-restricted fetus be delivered?

When it is felt that the risk of fetal death exceeds the risks of neonatal death. This is often difficult to determine. Non-reassuring fetal testing, lack of interval growth, and documentation of fetal lung maturity are possible indications for delivery.

FETAL MACROSOMIA

19. What is the difference between "large for gestational age" and macrosomia?

Large for gestational age refers to a birth weight equal to or greater than the 90th percentile for gestational age. Macrosomia is growth beyond a certain weight (usually 4000 or 4500 g), regardless of gestational age.

20. Are macrosomic infants at increased risk of perinatal complications?

Yes. Shoulder dystocia, clavicular fracture, Erb's palsy, decreased 5-minute Apgar, admission to neonatal intensive care unit, and obesity later in life are all more common with macrosomia.

21. What are the risk factors for the development of macrosomia?

Known risk factors in decreasing importance: prior history of a macrosomic infant, elevated maternal prepregnancy weight, excessive weight gain during pregnancy, multiparity, male fetus, gestational age > 40 weeks, ethnicity, maternal birth weight, maternal height, maternal age younger than 17 years, and a positive 1-hour glucose screen with negative 3-hour (100 g) glucose tolerance test. Both pregestational and gestational diabetes are also associated with fetal macrosomia.

22. How do macrosomic infants of diabetic mothers differ from those without diabetes?

Macrosomic infants of diabetics tend to have greater total body fat, greater shoulder and upper extremity skin fold measurements, and smaller head-to-abdominal circumference ratios. These factors may explain the associated elevated risk of shoulder dystocia.

23. How is macrosomia predicted?

Not very well. No combination of risk factors predicts macrosomia well enough to be used clinically. Clinical measurements (Leopold's maneuvers and fundal height measurement) have reported sensitivities of 10–43%, specificities of 99.0–99.8%, and positive predictive values of 28–53%. With fetal weight exceeding 4500 g (and no maternal diabetes), ultrasound biometry has a sensitivity of 22–44%, a specificity of 99%, and a positive predictive value of 30–44%. Interestingly, asking a parous woman to estimate the fetal weight may be as accurate as any of the above.

24. How should the diagnosis of probable fetal macrosomia affect the management of labor and delivery?

Pay close attention to the labor curve, and take time for careful consideration before performing an operative vaginal delivery (risk of shoulder dystocia is associated with assisted vaginal delivery). Note that fetal macrosomia is *not* a contraindication to an attempt at vaginal delivery following cesarean section.

CONTROVERSIES

25. When is cesarean delivery recommended for macrosomic fetuses?

It is known that the risk of birth trauma increases with birth weight, and that cesarean delivery greatly reduces this risk (but does not eliminate it). Nevertheless, the clinical efficacy of offering women with fetuses beyond a set estimated weight elective cesarean delivery has not yet been demonstrated in a prospective randomized trial. Studies to date reveal a non-significant reduction in shoulder dystocia with an associated increase in overall cesarean section rate. Additionally, studies in which women whose fetuses had an estimated weight over 4000 g were allowed a trial of labor document a very low risk of fetal injury. Despite this data, some physicians offer cesarean delivery when macrosomia is suspected.

26. Is there a role for induction of labor in cases of suspected or "impending" fetal macrosomia at term?

A role for induction of labor is not supported by cohort studies, which show the risk of cesarean to be at least doubled, while the risks of shoulder dystocia and neonatal morbidity are not decreased. These studies are faulted for small sample sizes and their retrospective nature. Despite the lack of scientific support, induction for this indication is common in most communities.

BIBLIOGRAPHY

1. American College of Obstetrics and Gynecology: Intrauterine growth restriction. ACOG Practice Bulletin No 12, 2000.
2. American College of Obstetrics and Gynecology: Fetal macrosomia. ACOG Practice Bulletin No. 22, 2000.
3. Bernstein PS, Divon MY: Etiologies of fetal growth restriction. Clin Obstet Gynecol 40(4).723–729.
4. Creasy RK, Resnick R: Intrauterine growth restriction. In Creasy RK, Resnick R (eds): Maternal-Fetal Medicine, 4th ed. Philadelphia, W.B. Saunders, 1999, pp 569–584.
5. Kramer WB, Weiner CP: Management of intrauterine growth restriction. Clin Obstet Gynecol 40(4):814–823, 1997.

57. DISORDERS OF AMNIOTIC FLUID

Sally Segel, M.D.

1. What is the origin of the amniotic fluid in the first trimester?

The origin of the amniotic fluid in the first trimester is uncertain. The two leading theories are: (1) a transudate of maternal plasma through the chorion/amnion, and (2) a transudate of fetal plasma through fetal skin prior to keratinization.

2. Describe the origin and dynamics of amniotic fluid in the second and third trimesters.

The amniotic fluid is a combination of fetal urine and lung liquid. The volume of amniotic fluid is a balance between fetal fluid production and fluid resorption. Resorption is a combination of fetal swallowing and flow across the fetal membranes to the fetal or maternal circulation.

Near term, the fetal lung produces 300–400 ml/day of lung fluid. This fluid helps to maintain lung expansion and allow for lung growth. During labor, several hormones act to decrease lung fluid and allow for the transition to spontaneous breathing.

Fetal urine is the major source of amniotic fluid. Near term, a fetus produces 400–1200 ml/day of urine. This production is dependent on fetal renal maturation. Fetal urine is normally hypotonic when compared to fetal or maternal plasma.

Fetal swallowing is the major source of amniotic fluid resorption. Near term, a fetus swallows 200–500 ml/day, primarily during active sleep states. Some intramembrane flow of amniotic fluid from the uterine cavity to the fetal placental vessels contributes to amniotic fluid resorption.

3. What is the overall trend in amniotic fluid volume during pregnancy?

The mean amniotic fluid volume increases from 250 to 800 ml between 16 and 32 weeks of gestation. This volume remains stable until 36 weeks' gestation; amniotic fluid then decreases to 500 ml at term. These changes in amniotic fluid volume are highly variable among individuals.

4. How is amniotic fluid volume measured?

Three techniques are commonly used to measure amniotic fluid volume; amniotic fluid index (AFI), single deepest pocket, and two-diameter pocket. Note that the umbilical cord and fetal extremities cannot be part of the pocket measured.

The **AFI** is measured by dividing the maternal abdomen into four quadrants. The umbilicus divides the uterus into upper and lower halves, and the linea nigra divides the uterus into right and left halves. With the transducer perpendicular to the floor, the deepest amniotic fluid pocket in each quadrant is identified. The AFI is the summation of the numbers obtained from each quadrant.

The **single deepest pocket** is measured by identifying the amniotic fluid pocket with the maximum vertical depth. The **two-diameter pocket** is measured by identifying the amniotic fluid pocket with the largest product of pocket depth multiplied by pocket width.

5. What is the significance of abnormal amniotic fluid?

Both oligohydramnios and polyhydramnios are associated with an increased maternal and perinatal morbidity and mortality.

OLIGOHYDRAMNIOS

6. What is the definition of oligohydramnios?

There are four definitions of oligohydramnios, and it is controversial as to which one is the best definition. The definitions are AFI < 5 cm, AFI < 5th percentile for a specific gestational age, single deepest pocket < 2 cm, and two-diameter pocket < 15cm^2.

7. Give the differential diagnosis for oligohydramnios.
- Fetal chromosomal/congenital anomalies
- Chronic fetal hypoxia (leading to low fetal plasma volume and decreased GFR)
- Posterm pregnancy
- Maternal dehydration
- Rupture of fetal membranes.

8. What congenital abnormalities cause oligohydramnios?

Renal agenesis and genitourinary obstructive uropathies (e.g., posterior urethral valves and urethral atresia) cause oligohydramnios.

9. What are the consequences of second-trimester oligohydramnios?

Second-trimester oligogyhydramnios can lead to fatal pulmonary hypoplasia.

10. Describe the management of oligohydramnios at term.

If the institutional definition of oligohydramnios is found in a term gravid patient, this is an indication for delivery. This practice is not well supported in the literature. There is some evidence to suggest that oligohydramnios at term and especially postdate pregnancy is associated with nonreassuring fetal heart rate testing and operative deliveries; however, there is no difference in perinatal outcome between postdate pregnancies with and without oligohydramnios.

POLYHYDRAMNIOS

11. What is the definition of polyhydramnios?

There are four definitions of polyhydramnios: AFI > 24 cm, AFI > 95% for a specific gestational age, single deepest pocket > 8 cm, and two-diameter pocket > 50 cm^2.

12. Give the differential diagnosis for polyhydramnios.
- Idiopathic
- Congenital anomalies
- Maternal diabetes (pregestational and gestational)
- Twin-twin transfusion syndrome
- Immune hydrops and nonimmune hydrops

Approximately two-thirds of all cases of polyhydramnios are idiopathic. There is some evidence to suggest that idiopathic polyhydramnios is associated with an increased risk for chromosomal aneuploidy.

13. What are the congenital anomalies associated with polyhydramnios?

They involve the central nervous system and the gastrointestinal system. The major CNS anomalies include anencephaly and primary neuromuscular disease. The major gastrointestinal anomalies include esophageal and duodenal atresia. Polyhydramnios can also be seen with a diaphragmatic hernia, cardiac valvular lesions, and arrhythmias.

14. What obstetric complications are caused by polyhydramnios?

Polyhydramnios can cause preterm labor and preterm premature rupture of fetal membranes, due to uterine overdistension or significantly increased uterine volume.

15. Rapid decompression of polyhydramnios leads to what obstetric complications?

Rapid decompression of polyhydramnios by either amniocentesis or rupture of fetal membranes can cause placental abruption.

BIBLIOGRAPHY

1. Brace RA, Resnik R: Dynamics and disorders of amniotic fluid. In Creasy R, Resnik R (eds): Maternal Fetal Medicine, 4th ed. Philadelphia, W.B. Saunders, 1999.
2. Called PW: Amniotic fluid: Its role in fetal health and disease. In Callen PW (ed): Ultrasonography in Obstetrics and Gynecology, 4th ed. Philadelphia, W.B. Saunders, 2000.
3. Magann EF, Sanderson M, Martin JN, Chauhan S: The amniotic fluid index, single deepest pocket, and two-diameter pocket in normal human pregnancy. Am J Obstet Gynecol 182:1581–1588, 2000.
4. Ross MG, Ervin MG, Novak D: Placental and fetal physiology. In Gabbe SG, Niebyl JR, Simpson JL (eds): Obstetrics—Normal and Problem Pregnancies, 4th ed. New York, Churchill Livingstone, 2002.

58. PATHOPHYSIOLOGY OF THE PLACENTA

Iraj Forouzan, M.D.

1. What is blastocyst and how it is formed?

Mitotic division of the zygote results in the production of *blastomeres*. As the blastomeres continue to divide, they form a solid ball of cells called a *morula*. Fluid gradually accumulates between the blastomeres of the morula to form a *blastocyst*. The blastocyst develops 96 hours after fertilization. At this time the conceptus is at a 58-cell stage, with a 5-cell inner mass and 53-cell trophoblasts.

2. When does implantation occur?

Six days after fertilization, the blastocyst initiates implantation into the maternal endometrium. The blastocyst is completely embedded in the endometrium at this time. By 9 days the trophoblastic cells are differentiated into two layers: the inner cytotrophoblasts (also called Langhans cell layer) and outer syncytiotrophoblasts. At this stage, these two layers of trophoblasts separate the maternal and conceptus circulations.

3. Why is the human placenta called hemochorial?

In the human being, maternal blood (hemo) directly surrounds the trophoblastic cells (chorial).

4. What is the origin of the fetal membrane?

The fetal membrane is composed of a chorion and an amnion. After implantation, the embedded blastocyst expands rapidly, which causes the surface of the endometrium, covering the blastocyst, to bulge into the endometrial cavity. This area of the blastocyst wall becomes the chorion laeve of the placenta. The amniotic membrane consists of a single layer of epithelial cell and a thin fibrous membrane. Its origin is from embryonic ectoderm.

5. What is the yolk sac?

It is a cavity formed from the endoderm layer of the embryo. Liver, gastrointestinal tract, and probably germ cells and hematopoietic cells differentiate from the yolk sac.

6. What are the functions of the human placenta?

The human placenta functions both as a transport organ and an endocrine organ. It transports nutrients from mother to fetus, and waste products from fetus to mother. Therefore, the placenta functions as kidney, lungs, and gut. Water exchange and oxygen transport also occur through the placenta. In addition, the human placenta produces certain important hormones.

7. What is the role of the placenta as an endocrine gland?

The **cytotrophoblast layer** of the placenta primarily produces neuropeptides, whereas the **syncytiotrophoblast** is responsible for producing the polypeptide hormones, such as human chorionic gonadotropin and human placental lactogen. It also produces the sex steroids (estrogen, progesterone).

8. What is human chorionic gonadotropin (hCG)?

HCG is a glycoprotein. It is one of the earliest secretions by the conceptus, and it is produced by the syncytiotrophoblast. Its production increases as the pregnancy continues, peaks at 8–10 weeks of gestation, and then plateaus. The function of hCG is to maintain the corpus luteum in early pregnancy, so that the corpus luteum continues to produce progesterone. HCG may also play a role in promoting the differentiation of cytotrophoblast into syncytiotrophoblast.

9. Explain the clinical utilities of hCG measurement.

The measurement of hCG levels during pregnancy has many clinical utilities. Maternal second-trimester hCG levels are elevated in pregnancies complicated with fetal chromosomal abnormalities. Higher than normal hCG levels may also indicate a molar pregnancy or multiple gestations. Low levels of hCG in early pregnancy indicate embryonic failure.

10. What is human placental lactogen (hPL)? What is its function?

HPL is a glycoprotein made by the syncytiotrophoblast throughout the pregnancy. It is also called human chorionic somatomamotropin. HPL is a polypeptide hormone with structural similarities to the human growth hormone and human prolactin. It plays a major role in fetal growth and maternal metabolism.

11. What is relaxin? Where is it produced?

Relaxin, a protein hormone, is produced in a number of sites, including the corpus luteum, the decidua, the atria of the heart, and the placenta. Its function in human pregnancy is not well understood.

12. What is a battledore placenta?

The umbilical cord normally inserts near the center of the placenta. When the umbilical cord inserts at the *margin* of the placenta, it is called a battledore placenta. Such marginal insertion is found in 7% of pregnant women; its incidence is higher in multi-fetal gestations. There is no clinical significance.

13. What is a velamentous placenta?

When the umbilical cord inserts into the fetal membranes away from the placenta disk, the placenta is referred to as velamentous. Such insertion occurs in 1% of singleton placentas. The portion of the placental blood vessel running from the insertion site to the placenta within the fetal membranes is unprotected by Wharton's jelly. If these blood vessels are positioned over the internal os, the condition is called **vasa previa**. Vasa previa can be a cause of third-trimester bleeding.

14. What are the physical measurements of a normal placenta?

The human placenta weighs between 450 and 550 grams. Its diameter is 20 cm, and its thickness is 2.5 cm.

15. Can the placental thickness be measured antenatally?

Placental thickness can be easily measured by ultrasound. The average ultrasonographic measurement during the third trimester is 3.4 cm. Conditions such as intrauterine fetal infections, diabetes mellitus, and immune and nonimmune hydrops are associated with a thickness > 4 cm.

16. What is Nitabuch's layer?

The layer of fibrinoid degeneration between the invading trophoblasts and the deciduas basalis is called Nitabuch's layer.

17. List the causes of third-trimester bleeding.

Third-trimester vaginal bleeding can be massive and life threatening to both mother and fetus. Causes are placenta previa, vasa previa, placental abruption, early labor, and local lesions of the lower genital tract. In most cases, the cause is unknown.

18. What is placenta previa?

When the placenta covers the internal os it is called placenta previa. The placenta may cover the os completely or only marginally. Placenta previa is more frequent at early gestation; as pregnancy progresses, most placenta previas resolve due to the differential growth of the upper and lower uterus.

19. What are the risk factors for placenta previa?
- Advanced maternal age
- Multiparity
- Previous cesarean delivery
- Prior suction curettage for spontaneous or induced abortion

20. What are placenta accreta, increta, and percreta?

Placenta *accreta* is the term used when the placental villi are attached to the myometrium as a result of partial or complete absence of the decidua basalis and faulty development of Nitabuch's layer. If placental villi invade the myometrium, it is called placental *increta*. When the invasion is through the myometrium, it is called *percreta*.

21. What are the risk factors for placenta accreta?
- Advanced maternal age
- Multiparity
- Placenta previa in patients with prior cesarean section (most important risk factor)

22. Describe placental abruption.

Placental abruption is a condition in which a normally implanted placenta separates prior to the birth of the fetus. The incidence of placental abruption is 1%. The incidence depends on the specifics of the population studied. Recent increase in cocaine use may explain the rise in incidence of placenta abruption.

23. What are the risk factors for placental abruption?
- Maternal hypertension
- Cigarette smoking
- Cocaine abuse
- Trauma
- Short umbilical cord
- Premature rupture of membranes

24. What is succentruate placenta?

Succentruate placenta is a condition when one or more extra lobes of the placenta are located distant from the main placenta. There is usually a vascular connection between the main placenta and the extra lobe. If not recognized at the time of delivery, this condition will cause postpartum bleeding and infection.

25. What is a placental polyp?

Placental polyps are degenerating villi usually covered by endometrium. Placental polyps are formed when parts of the placenta is retained within the endometrial cavity after delivery.

26. What are the different types of placentation in twin pregnancy?

There are three types of placentation in twin gestation: dichorionic-diamniotic (di-di), monochorionic-diamniotic (mono-di), and monochorionic-monoamniotic (mono-mono).

27. Why it is important to know the chorionicity of the placenta in twin gestations?

Perinatal mortality is much higher in mono-mono twins. Mono-di twins are also at increased risk for morbidity and mortality. There is always some vascular communication between twins in monochorionic pregnancies (mono-mono or mono-di). These vascular connections can lead to **twin transfusion syndrome** or **acardiac twin malformation**.

28. What is the significance of a single umbilical artery?

Normally there are three umbilical vessels: two arteries and one vein. The incidence of single umbilical artery (SUA) is approximately 1% of all singleton births. The incidence increases throughout gestation, indicating that in some cases a normally formed umbilical artery may atrophy as pregnancy progresses. The incidence is three to four times higher in twin gestations. It is frequently associated with intrauterine growth restriction. Twenty percent of infants with SUA have additional malformations.

BIBLIOGRAPHY

1. Benirschke K: Normal development. In Creasy R, Resnik R (eds): Maternal-Fetal Medicine, 4th ed. Philadelphia, W.B. Saunders, 1999.
2. Benirschke K: Twinning. In Knobil E, Neill JD (eds): Encyclopedia of Reproduction. Vol 4. San Diego, Academic Press, 1998, pp 887–891.
3. Heifetz SA: The umbilical cord: Obstetrically important lesions. Clinical Obstet Gynecol 39(3):571–587, 1996.
4. Liu JH, Rebar RW: Endocrinology of pregnancy. In Creasy R, Resnik R (eds): Maternal-Fetal Medicine, 4th ed. Philadelphia, W.B. Saunders, 1999.

59. ANTEPARTUM BLEEDING

Alfredo Gil, M.D.

PLACENTA PREVIA

1. What is a placenta previa?

A placenta previa is one that develops in the lower uterine segment, in the zone of dilatation, so that it cover or adjoins the internal os.

2. List the different types of placenta previa.

- Complete: The placenta completely covers the internal cervical os.
- Partial: The placenta partially covers the internal cervical os.
- Marginal: The edge of the placenta lies near, but does not cover, the internal cervical os.

With the advancement of ultrasound and our present ability to precisely define the distance between the edge of the placenta and the internal cervical os, older terms such as "low-lying placenta previa" are obsolete.

3. What is the incidence of placenta previa at term? In the second trimester?

The incidence at the time of delivery for placenta previa is 1/200 (0.5%). However, the incidence of placental tissue covering the internal cervical os at 18 weeks is 5–15%. Placenta previa seen in such early gestation has a 90% chance of resolution by term.

4. What are the risk factors for placenta previa?

Advancing maternal age (> 35)
Multiparity
Smoking
Cocaine use
Multi-fetal gestations
Prior history of placenta previa
Prior suction and curettage for induced or spontaneous abortion

5. Describe the role cigarette smoking plays in the risk of placenta previa.

Several studies have shown an increased risk of placenta previa among women who smoke. In fact, the risk of placenta previa is *doubled* in smokers compared to non-smokers. Reports of the relationship between risk and quantity and duration of smoking vary. One hypothesized mechanism is the relative carbon monoxide hypoxemia associated with smokers, which may result in compensatory placental hypertrophy with increased surface area more likely to cover the cervical os.

6. What are the potential maternal complications of placenta previa?

- Life-threatening maternal hemorrhage
- Cesarean delivery
- Increased risk of placenta accreta, necessitating a hysterectomy
- Increased risk of postpartum hemorrhage

7. What is a placenta accreta?

One of the most serious complications of a placenta previa is the development of a placenta accreta, which involves trophoblastic invasion past Nitabuch's layer. If the placenta invades into the uterine muscle, it is termed **placenta increta**; if it invades past the uterine serosa into the other pelvic structures (bladder, bowel, and vessels), it is termed **placenta percreta**. The risk of having a placenta accreta in the presence of a placenta previa is 1–5%; this increases to 25% with one prior cesarean section and 45% with two or more cesarean sections.

8. How does a placenta previa present?

The hallmark is the onset of painless vaginal bleeding in the late second or third trimester. The absence of uterine pain and contractions is the classic difference between placenta previa and abruptio placenta. Labor may precede the vaginal bleeding; therefore, the diagnosis of placenta previa must be excluded in every patient with complaints of vaginal bleeding in the second or third trimester. The initial episode of vaginal bleeding has a peak incidence in the early third trimester. The vaginal bleeding may start without any inciting factor (e.g., trauma, intercourse, labor, pelvic exam).

9. How is placenta previa diagnosed?

Vaginal bleeding in the second or third trimester is a contraindication to pelvic exam until the diagnosis of placenta previa is excluded. **Ultrasound** is the mainstay of diagnosis. Transabdominal ultrasound is highly accurate and sensitive for the diagnosis of placenta previa, with a false negative rate of 7%. The most common reason for missing the diagnosis is an obscured view due to the position of the fetal head or an overdistended bladder. *Transvaginal* and *translabial* ultrasound are both more sensitive than transabdominal ultrasound in some studies, identifying 100% of placenta previa. False positives and false negatives are only rarely reported.

10. How is placenta previa managed?

Maternal evaluation and stabilization are the first priorities. Secure a large-bore IV, type and cross for blood, check complete blood count, and obtain coagulation studies. If maternal resuscitation is necessary, begin aggressive fluid and blood replacement. Electronic fetal heart rate monitors can evaluate fetal condition simultaneously. If the pregnancy is > 37 weeks or fetal lung maturity has been documented by amniocentesis, then delivery by cesarean section is indicated. Delivery should also be undertaken in the presence of life-threatening maternal hemorrhage (regardless of fetal age) or if the pregnancy is > 24 weeks and there is fetal compromise. If the fetus is premature (< 37 weeks) and the vaginal bleeding is not considered life-threatening, then conservative management may be considered.

Steroids should be given to help accelerate fetal lung maturation. Tocolytics such as magnesium sulfate or β-mimetic may be used judiciously. Magnesium sulfate is the tocolytic of choice because of its minimal cardiac effects.

11. How can localization of the placenta facilitate choice of uterine incision when operative delivery is performed for placenta previa?

An anterior placenta previa is best managed with a low vertical or classic uterine incision, so as not to incise the placenta directly. With posterior or lateral localization of the previa, often a low transverse incision can be used if the lower uterine segment is sufficiently developed.

12. What is the risk of recurrence for placenta previa?

In one large study that had a baseline incidence of 0.3% for placenta previa at delivery, recurrence was 2.4%, an eight-fold increase over the general population.

13. What is a "double set-up" exam?

Double set-up refers to a pelvic exam for suspected placenta previa performed when the diagnosis is still unclear. The exam is done in the operating room with the patient prepped and draped for immediate surgery, adequate anesthesia administered, and the obstetrician scrubbed. Blood products should be readily available. Double set-up exams are less commonly done today because improvements in ultrasound have resulted in fewer instances where the diagnosis of placenta previa is still unclear.

14. List the predisposing factors for abnormal placental adherence.

- Placenta previa
- Uterine scars
- Submucosal leiomyomas
- Prior cesarean section
- Chronic endometritis
- Intrauterine synechiae

15. What are the complications of abnormal placental adherence?

Uterine rupture, uterine inversion during placental removal, and hysterectomy for incompletely removed placenta with maternal bleeding.

16. What is the relationship between maternal serum alpha feto-protein (MSAFP) and abnormal placentation?

Second-trimester elevations of MSAFP in women with ultrasound evidence of placenta previa are associated with an increased risk of placenta accreta, percreta, and increta. As MSAFP is governed by both fetal production and placental transference, abnormally deep invasion of the placenta results in elevations of MSAFP even in the second trimester.

17. What is placenta membranacea?

Placenta membranacea is a rare abnormality of placental development in which the chorion remains covered with villae instead of differentiating into chorion laeve and frondosum. If often presents clinically with vaginal bleeding. Ultrasound usually suggests a diffuse placenta occupying anterior and posterior uterine walls as well as previa location. The risk of postpartum hemorrhage and abnormal placental invasion requiring hysterectomy is high.

PLACENTAL ABRUPTION

18. What is placental abruption? What is its incidence?

Placental abruption is premature separation of a normally implanted placenta before delivery of the fetus. Placental abruption is initiated by hemorrhage into the decidua basalis. This hemorrhage can eventually lead to the formation of a hematoma, which can contribute to an expansion of the abruption. If vaginal bleeding accompanies the abruption, it is termed an external hemorrhage (90%). If abruption occurs without vaginal bleeding, the hemorrhage is said to be concealed (10%). The incidence of placental abruptions varies with the population studied but averages about 0.83% (1/120 deliveries).

19. What factors are associated with placental abruption?

Cocaine: a major risk factor for placental abruption, probably secondary to cocaine-induced vasospasm and hypertension

Trauma: accounts for only a small percentage of cases, and most occur in the initial 24 hours after the event

Smoking: increases risk by causing necrosis of the basalis layer

Increasing maternal age: an independent risk factor

Increasing parity: incidence is < 1% in primigravidas, 2.5% in grandmultiparas

Hypertension: either chronic or gestational

20. How does placental abruption present?

The clinical presentation varies, but the classic signs are vaginal bleeding (present in 90%), abdominal pain (present in 50%), uterine contractions (present in > 90%), uterine tenderness, and fetal demise.

21. Do pregnancies complicated by preterm premature rupture of the membranes (PPROM) have an increased risk of abruption?

In a recent study, expectant management of PPROM is associated with a five-fold higher rate of abruption, regardless of the gestational age at rupture of membranes or latency period to delivery.

Of note, vaginal bleeding before PPROM occurred significantly more often in pregnancies (15%) that subsequently had abruption.

22. Is the bleeding that occurs with an abruption maternal or fetal in origin?

Generally, most blood lost with an abruption comes from the mother. However, it may be either maternal or fetal in origin. Furthermore, it is common to underestimate actual blood loss on the basis of observation alone.

23. How is the diagnosis of placental abruption made?

The diagnosis is made on clinical suspicion in a patient that presents with vaginal bleeding, uterine contractions, and abdominal pain. Ultrasound is most useful to exclude a placenta previa as the cause of the vaginal bleeding. Ultrasound by itself is *not* sensitive enough to diagnose or to exclude the diagnosis of a placental abruption.

24. What is a Couvelaire uterus?

If there is widespread extravasation of blood into the uterine musculature and beneath the serosa, giving the uterus a bluish color at the time of laparotomy, this is termed a Couvelaire uterus. Such collections of blood rarely disrupt uterine contraction enough to cause postpartum hemorrhage and are not an indication for hysterectomy.

25. Which laboratory studies are helpful in the diagnosis and management of abruption?

Laboratory studies have limited utility in the diagnosis of abruption. Various studies, such as Kleihauer-Betke stain, D-dimer (a measure of fibrinolytic activity), and CA-125 have been proposed. Each, however, is limited by relatively poor sensitivity as well as the time required to obtain results.

Laboratory studies indicated for the management of abruption, however, often include maternal hematocrit, blood type, Kleihauer-Betke stain for determination of quantity of RhoGAM for Rh-negative mothers, and, in severe abruption, assessment for disseminated intravascular coagulation.

26. What are potential maternal complications of placental abruption?

Potential maternal complications include **hemorrhagic shock**: a healthy pregnant woman can lose 25% of her blood volume (1500 ml) before clinical signs of shock are evident. **Disseminated intravascular coagulation** (DIC) may be found in 10% of abruptions, and is more common in abruptions that lead to fetal death. DIC is thought to be due to entry of thromboplastins into the circulation from the site of placental injury, which initiates widespread activation of the clotting cascade. **Ischemic necrosis** of distal organs usually involves the kidneys, liver, adrenal glands, or pituitary gland. Ischemic necrosis of the kidney may take the form of **acute tubular necrosis** (ATN) or **bilateral cortical necrosis**. Both ATN and bilateral cortical necrosis are characterized by oliguria or anuria. However, bilateral cortical necrosis results in death from uremia within 1–2 weeks unless dialysis is instituted, whereas ATN usually resolves spontaneously.

27. What are potential fetal complications of placental abruption?

Fetal complications include hypoxia, anemia, growth retardation, increased incidence of anomalies (especially of the central nervous system), and death. Death of the fetus occurs in 4 of 1000 abruptions and accounts for 15% of all perinatal deaths. The major causes of perinatal death in abruption are anoxia, prematurity, and exsanguination. It is believed that early and more liberal use of abdominal delivery has lowered the perinatal mortality rate associated with abruption.

28. For low-birth-weight (LBW) infants (< 2500 g), do outcomes differ for infants delivered after abruption compared to other LBW infants?

For infants under 2500 g, neonatal and infant outcome appears to depend on severity of the abruption. Compared with infants delivered for other indications, preterm infants delivered due to a severe abruption have lower Apgar scores and higher rates of intraventricular hemorrhage. Follow-up at 2 years of age shows a similar significant increase in cerebral palsy. This difference remains even after correction for possible confounders of abruption and infant outcome, such as social class, level of education, gestational age, and birth weight.

29. How should placental abruptions be managed?

On presentation of significant abruption, initial measures include administration of intravenous fluids and supplemental oxygen. Type and cross match, usually for 4 units of packed red blood cells (RBCs), should be obtained. Placement of an indwelling urinary catheter allows close monitoring of urinary output. Finally, electronic fetal monitoring is recommended for continuous assessment of fetal well-being.

Hemorrhagic shock requires vigorous blood and volume replacement with packed RBCs and crystalloid. Goals of blood and volume replacement are to maintain the hematocrit at or above 30% and the urinary output ≥ 0.5 ml/kg/hr. Platelet count, fibrinogen level, and serum potassium level should be checked after each 4–6 units of packed RBCs administered. Invasive central monitoring (either central venous pressure or pulmonary capillary wedge pressure) is sometimes advisable.

The patient should be tested for **DIC** every 4 hours until delivery. Quantification of fibrin split products (FSPs) is the most sensitive lab test. However, once elevated, FSPs are not helpful in guiding therapy, and repeat testing is not necessary. Although normal results do not exclude DIC, fibrinogen levels and platelet counts are more indicative of the ongoing process and are more useful in terms of management. The ultimate therapy for DIC is delivery, which results in spontaneous resolution. Blood and volume replacement is all that is usually necessary until delivery. If a cesarean section needs to be performed and the platelet count is < 50,000 or the fibrinogen level is < 100 mg/100 ml, these components should be replaced individually. Fibrinogen may be replaced with fresh frozen plasma or cryoprecipitate. Heparin should not be used unless there is evidence of microvascular plugging (such as gangrene), which is rare.

30. When should a pregnancy complicated by abruption be delivered?

The method and timing of delivery depend on the gestational age of the fetus and the severity of abruption. If the pregnancy is at term and abruption is mild, vaginal delivery may be attempted. This may include cautious augmentation of labor with oxytocin, if needed. Amniotomy is generally considered to be advantageous because it may decrease extravasation of blood into the myometrium and entry of thromboplastic substances into the circulation. On the other hand, when the fetus is immature, mild abruptions may be managed expectantly and a trial of tocolysis considered. If distress occurs in a potentially viable fetus and vaginal delivery is not imminent, cesarean section should be performed immediately. Furthermore, severe maternal hemorrhage may necessitate immediate abdominal delivery. Finally, when a fetal demise has occurred, but the maternal condition is stable, vaginal delivery should be attempted.

31. What is the risk of recurrence with placental abruption?

It is estimated that 5.5%–16.6% of subsequent pregnancies will again be complicated by placental abruption. This risk increases to 25% during a third pregnancy if there have been two consecutive abruptions previously. Despite the significant risk of recurrence, it is impossible to predict which pregnancies will be affected and at what gestational age the abruption will occur. Therefore, a history of placental abruption with a prior pregnancy qualifies a present pregnancy as high risk.

BIBLIOGRAPHY

1. Besinger RE, Moniak CW, Paskiewicz LS, et al: The effect of tocolytic use in the management of symptomatic placenta previa. Am J Obstet Gynecol 172:1770–1775, 1995.
2. Combs CA, Nyberg DA, Mack LA, et al: Expectant management after sonographic diagnosis of placental abruption. Am J Perinatol 9:170–174, 1992.

3. Creasy RK, Resnik R (eds): Maternal-Fetal Medicine: Principles and Practice, 4rd ed. Philadelphia, W.B. Saunders, 1999.
4. Cunningham FG, Gant NF, Leveno KJ (eds): Williams Obstetrics, 21st ed. New York, McGraw Hill, 2001.
5. Farine D, Peisner DB, Timor-Tritsch IE: Placenta previa: Is the traditional diagnostic approach satisfactory? J Clin Ultrasound 18:328, 1990.
6. Handler AS, Mason ED, Rosenberg DL, Davis FG: The relationship between exposure during pregnancy to cigarette smoking and cocaine use and placenta previa. Am J Obstet Gynecol 170:884–889, 1994.
7. Hertzberg BS, Bowie JD, Caroll BA, et al: Diagnosis of placenta previa during the third trimester: Role of transperineal sonography. Am J Roentgenol 159:83–87, 1992.
8. Iyasu S, Saftlas AK, Rowly DL, er al: The epidemiology of placenta previa in the United States, 1979 though 1987. Am J Obstet Gynecol 168:1424, 1993.
9. Major CA, de Veciana M, Lewis DF, Morgan MA: Preterm premature rupture of membranes and abruptio placentae: Is there an association between these pregnancy complications? Am J Obstet Gynecol 172:672–676, 1995.
10. Monica G, Lilja C: Placenta previa, maternal smoking and recurrence risk. Acta Obstet Gynecol Scand 74:341–345, 1995.
11. Scott JR, Disaia PJ, Hammond CB, Spellacy WN (eds): Danforth's Obstetrics and Gynecology, 8th ed. Philadelphia, J.B. Lippincott, 1999.
12. Spinillo A, Fazzi E, Stronati M, et al: Severity of abruptio placentae and neurodevelopmental outcome in low birth weight infants. Early Hum Devel 35:45–54, 1993.
13. Taylor VM, Kramer MD, Vaughn TL, Peacock S: Placenta previa in relation to induced and spontaneous abortion: A population-based study. Obstet Gynecol 82:88, 1993.
14. Williams MA, Mittendorf R, Lieberman E, et al: Cigarette smoking during pregnancy in relation to placenta previa. Am J Obstet Gynecol 165:28–32, 1991.
15. Zelop C, Nadel A, Frigoletto FD, et al: Placenta accreta/percreta/increta: A cause of elevated maternal serum alpha fetoprotein. Obstet Gynecol 80(4):693–694, 1992

VII. Labor, Delivery, and Postpartum

60. PREMATURE CERVICAL DILATION

Iraj Forouzan, M.D.

1. What is premature cervical dilation?

Cervical dilation prior to the onset of labor is called premature cervical dilation (PCD).

2. What is the difference between premature cervical dilation and cervical incompetence?

Cervical incompetence is premature cervical dilation during the second trimester of the pregnancy that results in pregnancy loss. The classic definition of cervical incompetence requires two such occurrences consecutively. Therefore, incompetent cervix is a recurrent premature cervical dilation.

3. How common are premature cervical dilation and incompetent cervix?

The true incidence of premature cervical dilation is unknown, but reports indicate that the incidence of recurrent PCD (incompetent cervix) is 1% of all pregnancies. The recurrence rate for incompetent cervix is 20–30%. Women with classic incompetent cervix—who have had two consecutive mid-trimester pregnancy losses accompanied by painless cervical dilation—have a 70–75% chance of carrying their next pregnancy to term without intervention.

4. What causes premature cervical dilation?

The uterine cervix consists of fibrous connective tissue, muscular tissue, and blood vessels. The distribution of these tissues in the cervix is not even. There is more muscular tissue at the internal os, and more connective tissue at the lower end of the cervix. A defect in this tissue composition and arrangement has been regarded as the cause for incompetent cervix leading to premature cervical dilation.

5. How is premature cervical dilation diagnosed?

For many years, digital cervical length assessment has been the method of diagnosis. Recently, ultrasonographic examination of the cervix has gained popularity, and is rapidly becoming the method of choice for early detection of premature cervical dilation (see figure, top of next page). There is less inter-observer variation associated with ultrasound compared to digital exam. Ultrasound has the ability to measure the entire cervix compared to the digital exam, which only measures the vaginal portion of the cervix. Some studies have shown that short cervical length (< 2.5 cm) or funneling of the internal os at 24 weeks of gestation on transvaginal ultrasound is predictive of preterm delivery.

6. Is there a reliable diagnostic test for cervical incompetence?

The diagnosis of cervical incompetence is made primarily on the basis of history, but there are also a number of tests that can be performed. The ability to pass a no. 16 Foley catheter or no. 8 cervical dilator (positive Hegar test) through the cervix is suggestive of cervical incompetence. Hysterosalpingography is frequently used to study the intrauterine cavity when evaluating a patient with second-trimester pregnancy loss. Some clinicians regard an abnormally wide uterocervical canal (≥ 8 mm at the level of the internal os) on hysterosalpingography as a sign of an incompetent cervix.

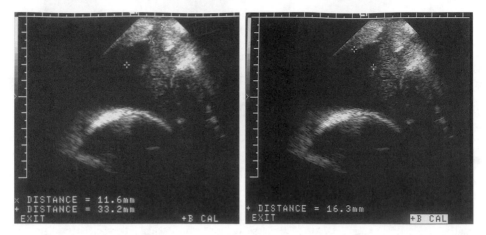

A transvaginal ultrasound image of the cervix in a patient with PCD and funneling. The entire cervical length is 33.2 mm, and the closed distal part of the cervix is 11.6 mm. The dilated portion's width is 16.3 mm.

7. What are the risk factors for premature cervical dilation?

The most common risk factor for premature cervical dilation is a history of previous PCD. Congenital cervical hypoplasia and intrauterine diethylstilbestrol (DES) exposure have been reported as risk factors for PCD. Acquired risk factors include previous trauma to the cervix. Cervical conization, amputation, obstetric laceration, and forceful dilatation are examples of such traumas.

8. What is the treatment for premature cervical dilation?

There are not many effective treatments. Treatments ranging from bed rest to tocolysis and cervical cerclage have been proposed.

9. Who is a candidate for cervical cerclage?

Women with proven cervical incompetence are candidates for cervical cerclage. The most important issue in selecting patients for cerclage is the absence of uterine contractions. The presence of uterine contractions is indicative of preterm labor. Cervical cerclage is not the appropriate treatment for preterm labor. Some clinicians argue that a prematurely dilated cervix may in turn provoke uterine contractions, subsequently making it difficult to distinguish between these two entities. Regardless of the sequence of events, the presence of uterine contractions is a *contraindication* to cervical cerclage.

10. How effective is cervical cerclage?

Cervical cerclage is indicated in patients with incompetent cervix, but its efficacy has not been proved in a large, randomized study. Most of the literature concerning cervical cerclage and its benefits are retrospective. Accurate diagnosis of an incompetent cervix is not possible in most cases, due to the lack of an objective diagnostic test. Usually the diagnosis is not clear, and the obstetrician is not certain as to the advisability of cerclage.

In 1993, the Royal College of Obstetricians and Gynecologists published its concluding report on a multicenter randomized study to address this issue. The most typical cases of incompetent cervix were excluded from the study. The study showed some benefit from cerclage. There were fewer deliveries in the cerclage group before 33 weeks of pregnancy (13% versus 17%).

11. Describe the most common techniques for cervical cerclage.

There are two common transvaginal cervical cerclage techniques: McDonald and Shirodkar. **McDonald cervical cerclage** is simple: a purse-string suture using no. 4 silk or nylon or Mersilene tape. Five or six deep bites are taken, and tied anteriorly. There is no mucosal dissection during the McDonald technique. Some clinicians prefer double sutures.

The **Shirodkar operation** was introduced in 1955. In this technique, vaginal mucosa is dissected away from the cervix before placing the suture.

12. What other techniques are available?

The **Wurm procedure** is a modification of the McDonald procedure. It was developed in 1959. The technique involves placement of interrupted mattress sutures using no. 3 heavy braided silk at the level of the internal os. One suture is placed from 12 to 6 o'clock and a second one from 3 to 9 o'clock. The **Lash operation** is basically repairing of cervical lacerations during the non-pregnant state. The **Emmet procedure** is also another type of trachelorrhaphy, performed during the non-pregnant state. The **Mann cerclage** and **Page techniques** are other methods of cervical cerclage.

13. When is the best time in gestation to place an elective (prophylactic) cerclage?

It is recommended that the cervical cerclage be placed at 13–16 weeks of pregnancy. There are situations when a patient may require cerclage later in gestation, either due to late initiation of prenatal care or unexpected premature cervical dilation. In these patients cerclage can be done until 23 weeks of pregnancy. Cerclage is not normally done after fetal viability.

14. Explain transabdominal cerclage (TAC).

In 1965, Benson and Durfee reported the TAC operation. Patients should be carefully selected, since the procedure has higher morbidity compared to the transvaginal cerclage. It requires laparotomy and subsequent delivery by cesarean. Transabdominal cerclage should be advised only to those patients in whom transvaginal cerclage is impossible.

15. Which cervical cerclage technique is best?

Some of the techniques are designed for particular patients such as those who have cervical lacerations, but there is no randomized study to compare the two most commonly employed techniques (McDonald and Shirodkar).

16. What are the contraindications to cervical cerclage?

The presence of uterine contractions (labor) is a contraindication to cervical cerclage. Ruptured fetal membranes, intrauterine infections, intrauterine fetal growth restriction, and major fetal anomalies are also contraindications.

17. PCD is diagnosed on routine second-trimester ultrasound in a patient with no risk factors. What is the optimal management of this patient?

Logically one would recommend cervical cerclage, but the literature is conflicting. More recent randomized studies show no benefit from cervical cerclage in patients with no history. Inform your patient of the ultrasound finding, and discuss the merits of prophylactic cerclage or simple bed rest.

18. What are the complications of cerclage?

The complications associated with cervical cerclage can be divided into two groups: those related directly to the procedure and those occurring later. Procedure-related risks include anesthetic risks, maternal soft tissue injury, bleeding, infection, rupture of fetal membranes, and abortion. Late complications are cervical laceration, fistulae formation, and increased incidence of cesarean section.

19. When should a cervical cerclage be removed?

Most clinicians advocate removal at 37–38 weeks of gestation, before labor starts, to reduce the risk of cervical damage and uterine rupture. In most cases the cerclage can be removed in the office, but occasionally it must be done in the operating room and under anesthesia.

20. What is the role of cervical cerclage in multi-fetal pregnancy?

In the past, some clinicians suggested cervical cerclage in these patients because multi-fetal pregnancies are at increased risk for preterm delivery. However, there is no evidence to support its usefulness.

BIBLIOGRAPHY

1. Benson RC, Durfee RB: Transabdominal cervicouterine cerclage during pregnancy for the treatment of cervical incompetence. Obstet Gynecol 25:145–155, 1965.
2. Danforth DN: The fibrous nature of the human cervix, and its relation to the isthmic segment in gravid and nongravid uteri. Am J Obstet Gynecol 53:541–560, 1947.
3. Goldberg J, Newman R, Rust P: Interobserver reliability of digital and endovaginal ultrasonographic cervical length measurements. Am J Obstet Gynecol 177:853–858, 1997.
4. Iams JD, Goldenberg RL, Meis PJ, et al: The length of the cervix and the risk of spontaneous premature delivery. N Engl J Med 334:567–572, 1996.
5. Iams JD, Johnson FF, Sonek J, et al: Cervical competence as a continuum: A study of ultrasonographic cervical length and obstetric performance. Am J Obstet Gynecol 172:1097–106, 1995.
6. McDonald IA: Suture of the cervix for inevitable miscarriage. J Obstet Gynecol Br Emp 64:346–350, 1957.
7. Medical Research Council/Royal College of Obstetricians and Gynecologists Multicentre Randomized Trial of Cervical Cerclage. MRC/RCOG working party on cervical cerclage. Br J Obstet Gynecol 100:516–523, 1993.
8. Norwitz ER, Goldstein DP: Transabdominal cervicoisthmic cerclage: Learning to tie the knot. J Gynecol Tech 2:49–54, 1996.
9. Rust O, Atlas R, Reed J, et al: Revisiting the clinical efficacy of cerclage in the treatment of second-trimester, sonographically detected premature cervical dilation of the internal os. Am J Obstet Gynecol 184(1):S3, 2001.
10. Shirodkar VN: A new method of operative treatment for habitual abortion in the second trimester of pregnancy. Antiseptic 52:299, 1955.
11. Tharakan T, Baxi L, Schwartz SJ: Cervical insufficiency. In O'Grady JP, Gimovsky ML, McIlhargie CJ (eds): Operative Obstetrics. Philadelphia, Williams & Wilkins, 1995, pp 41–54.
12. Wong GP, Farquharson DF, Dansereau J: Emergency cervical cerclage: A retrospective review of 51 cases. Am J Perinatol 10:341–347, 1993.

61. PRETERM LABOR

Hyagriv N. Simhan, M.D.

1. How is preterm labor defined?

Preterm labor is strictly defined as frequent uterine contractions with or without pain in the face of progressive cervical dilatation or effacement, occurring after the 20th week up to 37 weeks' gestation.

2. What are the common symptoms of preterm labor? How are they evaluated?

- Regular uterine contractions with or without pain more frequently than every 15 minutes, each more than 30–40 seconds long, for more than 1-hour duration
- Pelvic pressure
- Dull, constant back pain
- Change in vaginal discharge
- Intermittent abdominal cramping
- Spotting or vaginal bleeding

These symptoms may be evaluated with external tocodynamometry, which documents the frequency of contractions.

3. What causes preterm labor?

In the majority of cases, the cause of preterm labor is unknown. Because approximately 50% of patients who complain of preterm contractions do not deliver prior to term, the diagnosis, causes, and incidence of true preterm labor are difficult to assess accurately. Dehydration, urinary tract infection, systemic infection, vaginitis, or cervicitis may contribute or predispose to preterm labor.

4. What are the risk factors associated with preterm labor?

Previous induced abortion (two or more first-trimester or one second-trimester abortion)	Poor nutritional status
	Uterine anomalies
	Advanced maternal age
Low socioeconomic status	Maternal age less than 20
Smoking	Previous cervical surgery
Previous preterm delivery	Diethylstilbestrol (DES) exposure
Short interpregnancy interval	Urinary tract infection
Congenital anomalies	Bacterial vaginosis
Chorioamnionitis	Polyhydramnios
Preterm premature rupture of membranes	Serious systemic infection
Abruption	Multiple gestation
Fetal demise	Cocaine use
Placenta previa	Low prepregnancy weight

5. How frequently does preterm birth occur?

Preterm birth complicates 10–12% of all live births; this incidence varies with the population studied. Preterm labor occurs in 10–15% of all pregnancies.

6. What are the consequences of preterm labor?

Preterm birth is the major consequence, resulting in an increased risk of neonatal morbidity and death. Preterm birth accounts for approximately 100 neonatal deaths for every 100,000 live births in the U.S. The mobidity and mortality of preterm birth results from pulmonary immaturity, resulting in neonatal respiratory distress syndrome, persistent pulmonary hypertension, and bronchopulmonary dysplasia. Preterm babies also have an increased risk of intraventricular hemorrhage (IVH). IVH may result in seizures or permanent neurologic injury. Premature neonates are also at higher risk for sepsis, necrotizing enterocolitis, and apneic and bradycardic episodes. The majority of neonatal mortality occurs in infants born prior to 28 weeks' gestation.

7. What are key points in the initial evaluation and treatment of the patient with possible preterm labor?
- Baseline history for pregnancy complications, gestational age, symptoms of preterm premature rupture of the membranes (PROM), any infectious signs and symptoms (especially cystitis, pyelonephritis, or chorioamnionitis), hydration status, risk factors for preterm labor, and cardiac history
- Baseline physical exam with special attention to any fever, cardiac and respiratory exam, estimated fetal weight, uterine tenderness, any evidence of PROM, and cervical dilation and effacement; external monitoring of the fetus and uterine activity for confirmation of contractions, evidence of abruption, and fetal heart rate
- Baseline laboratory studies include a complete blood count for leukocytosis and hematocrit, urinalysis to assess degree of hydration and infection, cervical cultures for group B streptococcus, and ultrasound for gestational age, presentation, and evidence of rupture of membranes. A urine toxicology screen may be performed if indicated. If beta-mimetic tocolysis is contemplated, levels of potassium and glucose may also be measured. Isotonic intravenous fluids are begun (normal saline or lactated Ringer's), and the patient is put at bed rest and followed for contractions and cervical change.

8. What role does fibronectin play in the assessment of labor?
The appearance of fetal fibronectin in cervical samples correlates to a certain extent with the onset of labor in both term and preterm pregnancies. A fetal fibronectin assay has been proposed by some as an alternative risk stratification system to predict success of induction of term and post-term pregnancy.

As a predictor of preterm delivery, fetal fibronectin has been evaluated in several populations. As a screening tool in asymptomatic women (low-risk or high-risk populations), the efficacy of fibronectin assays is limited. Although sensitivity is low, negative predictive values (NPV), indicating true absence of preterm delivery in the absence of fibronectin, are high. The test is not recommended for screening of asymptomatic women.

Among pregnancies complicated by preterm contractions, some have advocated incorporating fetal fibronectin assays in management. Again, the negative predictive values are high, 76–83% for delivery before 37 weeks. In one study, a high NPV (99%) was noted for delivery within 7 days. In the same populations with premature contractions, positive predictive values for a preterm delivery were 60–80%. In a symptomatic woman, a negative test is fairly reassuring that delivery will not occur with the next 7 days. Therefore, costly and potentially morbid intervention such as tocolysis, admission, or bedrest may be avoided.

9. How is preterm labor treated?
Elimination of risk factors, bed rest, antenatal glucocorticoid treatment, and parenteral and oral tocolytics have been used. Tocolytics are routinely used at less than 34 weeks' gestation if there are no contraindications to treatment. Treatment is individualized from 34–37 weeks. Therefore, gestational age must be carefully documented prior to initiating tocolytic therapy. In the setting of intact membranes, antbiotics have not had any demonstrated benefit.

10. What are parenteral agents for treating preterm labor?
Intravenous beta agonists (ritodrine and terbutaline) have been used to treat premature labor. Ritodrine is the only medication approved by the U.S. Food and Drug Administration for tocolysis, but it is no longer commercially available in the U.S. Terbutaline is used as an infusion in

doses of 10–50 mg/min. It is begun at a low rate (2.5 mg/min) and increased in an incremental fashion every 10 minutes to achieve tocolysis. Intravenous magnesium sulfate is usually given in a 4–6 g bolus over 20 minutes and then continued at 2–4 g/hour as titrated to cessation of contractions. Infusions of **magnesium sulfate** and **beta agonists** are usually continued for up to 24 hours once tocolysis is achieved. Terbutaline has also been used subcutaneously in doses of 0.25 mg every 3–4 hours.

11. What are the oral tocolytic agents?
Terbutaline, 5 mg every 4–6 hours, has been employed, as has ritodrine, 10–20 mg every 4–6 hours. Oral magnesium preparations have also been used with minimal reported success. Each of these has side effects that may limit their tolerance.

Calcium channel blockers such as **nifedipine** and **verapamil** have been used with some success and are tolerated well by patients. Several human studies have confirmed the safety and efficacy of nifedipine for tocolysis. Nifedipine is given as a 40-mg load over 40 minutes followed by 10–30 mg every 3 to 6 hours. The dose and interval may be titrated based on contraction pattern and side effects.

Prostaglandin synthetase inhibitors such as **indomethacin** and **ibuprofen** have been used in standard doses, especially at less than 32 weeks' gestation. They are effective tocolytics. Their use appears to be complicated by oligohydramnios and possible premature closure of the ductus arteriosus. The maternal side effects are the same as those well known in the nonpregnant population.

12. What are relative contraindications to tocolysis?

Severe hemorrhage	Pulmonary hypertension
Abruption	Known intolerance to tocolytics
Severe preeclampsia	Fetal maturity
Eclampsia	Lethal fetal anomaly
Intrauterine fetal death	Chorioamnionitis
Severe intrauterine growth retardation	

13. Is tocolysis effective?
Clinical studies have shown effectiveness in prolonging gestation for 48 hours. The efficacy of maintenance oral tocolytic therapy is questionable. Currently, the most important benefit of tocolytic therapy is prolongation of gestation to provide maximal benefit of antenatal corticosteroid treatment.

14. What are the postulated mechanisms of action of the various tocolytics?
Beta-adrenergic agonists activate beta-adrenergic receptors and thus increase adenylate cyclase, with a concomitant increase in intracellular cyclic adenosine monophosphate (AMP). Cyclic AMP reduces intracellular calcium and the sensitivity of the myosin-actin contractile unit to calcium.

Magnesium sulfate has an unclear mechanism of action; according to one theory, it competes for calcium entry into muscle cells or calcium storage in muscle cell endoreticulum.

Calcium channel blockers interfere with influx of calcium into cells through voltage-mediated channels.

Prostaglandin synthetase inhibitors prevent formation of prostaglandins from arachidonic acid.

15. List the side effects of the usual tocolytics.
- Use of IV beta agonists may be complicated by hypotension, pulmonary edema, cardiac arrhythmias, chest pain, tachycardia, myocardial ischemia, hyperglycemia, glucose intolerance, and hypokalemia. Twin gestations are at greater risk of pulmonary edema secondary to tocolysis.
- Magnesium sulfate infusions may be complicated by hypotension, flushing, lethargy, hyporeflexia, pulmonary edema, and respiratory and cardiac depression and arrest. Neonatal suppression may also occur.

• Calcium channel blockers may cause flushing, headache, and maternal hypotension. The concomitant use of magnesium sulfate and calcium channel blockers should be avoided because of an increased risk of respiratory depression.
• Indomethacin may cause maternal gastric irritation and prolongation of bleeding time. Indomethacin may also cause decreased fetal renal perfusion and oligohydramnios, as well as premature closure of the ductus arteriosus.

16. How should patients on tocolytics be followed?

For patients on IV beta agonists, it is necessary initially to evaluate the hematocrit, potassium, and glucose. Each patient should be examined for a history of cardiac ischemia, valvular lesions, congestive heart failure, and arrhythmias, or for previous intolerance to these medications. Along with routine physical exam, perform a careful cardiac and pulmonary exam.

These patients should be followed with serial potassium and glucose every 6–24 hours or as symptoms require. Frequent physical examination and close monitoring of urine output is important for evidence of volume overload or pulmonary edema. Oral and parenteral fluids should be limited to not more than 100–125 cc/hr to decrease the risk of pulmonary edema. For complaints of chest pain, stop the infusion and obtain an electrocardiogram; if indicated, check cardiac enzymes.

Patients on magnesium sulfate should be followed with serial blood pressure evaluations and examined for deep tendon reflexes, alertness, and urine output. Strictly limit fluid intake in these patients. Serial magnesium and calcium levels may be followed to assess adequacy of infusion: 5–8 mg/dl is considered therapeutic; cardiac and respiratory depression may occur at > 10 mg/dl. Magnesium sulfate is renally excreted; therefore, renal function and adequate urine output must be assured.

If evidence of cardiac or respiratory depression occurs, stop the infusion and give 1 ampule of 10% calcium gluconate to competitively inhibit the elevated magnesium concentration.

17. Does home uterine activity monitoring (HUAM) decrease preterm deliveries?

No. In the early 1990s, there were strong advocates as well as opponents of this new technology. Initial studies that supported the ability of HUAM to decrease preterm labor and preterm birth and to improve neonatal outcomes were criticized for methodologic flaws. In addition, increased nursing contact with the patients in the group receiving twice-a-day HUAM played a role in their more favorable outcomes.

Other attempts to evaluate this question have reached varying conclusions. A meta-analysis of randomized studies in 1995 found statistically significant decreases in preterm labor with dilation > 2 cm and preterm birth in singleton pregnancies. These findings were not present in twin gestations. Additionally, no significant differences could be detected in infant referrals to the intensive care unit or in mean birth weights between the monitored and unmonitored groups. The 1995 Collaborative Home Uterine Monitoring Study (CHUMS) failed to find significant differences in gestational ages at delivery or neonatal outcomes in over 1000 patients at high risk for preterm labor who were randomized to monitoring vs. sham monitoring devices.

Thus, the available data do not support the use of HUAM for the prevention of preterm birth. Any potential benefit of HUAM is limited by effectiveness of treatment of preterm labor. No apparent benefit is derived from HUAM in assisting the provider in prescribing oral tocolytics.

18. What are general estimates for survival of the preterm infant?

Viability of a preterm gestation depends on several factors. Certainly immediate accessibility of neonatal support and the absence of congenital malformations are associated with better outcomes. Although gestational age is sometimes used as a marker of neonatal viability, birth weight is felt by some to be a more sensitive predictor. Generally infants weighing 1000–1500 g have > 90% survival. Below 1000 g, survival decreases 10–15% for each decrement of 100 g. Below 500 gm survival is rare, but has been documented (see table).

19. What are the short- and long-term complications of the early premature infant?

Neonatal complications include intraventricular hemorrhage (IVH), respiratory distress syndrome (RDS), sepsis, and necrotizing enterocolitis (NEC). In general, these complications of prematurity are more common and more severe at earlier gestational ages and smaller birth weights (Table 1).

Table 1. *Likelihood of Mortality and Morbidity in Preterm Babies by Birth Weight Category, 1995–1996*

	501–750 G	751–1000 G	1001–1250 G	1251–1500 G	501–1500 G
RDS	78%	63%	44%	26%	50%
Chronic lung disease	52%	34%	15%	7%	36%
IVH (grade III & IV)	26%	12%	8%	3%	11%
NEC	14%	9%	5%	3%	7%
Septicemia	48%	33%	18%	7%	24%
28-day mortality	40%	11%	5%	3%	14%

Data from Lemons JA, Bauer CR, Oh W, et al: Very low birth weight outcomes of the National Institute of Child Health and Human Development Neonatal Research Network, January 1995 through December 1996. Pediatrics 107:E1, 2001.

20. What are the complications in later preterm infants?

Both short-term and long-term complications decrease from 28 to 32 weeks. Developmental disability occurs in approximately 10% of survivors in the 28–30 week range, with retinal scarring in 2–3% and blindness in < 1%. Respiratory complications compromise approximately 50% of these neonates.

21. How can fetal lung maturity be assessed during preterm labor?

Various tests have been developed to analyze the components of fetal lung maturation. The ratio of lethicin to sphingomyelin or the appearance of phosphatidyglycerol are commonly employed as markers of fetal lung maturation. These tests are performed on amniotic fluid that is obtained via amniocentesis or, in the setting of rupture of membranes, from a vaginal pool.

22. In the classic studies of steroid use in preterm gestations, how was the incidence of hyaline membrane disease (HMD) altered?

The original findings of Liggins and Howie in 1972 have since been repeated in several studies and serve as a landmark contribution to the decreased mortality of premature neonates. Two doses of IM betamethasone 24 hours apart, with delivery 24 hours after the last dose and before 7 days from the first dose, were associated with a marked decrease in HMD. The findings were most significant for gestations of 30–34 weeks, with decreased effect for gestations of 27–30 weeks.

23. When does it appear that infants receive the greatest respiratory benefit from maternal betamethasone treatment?

Overall decrease in HMD is greatest in infants delivered between 1 and 7 days after maternal treatment. However, benefits are still derived if an infant is delivered within 24 hours of treatment (30% reduction in HMD) or at more than 7 days after treatment (40% reduction).

Currently, the gestational age at which infants benefit by reduction in HMD is not restricted to those at 30–34 weeks' gestation. Because few infants over 34 weeks develop HMD, benefits are difficult to ascertain; however, benefits to infants under 30 weeks appear equal to those in the 30–34 week range.

24. What other fetal benefits have been attributed to maternal steroid therapy?

Reduction in intraventricular hemorrhage by 60% and decrease in necrotizing enterocolitis by 65%. There is also a significant reduction in all-cause overall mortality in preterm neonates who have received antenatal steroids.

25. What fetal/neonatal and maternal complications have been ascribed to steroid administration?

No significant short-term fetal/neonatal complications have been definitely identified. Although an increased rate of neonatal infection has been suggested when steroids are administered in the presence of premature rupture of membranes, current estimates are imprecise. Twelve-year follow-ups of children treated in utero have shown no demonstrable effects on growth and development of the central nervous system. These studies have helped to alleviate initial concerns in animals for impaired myelination with third-trimester in utero steroid exposure.

Maternal complications include glucose intolerance with increased insulin requirements and the potential for increased pulmonary edema when steroids are used in conjunction with tocolytics. For increased pulmonary edema, the role of tocolysis vs. the combination of tocolysis plus steroids has been difficult to assess. A concern for possible increase in postpartum maternal infection remains unresolved.

26. What role does surfactant administration play in outcomes of premature infants?

Administered neonatally, synthetic surfactant has been shown to reduce neonatal morbidity and mortality. Initially used as a rescue treatment in markedly premature infants (< 1000 g), studies have also supported its efficacy as a prophylactic measure in extremely premature infants and as a rescue treatment in larger infants (< 2000 g). Debate continues about the greater efficacy of synthetic (Exosurf) vs. modified bovine surfactant extract (Survanta). Enhanced additive beneficial effects of maternal steroid administration (dexamethasone) and subsequent rescue surfactant use have been reported.

CONTROVERSY

27. Should steroids be administered one time or with multiple, repeated courses?

Steroids create a histologically detectable change in the developing lung about 48 hours after a dose. The duration of benefit is thought to be about a week. Thus, when steroid use first became popular, clinicians frequently gave "high-risk" women a course of steroids once a week, theoretically providing "constant" steroid benefit. There are small human studies and animal data that suggest some pulmonary benefit to repeated doses of steroids. However, over time, data has accumulated that suggests repeated dosing of antenatal steroids may result in smaller neonatal head circumference, increased risk of growth delay, increased risk of neonatal sepsis, and perhaps an increase in overall neonatal mortality. As this data has come forth, current clinical practice has shifted away from the routine use of weekly steroid treatment. In order to definitively resolve this controversy, a large, multi-center, prospective randomized controlled trial is underway.

PRETERM PREMATURE RUPTURE OF MEMBRANES

28. How is premature rupture of membranes (PROM) defined?

PROM is defined as rupture of membranes before the onset of labor.

29. How is *preterm* premature rupture of membranes (PPROM) defined?

PPROM is defined as rupture of membranes before the onset of labor in a gestation < 37 weeks.

30. What is prolonged rupture of membranes?

Ruptured membranes for > 24 hours before delivery.

31. How is PROM diagnosed?

History of fluid leaking through the vagina is the most common symptom. Urinary incontinence, excessive vaginal discharge, and mucus discharge are in the differential diagnosis.

32. What is the work-up for PROM?

- *Never do a digital exam*, because even one digital exam can increase the chance of infection by carrying vaginal organisms into the cervix and uterus.
- Do a sterile speculum exam to look for pooling of amniotic fluid and to assess the cervix.
- Confirm the diagnosis by testing the fluid for pH using nitrazine paper. The pH of the vagina in pregnancy is 4.5–5.5. Nitrazine paper changes from yellow to blue at a pH above 6. Since the pH of amniotic fluid is about 7, the nitrazine paper turns blue if there is amniotic fluid in the vagina. False-positive nitrazine tests may occur from semen, blood or serum, trichomonas or bacterial vaginitis infections, or soap. False-negative tests occur in < 10% of cases.
- Do a fern test. A swab from the posterior vaginal fornix should be rolled on a slide and allowed to *air dry* for at least 10 minutes. Under the microscope a typical arborization or "fern" pattern will appear if amniotic fluid is present. False-positive tests have been attributed to fingerprints, talc, and semen.
- Ultrasound often shows decreased amniotic fluid volume.
- A definitive diagnosis can be made when the above tests are equivocal by injecting indigo carmine dye into the amniotic cavity under ultrasound guidance via amniocentesis. A tampon is placed in the vagina, left for 2 hours, and then removed. If the membranes are ruptured, the tampon will turn blue from the colored amniotic fluid. Methylene blue dye should be avoided because of the risk of fetal methemoglobinemia.

33. What is the latency period?

The interval between rupture of membranes and the onset of labor.

34. What is the incidence of premature rupture of membranes?

PROM occurs in 10–15% of all pregnancies, including 10% of term pregnancies. Preterm PROM complicates 2–4% of preterm pregnancies.

35. What is the major complication of preterm PROM?

Preterm birth. Preterm PROM is associated with 30–40% of preterm births and 10% of all perinatal mortality.

36. List the other complications of preterm PROM.

- Cord prolapse, especially in nonvertex presentations
- Increased number of cesarean sections because of nonvertex presentations
- Fetal pulmonary hypoplasia and orthopedic deformations with severe, *early*, and prolonged oligohydramnios/anhydramnios
- Placental abruption

37. What causes preterm PROM?

Preterm PROM probably occurs because several factors act to weaken the chorioamnion. Physical stress, bacteria, and macrophages produce proteases, elastases, phospholipases, cytokines, and eicosanoids that produce uterine irritability, cervical ripening, and membrane weakness and rupture. In the majority of cases, it is likely an inflammatory process that causes rupture "biochemically" rather than physically.

38. List the risk factors for preterm PROM.

- History of premature PROM (most common risk factor)
- Cervicovaginitis: sexually transmitted diseases, including gonorrhea, trichomonas, bacterial vaginosis, group B β-hemolytic streptococcus
- Incompetent cervix
- Cigarette smoking
- Amniocentesis

• Prior cervical surgery
• Vaginal bleeding in the first or second trimester
• Polyhydramnios
• Connective tissue disease such as Ehlers-Danlos syndrome
• Chronic steroid use

39. What is the recurrence rate for preterm PROM?

The PROM recurrence rate is 20–30%, compared with a 4% incidence if the prior pregnancy was an uncomplicated term pregnancy.

40. Which characteristics are no longer believed to be risk factors for premature PROM?

Coitus   Maternal exercise
Cervical exams   Vitamin or mineral deficiencies
Changes in barometric pressure   Parity
Male fetal sex

41. How soon does labor follow PROM?

• 80–90% of term patients are in labor within 24–48 hours of membrane rupture.
• 50% of preterm patients are in labor within 24–48 hours.
• 70% of preterm patients are in labor within 7 days.

In some, but not all, studies there is an inverse relationship between gestational age at PROM and latency period, with very early preterm PROM having a longer latency.

42. What is the major neonatal complication of preterm delivery in patients with preterm PROM?

Hyaline membrane disease occurs in 10–40% of deliveries and is responsible for 30–70% of neonatal deaths.

43. What is the second most common complication of preterm PROM after preterm labor?

Infection occurs in 15–30% of patients, including choriamnionitis, fetal infection, and endometritis. Neonatal sepsis accounts for 3–20% of neonatal deaths. Infection and inflammation in the fetus and newborn is thought to be most important predisposing factor in the development of cerebral palsy.

44. What organisms have been cultured from infected amniotic fluid in patients with preterm PROM?

Infections are usually polymicrobial. Cultured organisms include *Ureaplasma* spp., *Mycoplasma* spp., group B β-hemolytic streptococci, peptostreptococci, *Fusobacteria* spp., *Gardnerella vaginalis*, *Escherichia coli*, enterococci, *Bacteroides* spp., and others (more rarely).

45. Are corticosteroids to accelerate fetal lung maturation contraindicated in pregnancies complicated by preterm PROM?

No. They are indicated in pregnancies < 32 weeks to reduce the incidence and severity of hyaline membrane disease, intraventricular hemorrhage, and necrotizing enterocolitis in the event of preterm delivery. They do not increase the risk of chorioamnionitis or neonatal sepsis, but may increase the risk for postpartum endometritis.

46. Can ruptured membranes seal again?

Resealing can happen, but is rare. Membrane rupture that occurs after physical disruption, such as after genetic amniocentesis, is more likely to reseal. The chronic inflammatory process that contributes to PPROM is not likely to spontaneously resolve.

47. What are the management options for patients with preterm PROM?

• Expectant management with delivery in presence of labor, infection, or nonreassuring fetal status

• Delivery when fetal lung maturity is documented, regardless of gestational age
• Delivery when the risks of prematurity are small compared with the risk of infection. The gestational age at which this tradeoff is most reasonable is probably in the 32–34 week range

48. What are the serious complications of chorioamnionitis?
• Fourfold increase in neonatal mortality
• Threefold increase in neonatal morbidity from hyaline membrane disease, sepsis, and intraventricular hemorrhage

49. How does the incidence of chorioamnionitis differ between term and preterm PROM?
1% at term, 20–40% preterm

50. What is the outcome of preterm PROM before 26 weeks?
Most of the adverse neonatal outcome is due to prematurity; the longer the latency period and the greater the gestational age at delivery, the better the prognosis. Overall outcome: chorioamnionitis, 40%; neonatal survival, 46%; normal child at long-term follow-up, 60% of survivors.

51. At what gestational age do the complications of prematurity become so low that one might consider delivery to avoid potential problems from sepsis or cord prolapse?
32 to 34 weeks

52. Other than confirming the diagnosis of PROM, what information is available from a sterile speculum exam?
• Presence of cord prolapse or fetal part can be determined.
• The dilatation and effacement of the cervix can be estimated.
• Amniotic fluid can be aspirated from the vagina for lung maturity testing.
• Cultures for gonorrhea, chlamydia, and group B streptococci can be obtained.

53. Why is PROM associated with a high prevalence of nonreassuring fetal tracings in labor?
Umbilical cord compression is more common among fetuses with oligohydramnios. This may result in repetitive, moderate to severe variable decelerations associated with uterine contractions. Also, placental abruption is more common in pregnancies complicated by PROM. This may result in repetitive late decelerations, fetal tachycardia, prolonged decelerations, or bradycardia.

54. What procedure may decrease the number and severity of variable decelerations on the fetal heart rate tracing?
Transcervical amnioinfusion with saline using an intrauterine pressure catheter may be performed in the setting of labor.

CONTROVERSIES

55. Do antibiotics prolong the latency period and prevent infection?
There is some evidence to suggest that certain antibiotic regimens may prolong the latency period and reduce neonatal morbidity. The largest trial in the U.S. to date suggests the use of ampicillin/amoxicillin and erythromycin for 1 week prolongs latency and reduces composite neonatal morbidity. A recent large multicenter international trial suggests that erythromycin prolongs latency while the addition of amoxicillin/clavulanic acid may increase the risk of neonatal necrotizing enterocolitis.

56. Are tocolytics useful to prolong pregnancy when preterm labor complicates preterm PROM?

Tocolytics may be helpful at very early gestational ages to prolong gestation to achieve time for steroid benefit. Many experts, however, believe tocolytics are *not* effective in prolonging pregnancy in the setting of PROM and are more effective for prolonging pregnancy in preterm labor with intact membranes.

BIBLIOGRAPHY

1. Anonymous: ACOG committee opinion. Home uterine activity monitoring. Number 172. May 1996 (replaces number 115, September 1992). Committee on Obstetric Practice. American College of Obstetricians and Gynecologists. Int J Gynaecol Obstet 54:71–77, 1996.
2. Anonymous: Preterm singleton births—United States, 1989–1996. MMWR 48:185–189, 1999.
3. Ferguson JEd, Dyson DC, Schutz T, Stevenson DK: A comparison of tocolysis with nifedipine or ritodrine: Analysis of efficacy and maternal, fetal, and neonatal outcome. American Journal of Obstetrics & Gynecology 163:105–11, 1990.
4. Goldenberg RL, Hauth JC, Andrews WW: Mechanisms of disease: Intrauterine infection and preterm delivery. N Engl J Med 342:1500–1507, 2000.
5. Hellemans P, Gerris J, Verdonk P: Fetal fibronectin detection for prediction of preterm birth in low risk women. Br J Obstet Gynaecol 102:207–212, 1995.
6. Hollander DI, Nagey DA, Pupkin MJ: Magnesium sulfate and ritodrine hydrochloride: A randomized comparison. American Journal of Obstetrics & Gynecology 156:631–637, 1987.
7. Iams JD, Casal D, McGregor JA, et al: Fetal fibronectin improves the accuracy of diagnosis of preterm labor. Am J Obstet Gynecol 173:141–145, 1995.
8. Kari MA, Hallman M, Eronen M, et al: Prenatal dexamethasone treatment in conjunction with rescue therapy of human surfactant: A randomized placebo-controlled multicenter study. Pediatrics 93:730–736, 1994.
9. Kenyon SL, Taylor DJ, Tarnow-Mordi W, Group OC: Broad-spectrum antibiotics for preterm, prelabour rupture of fetal membranes: The ORACLE I randomised trial. ORACLE Collaborative Group. Lancet 357:979–988, 2001.
10. Lemons JA, Bauer CR, Oh W, et al: Very low birth weight outcomes of the National Institute of Child Health and Human Development Neonatal Research Network, January 1995 through December 1996. Pediatrics 107:E1, 2001.
11. Lockwood CJ, Wein R, Lapinski R, et al: The presence of cervical and vaginal fetal fibronectin predicts preterm delivery in an inner-city obstetric population. Am J Obstet Gynecol 169:798–804, 1993.
12. Matsuda Y, Ikenoue T, Hokanishi H: Premature rupture of the membranes—Aggressive versus conservative approach. Effect of tocolytic and antibiotic therapy. Gynecol Obstet Invest 36:102–107, 1993.
13. Mercer BM, Miodovnik M, Thurnau GR, et al: Antibiotic therapy for reduction of infant morbidity after preterm premature rupture of the membranes. A randomized controlled trial. National Institute of Child Health and Human Development Maternal-Fetal Medicine Units Network [see comment]. JAMA 278:989–995, 1997.
14. NIH Consensus Developmental Panel: The effect of corticosteroids for fetal maturation on perinatal outcomes. JAMA 273:413, 1995.
15. Parry S, Strauss III JF: Premature rupture of the fetal membranes. New Engl J Med 338:663–670, 1998.

62. MALPRESENTATION

Thomas J. Bader, M.D., and Robert J. Wester, M.D.

1. What are the various types of fetal presentations?

The "lie" of the fetus refers to the orientation of the fetus with regard to the maternal abdomen. The lie can be **longitudinal** (where the fetal breech or fetal head are presenting), **transverse**, or **oblique**. Fetal lie is further described by identifying the fetal "presenting part." The presenting part is the point on the fetus closest to the cervix.

Longitudinal lies are further classified based on whether the fetal breech or fetal head (cephalic presentation) is the presenting part. Finally, *fetal breech* presentations are then subclassified based on the position of the fetal legs, and *cephalic* presentations are subclassified based on the part of the head that is presenting.

2. Describe the different breech presentations.

A **frank** breech presentation is the most common type of breech presentation. In this position, both hips are flexed and both knees are extended. If one or both knees are flexed, it is termed a **complete** breech. If either hip is extended—leading to a foot or knee presentation—there is an **incomplete** breech.

3. What are the different cephalic presentations?

Nearly all cephalic presentations are **vertex** (the "back" of the fetal head). However, in unusual circumstances the **fetal face** can be the presenting part. A **brow** presentation is intermediate between a face presentation and a vertex presentation. This is an unstable presentation and will usually convert to either a face or a vertex presentation.

4. How is position determined?

By abdominal exam (Leopold's maneuvers), vaginal examination, and ultrasonography. The point on the abdomen where fetal heart tones are best auscultated can also provide a clue to the fetal lie.

5. What is the definition of malpresentation?

Any presentation other than vertex (i.e., a longitudinal lie, cephalic presentation, with the vertex as the presenting part) is a malpresentation.

6. How frequently does malpresentation occur?

Early in pregnancy, malpresentation is fairly common. For example, at 20 weeks up to a third of fetuses are breech. At term, however, only 3% of singleton fetuses have a non-vertex presentation. Of these, the vast majority are one form or another of breech presentation. Thus 99% of term singleton fetuses are in a longitudinal lie.

7. Which factors increase the likelihood of breech presentation or malpresentation?

- Maternal: uterine anomalies, multiparity, pelvic tumors
- Fetal: anomalies (anencephaly), macrocephaly, neuromuscular disorders, polyhydramnios, oligohydramnios
- Placental: placenta previa (placenta over the internal cervical os)

8. Is there an increased incidence of congenital anomalies in babies that are breech at term compared to babies that are vertex at term?

Yes. Term breech fetuses have an increased incidence of fetal anomalies and greater perinatal morbidity and mortality compared with vertex fetuses.

9. Is vaginal delivery safe for breech fetuses?

It has long been recognized that breech vaginal delivery is a high-risk situation requiring careful patient selection and experienced operators. A recent randomized, controlled study found an increased risk of neonatal morbidity and mortality with attempted vaginal delivery compared to planned cesarean section in fetuses at term in a breech presentation. Because of this study, vaginal delivery is no longer considered an appropriate method of delivery except under unusual circumstances. These circumstances include: babies born at the limits of survivability (22–26 weeks); cases of severe or even lethal fetal anomalies; delivery of a second, non-vertex twin; or cases of advanced labor with a breech presentation.

10. What is the appropriate management of a breech presentation at term?

There are two basic options for management: (1) somehow effecting conversion to a vertex presentation and then allowing labor, or (2) performing a cesarean section. Vaginal delivery of a breech baby is no longer considered standard of care.

11. What is external version?

In this technique one or two people attempt to maneuver the fetus into a cephalic presentation by applying pressure to the maternal abdomen. This technique is performed under ultrasound guidance to assist the operators and to help monitor the fetus. In the hope of improving success, tocolytic agents to relax the uterus and regional anesthesia to ensure patient comfort are sometimes employed.

12. List the contraindications to external version.

- Absolute: placenta previa or abruption
- Relative: labor, oligohydramios, evidence of fetal compromise (e.g., fetal growth restriction, non-reassuring fetal testing)

Note: Prior cesarean section is *not* a contraindication to version.

13. What are the potential complications?

Placental abruption, uterine rupture, amniotic fluid embolism, preterm labor, fetal compromise, and even fetal demise have been reported. Any of these events can lead to urgent or emergent cesarean section.

Rh negative mothers should receive Rhogam to prevent isoimmunization.

14. When is external version usually performed?

The procedure is usually done around 36 or 37 weeks of gestation. *Earlier* attempts may be unnecessary (because the fetus still has time to convert spontaneously), increase the risk of conversion back to breech, and put the fetus at risk of iatrogenic premature delivery. *Later* attempts may have a lower success rate (because of a relative increase in the size of the fetus and the volume of amniotic fluid), and there is also a risk that labor will begin before the version can be attempted.

15. What is the success rate of external version?

There is a wide range of success rates, from 35% to 85%. Success is greater when attempted earlier in pregnancy. Careful patient selection (parous women, no fetal engagement, adequate amniotic fluid) can also affect the success rate.

16. What are other methods for converting the fetus to vertex?

Two other methods are breech maneuvers and moxibustion. **Breech maneuvers** use maternal position and gravity to attempt to facilitate fetal movement into a cephalic presentation. The mother is advised to perform these maneuvers one or more times each day.

Moxibustion is the practice of burning herbs near the foot to stimulate fetal movement and conversion to cephalic presentation. One randomized, controlled study found it more effective than placebo.

17. Do breech babies born by cesarean section have the same neonatal outcomes as vertex babies born by vaginal delivery or cesarean section?

No. Babies that are breech at term have more neonatal complications and more poor outcomes than babies that are vertex at term—regardless of the route of delivery.

18. If vaginal breech deliveries are no longer standard of care, is it important to understand the proper technique for breech delivery?

Yes. The same or similar maneuvers are performed during most deliveries of the fetus via cesarean section. In addition, there are still unusual circumstances when a woman and her obstetrician will decide to attempt a vaginal breech delivery. These include extreme prematurity, delivery of a non-vertex second twin, and refusal of cesarean section. Finally, even with the most careful planning, undiagnosed vaginal breech deliveries may present in an advanced stage of labor, so every obstetrician should be familiar with the proper method of breech delivery.

19. What are the important elements in effecting a successful vaginal breech?

- Allowing spontaneous delivery to the level of the umbilicus
- Delivery of the fetal legs by abducting the thighs
- Rotation of the fetal trunk so the sacrum is anterior
- Gentle traction on the fetal bony pelvis until the scapulae are visible
- Rotation of the fetal trunk to allow the arms to be delivered by drawing the elbow across the fetal chest
- Careful manipulation of the head and shoulders (Mauriceau-Smellie-Veit maneuver) to maintain head flexion during delivery of the head.

20. What is a variable lie?

As the name implies, a variable lie is one where the fetal position is inconsistent.

21. How is a variable lie managed?

Usually a variable lie is managed expectantly. Sometimes at term, the obstetrician will induce labor or perform an external version and induce labor. This option is more attractive if the cervix is favorable for induction of labor.

22. How is a transverse or oblique lie managed?

Transverse and oblique lies are unstable and will eventually convert to a longitudinal (cephalic or vertex) lie. Some providers will perform an external version, but the benefit of this approach is uncertain.

23. What is the incidence of face presentation at term?

Approximately 1 in 2000.

24. Is face presentation associated with increased neonatal morbidity or mortality?

Face presentations pose unique challenges requiring experienced operators and careful intrapartum and neonatal surveillance. However, with such preparation there does not appear to be an increased rate of neonatal complications.

25. How is face presentation managed?

Initial management is expectant. Occassionally a face presentation will spontaneously convert to a vertex presentation. If the face presentation persists, the face must rotate so the chin is under the pubic bone (mentum anterior). This position allows delivery of the fetal head by flexion. Further hyperextension (which would be required with a mentum posterior position) is not possible.

BIBLIOGRAPHY

1. American College of Obstetricians and Gynecologists: External cephalic version. ACOG Practice Bulletin No. 13, February 2000.

2. American College of Obstetricians and Gynecologists: Mode of term singleton breech delivery. ACOG Committee Opinion No. 265, December 2001.
3. Cardini F, Weixin H: Moxibustion for correction of breech presentation: A randomized controlled trial. JAMA 280:1580, 1998.
4. Cunningham FG, et al (ed): Williams Obstetrics, 21st ed. New York, McGraw-Hill, 2001.
5. Duff P: Diagnosis and management of face presentation. Obstet Gynecol 57(1):105–112, 1981.
6. Hannah ME, Hannah WJ, Hewson SA, et al: Planned caesarean section versus planned vaginal birth for breech presentation at term: A randomised multicentre trial. Term Breech Trial Collaborative Group. Lancet 356:1375–1383, 2000.
7. Schutte MF, van Hemel OJS, van de Berg C, van de Pol A: Perinatal mortality in breech presentations as compared to vertex presentations in singleton pregnancies: An analysis based upon 57,819 computer-registered pregnancies in the Netherlands. Eur J Obstet Gynecol Reprod Biol 19:391, 1985.

63. ANTEPARTUM FETAL SURVEILLANCE

Kent Heyborne, M.D.

1. What is antepartum fetal surveillance? What is its purpose? What is its rationale?

Antepartum fetal surveillance (AFS) refers to the assessment of in utero fetal well-being prior to the onset of labor. AFS is intended to identify those fetuses that may be at risk for in utero death or hypoxic injury, so that they can be delivered before death or injury occurs. It is based upon the rationale that progressive fetal hypoxemia can be detected by changes in the fetal heart rate, amniotic fluid volume, fetal behavior, and fetal umbilical artery blood velocity.

2. What type(s) of fetal compromise is antepartum fetal surveillance designed to detect?

AFS is designed to detect those fetuses at risk due to uteroplacental insufficiency. It is less effective in detecting other types of fetal risk, such as sudden occlusion of the umbilical cord ("cord accident") or infection, but is still useful.

3. Which patients should receive antepartum fetal surveillance?

Any patient with an increased chance of fetal compromise due to uteroplacental insufficiency is a candidate. Examples include present pregnancy complications (preeclampsia, fetal growth restriction, oligohydramnios, post-dates pregnancy), maternal medical illness (insulin-dependent diabetes, hypertension, renal disease, systemic lupus erythematosus), and previous in utero demise.

4. In what other clinical situations is antepartum fetal surveillance used?

AFS is also used to evaluate patients who perceive decreased fetal movement, to detect umbilical cord compression in patients with decreased amniotic fluid volume, and to help diagnose intra-amniotic infection in patients with ruptured fetal membranes.

5. Describe in general terms the tests used for antepartum fetal surveillance.

Fetal movement record (FMR)—quantitation by the mother of the number of fetal movements perceived within a given time frame.

Nonstress test (NST)—external fetal heart rate monitoring allows evaluation of the fetal heart rate, including baseline heart rate, variability, and response to fetal movement.

Contraction stress test (CST)—external fetal cardiac and uterine contraction monitoring allows evaluation of the fetal heart rate in response to uterine contractions.

Biophysical profile (BPP)—an NST coupled with an ultrasound evaluation of several fetal biophysical parameters provides more comprehensive evaluation of fetal well-being.

Amniotic fluid index (AFI)—ultrasound estimation of amniotic fluid volume.

Doppler velocimetry—Doppler ultrasound evaluation of blood flow velocity in various fetal vessels.

6. Which patients should record an fetal movement record? How is it done? What are its advantages and disadvantages?

Based on its low cost and ease of performance, all pregnant women should be instructed in keeping at least an informal FMR. Fetal movement is recorded daily. A daily total below a set threshold (10–15 total movements) or any drastic change in fetal activity perceived by the mother prompts further evaluation.

The FMR is cheap, simple, and noninvasive, and it actively involves the patient in the assessment of her fetus. The FMR's main disadvantage is its high false-positive rate. At least 90% of fetuses with perceived decreased movement are found to be well on further testing.

7. What should be done if the patient perceives decreased fetal movement?

An NST should be preformed as promptly as possible.

8. How is a nonstress test performed and interpreted?

The fetal heart rate is recorded with an external monitor for 20–40 minutes. Three components of the heart rate are assessed: baseline, variability, and response to fetal movement. To achieve a reactive NST, there must be a normal baseline (120–160 bpm); heart rate variability of 6–10 bpm; and two to four accelerations of the fetal heart rate, with a peak of at least 15 bpm above baseline, lasting for at least 15 seconds and associated with fetal movement. Because of central nervous system immaturity, the NST may be nonreactive before 30–32 weeks.

9. Describe fetal acoustic stimulation testing (FAST). What is its role during a nonstress test?

Many NSTs are nonreactive by the criteria described previously, perhaps owing to a fetal sleep cycle. FAST causes the fetus to wake up and potentially enter a more active state. FAST can be performed with an artificial larynx or an electric toothbrush held briefly to the maternal abdomen. FAST has been shown to shorten the amount of time necessary to obtain an NST. The NST also has a high false-positive rate (50%); FAST can decrease the number of falsely nonreactive NSTs.

10. How should a nonreactive nonstress test be evaluated?

In most cases, a BPP or CST should be performed. Depending on the clinical situation, it might be more appropriate to proceed directly with delivery.

11. How is the contraction stress test performed and interpreted?

Uterine contractions and fetal heart rate are monitored with the patient in a left lateral recumbent position. Uterine contractions may be spontaneous or induced with maternal nipple stimulation or intravenous oxytocin. Three moderate contractions in 10 minutes must be achieved for an adequate CST.

The CST is interpreted as follows:

• **Positive CST**—late decelerations of fetal heart rate with more than half of the uterine contractions
• **Negative CST**—no late decelerations
• **Equivocal CST**—decelerations with uterine hyperstimulation, isolated late decelerations, or technical problems such as inability to achieve adequate contractions

At least 50% of patients with a positive CST are later deemed to have a healthy fetus (false positive test).

12. In what sequence do fetal tone, fetal movement, and fetal breathing appear in the developing fetus? In what sequence do they disappear in the compromised fetus?

Fetal tone appears first, followed by fetal movement, then fetal breathing. In the compromised fetus, they disappear in the reverse order (breathing first, tone last).

13. How is a biophysical profile done?

In addition to an NST, the BPP measures fetal breathing, fetal body and extremity movement, fetal tone, and amniotic fluid volume. Some physicians use placental grade (maturity) as a fifth component. A standard scoring system is available, with points given in each category; the overall score is then interpreted as an indicator of fetal well-being.

14. What are the advantages and disadvantages of the biphysical profile as compared to the nonstress test?

BPP can potentially diagnose disorders of amniotic fluid volume and fetal anomalies. It appears to have a lower false-positive rate than the NST. However, the BPP is more time consuming, requires more expensive equipment (ultrasound machine), and requires more skilled personnel to perform.

15. What is a modified biophysical profile? What are its advantages?

A modified BPP consists of an NST and AFI. It is quicker than a complete BPP and appears to have the same sensitivity for detecting fetal compromise. If the NST is nonreactive, a complete BPP should be done.

16. How is an amniotic fluid index performed? Why does the compromised fetus have a decreased amniotic fluid volume?

The depths of the deepest amniotic fluid volume pockets (in cm) in each of the four uterine quadrants are summed. The normal range for the AFI varies slightly with gestational age. In general:

AFI < 5 cm = oligohydramnios
AFI 5–10 cm = decreased fluid
AFI 10–25 cm = normal
AFI > 25 cm = polyhydramnios

Shunting of blood away from the kidneys and towards the heart and brain causes a decreased amniotic fluid volume in the compromised fetus.

17. How is the Doppler principle applied to antepartum fetal surveillance?

The Doppler shift phenomenon is used to approximate velocity of blood flow during systole and diastole in the fetal umbilical artery. Increased ratios of systolic-to-diastolic velocity (S/D ratio) correlate with high resistance in the placental vasculature.

18. What is meant by false-positive rate and false-negative rate? How do the nonstress test and the biophysical profile compare in terms of false-positive and false-negative rates?

The false-positive rate is the proportion of non-reassuring tests when the fetus is in fact well. The false-negative rate is the proportion of reassuring tests when the fetus is at imminent risk.

The NST has a 50% false-positive rate. The BPP may have a false-positive rate as low as 20%. The NST has a false-negative rate of 1.4 per 1000 tests. The BPP has a slightly lower false-negative rate of 0.6 per 1000.

19. In which patients have a false-negative nonstress tests and/or biphysical profiles been most commonly observed (i.e., reassuring test within 1 week of fetal death in utero)? What implication does this have for fetal surveillance?

False-negative tests occur most commonly in association with insulin-dependent diabetes, postdate pregnancies, and preeclampsia with intrauterine growth retardation. For this reason, twice-weekly monitoring has been advocated in such situations.

20. How is an antepartum fetal surveillance plan formulated?

Antepartum fetal surveillance is often initiated at least 1–2 weeks before fetal risk is perceived to begin. Patients at relatively low risk might receive a daily FMR and weekly NSTs. Patients at higher risk might receive a daily FMR, twice weekly NSTs, and a weekly AFI. BPP and/or Doppler velocimetry can be added for patients at very high risk. Patients beyond 40 weeks' gestation are typically followed with twice weekly NST and weekly AFI, starting at or before 41 weeks gestation.

POST-TERM PREGNANCY

21. What is the definition of post-term pregnancy?

Postdate pregnancy is defined as a gestation that has entered in its 42nd week (294 days) from the last menstrual period. Post-term pregnancy can only be diagnosed when accurate dating criteria, such as an early ultrasound examination, are available.

22. What is the incidence of post-term pregnancy?

Without intervention, approximately 7–12% of pregnancies proceed past 42 weeks, and 4% proceed beyond 43 weeks. However, many pregnancies suspected of being post-term are actually incorrectly dated. When strict dating criteria are applied, the incidence of post-term pregnancy falls to 1–3%. As such, accurate dating criteria are required for the precise diagnosis of post-term pregnancy. This problem is especially acute in populations of women with poor and/or late pre-natal care, where such accurate dating criteria may be unavailable.

23. What is the clinical significance of post-term pregnancy?

Post-term gestations are at risk for two distinct clinical problems: "dysmaturity" and macro-somia. While macrosomia is more common than dysmaturity, the latter is of more concern due to its association with fetal death.

24. Define the term dysmaturity.

Dysmaturity refers to the post-term fetus suffering from placental insufficiency related to pla-cental aging. Such fetuses are characterized by a wasted appearance, lack of subcutaneous fat, meconium-stained amniotic fluid and skin, and peeling skin. These fetuses are at risk for meconium aspiration syndrome, fetal distress, and/or intrauterine fetal death due to placental insufficiency.

25. True or false: The cause of postdate pregnancy is unknown.

Mostly true. The cause of the majority of cases is unknown. Rarely associated disorders are anencephaly, fetal adrenal hypoplasia, placental sulfatase deficiency, and extrauterine pregnancy. Most postdate pregnancies occur in perfectly healthy and normal gestations.

26. Your first step after the diagnosis of post-term pregnancy has been made is . . . . . ?

Any patient reaching 40–41 weeks' gestation should be evaluated with baseline fetal surveil-lance. The most common evaluation includes a daily fetal activity monitoring, weekly measure-ments of amniotic fluid volume (AFI), and twice-weekly nonstress tests (NSTs). Any abnormal results from these tests should result in prompt delivery. Variable decelerations on an NST, even if it is reactive, are an indication for delivery.

27. Do patients with postdate pregnancy have a higher cesarean section rate?

Yes. The cesarean section rate in women induced at 41–42 weeks is around 20%. In those women managed expectantly, it may approach 40%. A cesarean section may be due to either fetal distress secondary to placental insufficiency, or obstructed labor resulting from macrosomia.

CONTROVERSIES

28. How are the contraction stress test and biophysical profile used in clinical practice?

The CST is quite cumbersome to perform in practice, and has been largely replaced by the BPP.

29. What are the current clinical applications of Doppler velocimetry?

Despite several years of study, the role for Doppler waveform analysis in the care of the pregnant patient remains unclear. Doppler analysis of multiple fetal vessels (cerebral, renal, he-patic, splenic, etc.) is being investigated in cases of fetal growth restriction, isoimmunization, and other fetal disorders. The only well-accepted use of Doppler velocimetry is in the discrimination of the small-for-gestational-age fetus ("small but well") from the growth-restricted fetus (small due to placental insufficiency). This is a common clinical problem, and Doppler velocimetry is very useful in this setting.

Doppler velocimetry is also used as an adjunct in other clinical scenarios that may result from placental insufficiency. It has the advantage of becoming abnormal prior to other testing (NST, BPP), so that increased scrutiny can be directed at the proper fetuses.

30. What is the significance of absent end-diastolic velocity in Doppler analysis?

Although the predictive value of decreased diastolic velocity in the umbilical artery remains controversial, the finding of absent end-diastolic velocity (AEDV) or, in severe cases, reversed end-diastolic velocity (REDV) indicates current or impending fetal distress. Fetuses with AEDV or REDV warrant intensive inpatient surveillance and delivery by cesarean birth.

31. What if testing is normal in a postdate pregnancy?

While this is somewhat controversial, most studies have shown improved outcomes, especially in terms of a reduced cesarean section rate, when labor is induced at 41–42 weeks' gestation. Induction of labor is clearly the preferred protocol if the cervix is favorable (i.e., dilated and effaced).

BIBLIOGRAPHY

1. Anon. Management of Post-term Pregnancy. ACOG Practice Patterns, 1997, pp 1–6.
2. Chamberlain PF, Manning FA, Morrison I, at al: Ultrasound evaluation of amniotic fluid volume. I. The relationship of marginal and decreased amniotic fluid volumes to perinatal outcome. Am J Obstet Gynecol 150(3):245–249, 1984.
3. Clark SL, Sabey P, Jolley K: Nonstress testing with acoustic stimulation and amniotic fluid volume assessment: 5973 tests without unexpected fetal death. Am J Obstet Gynecol 160(3):694–697, 1989.
4. Devoe LD, Castillo RA, Sherline DM: The nonstress test as a diagnostic test: A critical reappraisal. Am J Obstet Gynecol 152(8):1047–1053, 1985.
5. Dyson DC, Miller PD, Armstrong MA: Management of prolonged pregnancy: Induction of labor versus antepartum fetal testing. Am J Obstet Gynecol 156(4):928–934, 1987.
6. Erskine RL, Ritchie JW: Umbilical artery blood flow characteristics in normal and growth-retarded fetuses. Br J Obstet Gynaecol 92(6):605–610, 1985.
7. Freeman RK: The use of the oxytocin challenge test for antepartum clinical evaluation of uteroplacental respiratory function. Am J Obstet Gynecol 121(4):481–489, 1975.
8. Hannah ME, Hannah WJ, Hellmann J, et al: Induction of labor as compared with serial antenatal monitoring in post-term pregnancy. A randomized controlled trial. The Canadian Multicenter Post-term Pregnancy Trial Group. N Engl J Med 326(24):1587–1592, 1992.
9. Manning FA, Morrison I, Harman CR, et al: Fetal assessment based on fetal biophysical profile scoring: Experience in 19,221 referred high-risk pregnancies. II. An analysis of false-negative fetal deaths. Am J Obstet Gynecol 157(4 Pt 1):880–884, 1987.
10. Moore TR, Cayle JE: The amniotic fluid index in normal human pregnancy. Am J Obstet Gynecol 162(5):1168–1173, 1990.
11. Moore TR, Piacquadio K: A prospective evaluation of fetal movement screening to reduce the incidence of antepartum fetal death. Am J Obstet Gynecol 160(5 Pt 1):1075–1080, 1989.
12. Nicolaides KH, Bilardo CM, Soothill PW, Campbell S: Absence of end diastolic frequencies in umbilical artery: A sign of fetal hypoxia and acidosis. BMJ 297(6655):1026–1027, 1988.
13. Resnik R: Post-term Pregnancy. In Creasy RK, Resnik R, (eds): Maternal-Fetal Medicine: Principles and Practice, 3rd ed. Philadelphia, W.B. Saunders, 1994, pp 521–526.
14. Sachs BP, Friedman EA: Results of an epidemiologic study of postdate pregnancy. J Reprod Med 31(3):162–166, 1986.
15. Small ML, Phelan JP, Smith CV, Paul RH: An active management approach to the postdate fetus with a reactive nonstress test and fetal heart rate decelerations. Obstet Gynecol 70(4):636–640, 1987.
16. Thacker SB, Berkelman RL. Assessing the diagnostic accuracy and efficacy of selected antepartum fetal surveillance techniques. Obstet Gynecol Surv 41(3):121–141, 1986.

64. INTRAPARTUM FETAL SURVEILLANCE

Emmanuelle Paré, M.D., FRCSC

1. What was the purpose of intrapartum fetal heart rate (FHR) monitoring when it was introduced?

The purpose was to detect asphyxia early enough to prevent intrapartum fetal death and asphyxia-induced brain damage (such as cerebral palsy). While intrapartum stillbirths virtually disappeared after FHR monitoring was introduced, long-term neurologic impairment and cerebral palsy have not been prevented, despite an increase in cesarean section rate.

2. What are our tools to monitor fetal well-being in labor?

Intermittent auscultation by Doppler or stethoscope
Continuous electronic FHR monitoring
Fetal scalp pH
Fetal pulse oximetry (investigational)

3. Which is superior: electronic FHR monitoring or intermittent auscultation?

Neither. Fetal heart monitoring is equally effective whether done electronically or by auscultation.

4. How is intermittent auscultation performed?

The nurse-to-patient ratio should be 1:1, and intermittent auscultation should be performed by trained and experienced personnel. The fetal heart is auscultated during and after a uterine contraction to detect decelerations, and the FHR is recorded in the chart after every observation.

Auscultation should occur at regular intervals: (1) in the presence of risk factors, at least every 15 minutes during the active phase of the first stage of labor, and at least every 5 minutes during the second stage of labor; (2) in the absence of risk factors, no data determine the optimal frequency of auscultation. One method is to auscultate the fetal heart at least every 30 minutes during the active phase of the first stage of labor, and at least every 15 minutes during the second stage of labor.

5. How should electronic FHR monitoring be performed?

The FHR tracing should be evaluated and recorded in the chart at regular intervals. In the presence of risk factors, it should be evaluated at least every 15 minutes during the active phase of the first stage of labor and at least every 5 minutes during the second stage of labor.

6. List the risk factors warranting more intense fetal surveillance in labor.

No validated, clear definition or exhaustive list of such risk factors exists. However, it is prudent to consider the following conditions as risk factors warranting more intense fetal surveillance in labor:

- Antepartum risk factors—pre-eclampsia, chronic hypertension, maternal diabetes, intrauterine growth restriction, multiple gestation
- Intrapartum risk factors—placental abruption, induction for non-reassuring fetal status, prematurity, meconium-stained amniotic fluid, chorioamnionitis, documentation of non-reassuring FHR patterns when using the low-risk auscultation protocol
- Intervention in labor—use of analgesia or anesthesia, use of oxytocin

7. What is the sensitivity of continuous electronic FHR monitoring in detecting true hypoxia with metabolic acidosis? What is its specificity?

Continuous electronic FHR monitoring has very good sensitivity in detecting fetuses at risk for asphyxia (hypoxia with metabolic acidosis). False-negatives are rare, which means that a normal FHR tracing confirms reassuring fetal well-being in almost all cases.

However, specificity of continuous electronic FHR monitoring is poor. The false-positive rate is high ($\geq$ 50%) and most fetuses with abnormal FHR tracings do not suffer from asphyxia (hypoxia with metabolic acidosis) at birth.

8. What is the largest risk associated with continuous FHR monitoring?

An increase in the cesarean section rate. Most studies (retrospective as well as randomized controlled trials) have reported this effect. Continuous FHR monitoring has increased the frequency of abnormal fetal heart rate patterns observed during labor. The majority of abnormal patterns are false positives (see Question 7) and do not reflect true fetal asphyxia (hypoxia with metabolic acidosis). Some believe that more accurate and standardized interpretation of continuous FHR monitoring and the use of adjunct techniques such as fetal scalp blood pH monitoring, scalp or vibroacoustic stimulation, or amnioinfusion can reduced the number of cesarean sections.

10. What are the two common methods for performing continuous FHR monitoring in labor?

External FHR monitoring uses a Doppler device to detect movement of the fetal cardiac valves (ideally) or movement of blood in the fetal heart and vessels. These "movement" signals are then interpreted and counted by computerized logic.

Internal FHR monitoring uses a small electrode, which is a spiral wire, directly applied to the fetal scalp (or other presenting part). A fetal electrocardiogram is obtained: R-R intervals are calculated and the fetal heart rate is derived.

11. What are the advantages and disadvantages of internal FHR monitoring, as compared to external FHR monitoring?

Advantages—always represents fetal heart rate (except in rare cases of fetal death); truer representation of beat-to-beat variability; technically easier to obtain FHR tracings uninterrupted by maternal or fetal movement

Disadvantages— requires minimal cervical dilation as well as ruptured membranes for placement; small risk of fetal infection from the electrode; increased risk of perinatal transmission of maternal infections such as HIV, hepatitis B, hepatitis C, and herpes; small increase in risk of chorioamnionitis and endometritis

12. What are the two common methods to monitor uterine contractions in labor?

External tocodynamometers evaluate the uterine activity in a nonquantitative way. They detect the change in shape and rigidity of the uterus associated with contractions. External uterine monitoring can be accurate for *frequency* and, to some extent, *duration* of contractions, but does not reflect the *intensity* of the contractions. Clinical palpation of the uterus is probably as good as external uterine monitoring, and is even better for measure of intensity.

Intrauterine pressure-monitoring catheters accurately detect the intensity (in mmHg) as well as the frequency and duration of contractions.

13. What are the advantages and the disadvantages of internal uterine contraction monitors, as compared to external uterine contraction monitors?

Advantages—intensity of uterine contractions is recorded; overall more accurate for frequency and duration of uterine contractions; intrauterine catheter can also be used for amnioinfusion (i.e., the therapeutic introduction of fluid into the uterine cavity); less sensitive to maternal movements in terms of displacement of the transducer and loss of signal

Disadvantages—requires minimal cervical dilation and ruptured membranes for placement; small risk of uterine perforation and placental abruption from the intrauterine catheter; increased risk of chorioamnionitis and endometritis

14. Which parameters should be evaluated and recorded when FHR monitoring is performed and interpreted in labor?

- Baseline rate
- Baseline FHR variability

- Presence of FHR accelerations
- Periodic or episodic FHR decelerations
- Change or trends of FHR patterns over time

15. How is baseline FHR defined? How is it evaluated? What is normal and abnormal baseline FHR?

Baseline FHR is the approximate mean FHR rounded to increments of 5 beats/min during a 10-minute segment, excluding: periodic or episodic changes, periods of marked FHR variability, and segments of the baseline that differ by more than 25 beats/min. In order to establish baseline FHR, the minimum baseline duration must be 2 minutes out of the 10-minute segment, or the baseline for that period is indeterminate.

Normal baseline FHR is 110–160 beats/min. Bradycardia defines baseline FHR < 110 beats/min. Tachycardia defines baseline FHR > 160 beats/min.

16. How is baseline FHR variability defined? How is it evaluated?

Baseline FHR variability is fluctuations in the baseline FHR of two cycles per minute or greater. These fluctuations are irregular in amplitude and frequency. They are visually quantitated as the amplitude of the peak-to-trough in beats/min and defined as follows:

Absent FHR variability: amplitude range undetectable

Minimal FHR variability: amplitude range > undetectable and ≤ 5 beats/min

Moderate FHR variability: amplitude range 6–25 beats/min

Marked FHR variability: amplitude range > 25 beats/min

17. How are FHR accelerations defined?

An acceleration is defined as a visually apparent, abrupt increase (onset of acceleration to peak in less than 30 seconds) in FHR above the baseline. The peak is ≥ 15 beats/min above the baseline, and the acceleration lasts ≥ 15 seconds and < 2 minutes from the onset to return to baseline. Before 32 weeks of gestation, accelerations are defined as having a peak ≥ 10 beats/min and a duration ≥ 10 seconds.

A prolonged acceleration lasts ≥ 2 minutes and < 10 minutes. An acceleration that lasts ≥ 10 minutes is a change in the baseline.

18. What are the types of FHR decelerations? How are they defined?

Early—An early FHR deceleration is a visually apparent, *gradual* decrease (onset of deceleration to nadir ≥ **30 seconds**) and return to baseline FHR associated with a uterine contraction. The nadir of the deceleration occurs *at the same time* as the peak of the contraction. In most cases, the onset, nadir, and recovery of the deceleration *are coincident with* the beginning, peak, and ending of the contraction, respectively.

Late—A late deceleration is similar to an early deceleration EXCEPT the deceleration is delayed in timing, and the nadir of deceleration occurs *after* the peak of the contraction. In most cases, the onset, nadir, and recovery of the deceleration *occur after* the beginning, peak and ending of the contraction, respectively.

Variable—A variable FHR deceleration is a visually apparent, *abrupt* decrease (onset of deceleration to beginning of nadir **< 30 seconds**) in FHR below the baseline. This decrease in FHR below the baseline is ≥ 15 beats/min and lasts ≥ 15 seconds but < 2 minutes from onset to return to baseline. Variable decelerations are *not always associated* with uterine contractions, and when they are, their onset, depth, and duration vary with successive uterine contractions.

Prolonged—A prolonged FHR deceleration is a visually apparent decrease in FHR below the baseline. The decrease is ≥ 15 beats/min and lasts ≥ 2 minutes but < 10 minutes from onset to return to baseline. A deceleration that lasts ≥ 10 minutes is a change in the baseline.

19. What are the causes of fetal bradycardia? What are the causes of fetal tachycardia?

- Bradycardia—acute cord occlusion (including prolapse), uterine hyperstimulation (often iatrogenic [oxytocin and prostaglandins]), persistent maternal hypotension, congenital heart block, inadvertent measurement of the maternal pulse

• Tachycardia—chorioamnionitis, fetal anemia, maternal fever, fetal hypoxia, sympath-omimetic drugs (e.g., terbutaline), fetal tachyarrythmias

20. What are the causes of minimal or absent FHR variability?

Fetal hypoxia
Narcotics
Magnesium sulfate
Congenital anomalies (of the central nervous system)
Fetal sleep cycles
Extreme prematurity
Preexisting neurologic injury

21. What is a sinusoidal FHR pattern? What are its causes?

A sinusoidal FHR pattern is a smooth wave-like pattern of regular frequency (usually 3–5 cycles per minute) and amplitude (usually 5–20 beats/min). Short episodes (< 5–10 minutes) of a sinusoidal pattern may be a variant of normal. A prolonged period of a sinusoidal FHR pattern has been associated with moderate to severe fetal anemia (allo-immunization or fetomaternal hemorrhage) and severe fetal hypoxia. Maternal narcotics can also lead to a sinusoidal FHR pattern; in this circumstance, the pattern is *not* an indication of fetal compromise.

22. What are the causes and significance of decelerations?

Early—Early decelerations are thought to be caused by fetal head compression leading to a vagal response. Early decelerations are not associated with fetal hypoxia or acidosis. Since they are presumed to be benign, no intervention is required when they are present.

Late—Late decelerations are thought to be caused by hypoxia and acidosis due to utero-placental insufficiency. Two mechanisms lead to late decelerations: (1) central reflex caused by hypoxia, and (2) direct myocardial depression caused by acidosis. When late decelerations are recurrent (occur with 50% or more of uterine contractions), suspect fetal hypoxia and/or acidosis, despite the high false-positive rate of FHR monitoring. Consider further testing (e.g., fetal scalp pH) and/or intervention (e.g., delivery).

Variable—Variable decelerations are thought to be caused by umbilical cord compression, usually due to uterine contraction or fetal movement. They are the most common decelerations seen in labor, especially during the second stage of labor. Variable decelerations are usually not ominous when isolated, but fetal hypoxia and/or acidosis should be suspected when they are associated with non-reassuring changes on FHR tracings (such as decreased FHR variability and tachycardia). Consider further testing and/or intervention if the overall FHR tracing is non-reassuring.

Prolonged—Prolonged decelerations are usually caused by prolonged umbilical cord compression (hyperstimulation, umbilical cord prolapse) or fetal hypoxia (maternal hypotension). They can also be seen on occasion with rapid descent of the fetal head during the second stage. If isolated, they might not require intervention; however, other FHR pattern changes are often seen with prolonged decelerations (recovery tachycardia and decreased variability) and usually warrant intervention.

23. What is the significance of accelerations?

Accelerations can occur spontaneously or be associated with fetal movements or uterine contractions. The presence of accelerations means an intact central nervous system and a normal pH. Therefore, they are reassuring. However, their absence is not a sign of fetal compromise as long as other reassuring parameters are present, such as moderate variability.

24. What is a reassuring FHR tracing? What is a non-reassuring FHR tracing?

• Reassuring—normal baseline rate, moderate FHR variability, absence of late decelerations, presence of accelerations (not required)

• Non-reassuring—tachycardia or bradycardia, minimal or absent FHR variability, late decelerations, repetitive variable decelerations (especially if associated with changes in baseline FHR and FHR variability), absence of accelerations (spontaneous or elicited)

25. What should be done when the FHR tracing is non-reassuring?

Undertake general measures to improve uterine blood flow and fetal oxygenation (i.e., intrauterine resuscitation measures), such as lateral recumbent position (either side), maternal oxygen administration, increase in intravenous hydration, and discontinuation of oxytocin infusion.

If an etiology for a non-reassuring FHR tracing can be identified, then attempt to correct this etiology (such as amnioinfusion for recurrent moderate or severe variables, terbutaline for uterine hyperstimulation).

Also attempt to further assess fetal well-being, with fetal scalp stimulation, vibroacoustic stimulation, or fetal scalp pH.

Finally, if the FHR pattern is ominous (bradycardia), if the fetus does not respond to intrauterine resuscitation measures, or if the fetal well-being is still non-reassuring with further testing, the fetus should be delivered promptly by cesarean section or assisted vaginal delivery.

26. What is amnioinfusion? What are the indications for its use?

Amnioinfusion is a process where sterile fluid is introduced into the uterine cavity during labor. It is used principally to deal with two clinical problems: moderate or severe variable decelerations, and meconium in the amniotic fluid. In the setting of variable decelerations, amnioinfusion decreases the frequency and the severity of the decelerations (likely by relieving umbilical cord compression) as well as the risk of cesarean section for non-reassuring FHR tracing.

In the setting of moderate to thick meconium, amnioinfusion decreases the risk of meconium aspiration syndrome, probably via its dilutional effect and by preventing in utero fetal gasping associated with episodes of hypoxia.

27. How is amnioinfusion performed?

With a catheter inserted into the uterine cavity. Both bolus and continuous infusions can be given, and normal saline or lactated Ringer can be used. Bolus infusion of up to 800 ml can be given at 10–15 ml/min and additional 250-ml boluses can be given at intervals thereafter. Continuous infusion can be initiated with 10 ml/min for 1 hour and a maintenance level of 3 ml/min. Warmed infusion does not appear to have any benefit over infusion at room temperature.

28. When and how should tocolytic agents be used in the setting of non-reassuring FHR tracing?

Terbutaline should be used when the non-reassuring FHR pattern is thought to be caused by excessive uterine activity (i.e., tachysystoly or hypertonia). Terbutaline, 0.25 mg subcutaneously or 0.125–0.25 mg intravenously, may be administered. A response to terbutaline allows time for continued observation, transport to another hospital, or preparation for cesarean delivery. Note that the use of terbutaline should not delay an otherwise appropriate intervention.

29. How is fetal scalp stimulation or vibroacoustic stimulation used in the setting of non-reassuring FHR tracing?

The presence of acceleration in response to either stimulus indicates the absence of fetal acidosis. If the FHR pattern remains non-reassuring, fetal scalp or vibroacoustic stimulation should be repeated every 20–30 minutes for continued reassurance with elicited accelerations. Failure to elicit acceleration does not always mean fetal acidosis, given the high false-positive rate for these maneuvers. Fetal scalp blood sampling might be considered in that situation.

30. How is fetal scalp blood sampling performed and interpreted?

Fetal scalp blood sampling is performed with the patient in the lithotomy position. Under direct visualization, the fetal scalp is punctured and capillary blood obtained for pH assessment.

Guidelines for interpretation and management are as follow: pH > 7.25, reassuring—no immediate intervention required; pH ≤ 7.25 and ≥ 7.20, indeterminate—fetal scalp blood pH should be repeated immediately to confirm the value; pH < 7.20, non-reassuring—delivery. If the FHR pattern remains non-reassuring, fetal scalp blood sampling should be repeated every 20–30 minutes.

31. What is fetal pulse oximetry? What is its role in intrapartum fetal surveillance?

Fetal pulse oximetry uses a sensor placed on the fetus' cheek to determine fetal blood oxygen saturation. Ruptured membranes are required for its placement. Reliable readings are obtained 60–70% of the time. Fetal pulse oximetry was shown to assess fetal oxygenation safely and effectively. However, when used as an adjunct to FHR monitoring when FHR tracing was non-reassuring, fetal pulse oximetry did not lead to a decrease in the overall cesarean section rate despite a decrease in the rate of cesarean section for non-reassuring FHR tracing. Therefore, the American College of Obstetricians and Gynecologists does not endorse its adoption in clinical practice.

BIBLIOGRAPHY

1. American College of Obstetricians and Gynecologists. Fetal heart rate patterns: Monitoring, interpretation, and management. ACOG Technical Bulletin 207, 1995.
2. American College of Obstetricians and Gynecologists. Fetal pulse oximetry. ACOG Committee Opinion 258, 2001.
3. Freeman RK, Garite TJ, Nageotte MP. Fetal Heart Rate Monitoring, 2nd ed. Baltimore, Williams & Wilkins, 1991.
4. National Institute of Child Health and Human Development Research Planning Workshop. Electronic fetal heart rate monitoring. Research guidelines for interpretation. Am J Obstet Gynecol 177:1385, 1997.
5. Parer JT, King T. Fetal heart rate monitoring: Is it salvageable? Am J Obstet Gynecol 182:982, 2000.
6. Society of Obstetricians and Gynecologists of Canada. Fetal health surveillance in labor. J Soc Obstet Gynaecol Can 17:865, 1995.

65. LABOR AND VAGINAL DELIVERY

Peter J. Chen, M.D.

1. What is the definition of labor?

Labor begins when uterine contractions of sufficient frequency, intensity, and duration are attained to bring about effacement and progressive dilatation of the cervix.

2. What two steps are theorized to be crucial to the initiation of labor in human pregnancy?

Retreat from pregnancy maintenance and uterotonic induction are the two simplistic speculations. Despite extensive investigations into both the physiologic and biochemical changes associated with the onset of labor, the physiological processes in human pregnancy that result in the onset of labor are still not defined.

3. In which situations is induction of labor considered?

Awaiting the onset of normal labor may not be an option in certain circumstances. In preterm gestations, indications for labor induction include severe pre-eclampsia, fetal growth restriction or other evidence of fetal compromise, and deteriorations of maternal disease so that continuation of pregnancy is believed to be detrimental. In the term (37–42 weeks) or post-term ($\geq$ 42 weeks) pregnancy, induction of labor is often undertaken after rupture of membranes without labor (premature rupture of membranes).

The overall rate of labor induction in the United States has increased from 90 per 1000 live births in 1989 to 184 per 1000 live births in 1997.

4. What methods are available for cervical ripening?

Mechanical cervical ripening methods include placement of a large 24-French Foley catheter with an inflated balloon in the cervical canal and use of osmotic dilators (laminaria). However, osmotic dilators have been associated in some studies with higher rates of maternal and neonatal infection. Other options include nipple stimulation, amniotomy, low-dose oxytocin, prostaglandin E_2 (dinoprostone), and prostaglandin E_1 (misoprostol). Prostaglandin E_1 can be administered intravaginally or orally. Prostaglandin E_2 can be applied within the vagina in either gel or suppository form, and lower doses have been used intracervically.

5. Is cervical ripening contraindicated in any particular group of patients?

Generally, the contraindications to labor induction are the same as those for spontaneous labor and vaginal delivery. They include, but are not limited to, vasa previa or complete placenta previa, transverse fetal lie, umbilical cord prolapse, and previous transfundal uterine surgery. Initial concerns about the risk of uterine rupture during induction of labor with prostaglandin among women with previous low-transverse cesarean sections, who are attempting vaginal birth after cesarean section (VBAC), have been supported in a recent study. Although the population reviewed was a selective one, the study noted a 15-fold increased risk of uterine rupture in women attempting VBAC who were induced with prostaglandin, compared to those with an elective repeat cesarean section who experienced no labor.

6. What is Bishop's score? How is it used?

Bishop's score is a quantifiable method for assessment of inducibility. Elements of the Bishop score, as assessed by internal exam, include dilatation, effacement, station, consistence, and position of the cervix (see table). Induction to active labor is usually successful with a score of 9 or greater and is less successful with lower scores.

Bishop Scoring System For Assessment of Inducibility

SCORE	DILATATION (CM)	EFFACEMENT (%)	STATION (−3 TO +3 SCALE)	CERVICAL CONSISTENCY	CERVICAL POSITION
0	Closed	0–30	−3	Firm	Posterior
1	1–2	40–50	−2	Medium	Midposition
2	3–4	60–70	−1, 0	Soft	Anterior
3	≥ 5	≥ 80	+1, +2	—	—

7. How is the pelvis assessed clinically?

The **pelvic inlet** is bounded by the sacral promontory and the pubic symphysis in the anterior-posterior dimension (obstetric conjugate) and laterally by the linea terminalis. An estimate of the inlet can be obtained by palpating the sacral promontory, which provides the measurement for the diagonal conjugate. The diagonal conjugate is approximately 1.5 to 2 cm greater than the obstetric conjugate.

The **pelvic mid plane** is bounded laterally by the inferior margins of the ischial spines, anteriorly by the lower margin of the symphysis pubis, and posteriorly by the sacrum (usually S4 or S5).

The **pelvic outlet** consists of two triangular areas not in the same plane but sharing a common base, which is a line drawn between the two ischial tuberosities. The apex of the posterior triangle is at the tip of the sacrum. The anterior triangle is formed by the area under the pubic arch (Fig. 1).

Assessment of clinical pelvimetry provides information about a patient's overall pelvic dimensions and configuration. Most patients have an intermediate form of the four classically described pelvic types (see Fig. 2; top of next page).

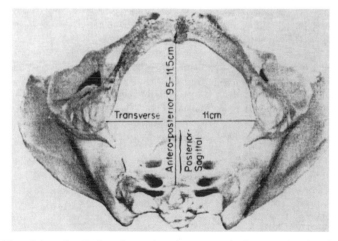

FIGURE 1. The pelvic outlet consists of two triangular areas not in the same plane but sharing a common base, which is a line drawn between the two ischial tuberosities. The apex of the posterior triangle is at the tip of the sacrum. The anterior triangle is formed by the area under the pubic arch. (From Anatomy of the reproductive tract. In Cunningham FG, et al [eds]: Williams Obstetrics, 21st ed. New York, McGraw-Hill, 2001, p 56; with permission.)

8. How are the three stages of labor defined?

The first stage begins with the onset of labor and ends when the cervix is fully dilated (about 10 cm). The second stage begins when dilatation of the cervix is complete and ends with delivery of the fetus. The third stage begins immediately after delivery of the fetus and ends with delivery of the placenta.

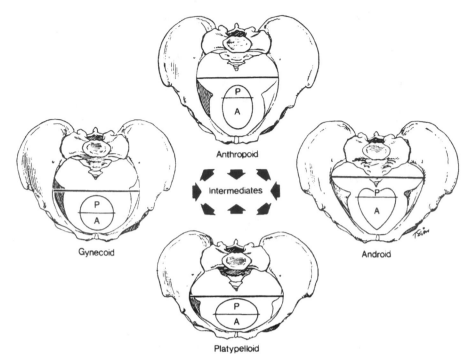

Anthropoid

Intermediates

Gynecoid

Android

Platypelloid

FIGURE 2.   The four parent pelvic types of the Caldwell-Moloy classification. A line passing through the widest transverse diameter divides the inlet into posterior (P) and anterior (A) segments. (From Anatomy of the reproductive tract. In Cunningham FG, et al [eds]: Williams Obstetrics, 21st ed. New York, McGraw-Hill, 2001, p 57; with permission.)

9. The first stage of labor is further divided into what two phases?

The first stage is divided into a relatively flat **latent phase** and a rapidly progressive **active phase**. The duration of the latent phase is more variable and subject to change by extraneous factors such as sedation and myometrial stimulation. The duration of the latent phase has little bearing on the subsequent course of labor, whereas the characteristics of the accelerated active phase are usually predictive of the outcome of a particular labor.

10. What are Friedman curves?

Emanuel A. Friedman popularized the use of an objective measure of labor progression over 30 years ago. Friedman curves plot cervical dilatation against time passed, with varying expectations for nulliparous and multiparous patients. Used in conjunction with fetal descent, the curves provide clinical feedback about the normalcy of the parturient's progress in labor.

11. What cervical changes generally take place during the latent phase?

Cervical ripening in the latent phase generally includes palpable softening, effacement, and anterior rotation of the cervix in the pelvic axis. Although little cervical dilatation occurs during this time, considerable changes take place in the extracellular matrix (collagen and other connective tissue components) of the cervix.

12. When does conversion from latent to active phase occur?

This assessment can be best made only retrospectively. During labor, the transition is characterized by increased regularity and intensity of contractions, accompanied by progressive and predictable cervical change. In nulliparous patients, the latent phase is generally longer, with active labor present at relatively minimal cervical dilatations (3 cm). In multiparous patients the latent phase may be shorter, with the active phase not initiated until 5cm; many multiparous patients have baseline cervical dilatation of 3 cm at term even before the latent phase.

13. What is the average duration of the first stage of labor in nulliparous women and in parous women?

The average duration of the first stage of labor in nulliparous women is about 7 hours and in parous women about 4 hours. However, there are marked individual variations.

14. What is a prolonged latent phase?

In nulliparous women, a prolonged latent phase is > 20 hours; in multiparous women, > 14 hours. It occurs in 5% of patients and is considered the dysfunctional labor pattern in the latent phase.

15. Describe the treatment of prolonged latent phase.

Two options are available—maternal sedation (therapeutic morphine rest) and oxytocin stimulation of contractions. Eighty-five percent of patients in prolonged latent phase go into active-phase labor after maternal sedation; 5% of them wake up without any more contractions; and the remaining 10% still with painful, irregular contractions necessitating oxytocin stimulation to go into active-phase labor.

16. What are abnormalities of the active phase? How are they treated?

Two dysfunctional labor patterns are described in this phase: protracted active phase and arrest of active phase. In general, **protracted active phase** is defined as dilatation that occurs at a rate less than the 5th percentile. This value is 1.2 cm/hr in nulliparas and 1.5 cm/hr in multiparas. The treatment for protracted active phase is simply observation. Careful maternal and fetal surveillance is required for these patients because protracted active phase is recognized as a risk factor for perinatal mortality.

Arrest of active phase is defined as cessation of a previously normal dilatation after a uterine contraction pattern of 200 montevideo units or more in a 10-minute period has been present for 2 hours. Management of arrest in the active phase depends on its etiology. If inadequate uterine contractions are observed, oxytocin augmentation may be used with a high degree of success and safety. Cesarean section is indicated in cases of fetal malpresentation and cephalopelvic disproportion

17. How many centimeters is considered full dilatation?

Generally, 10 cm is considered full dilatation, because it is approximately the diameter of the fetal vertex at term. For preterm infants, however, full dilatation may be < 10 cm, given the smaller presenting vertex and the fact that the cervix will not dilate past the maximal point of the presenting part.

18. What are abnormalities of the second stage of labor?

Two dysfunctional labor patterns are described in this stage: protraction of descent and arrest of descent. Although protraction of descent has been defined as descent occurring at < 1 cm/hr in nulliparas and < 2 cm/hr in multiparas, it is not useful clinically. Arrest of descent, on the other hand, requires prompt re-evaluation of uterine contractility, maternal and fetal well-being, and cephalopelvic relationships. For patients in whom operative delivery is possible, this is the procedure of choice. When operative delivery is not possible, cesarean section is indicated.

19. What is "active management" of labor?

O'Driscoll and colleagues working in Dublin described a protocol for active management of labor in nulliparous women. Their protocol includes: strict criteria for admission to the labor suite, early amniotomy, hourly cervical examinations, oxytocin administration for dilatation rates < 1 cm/hr, high concentrations of oxytocin in patients requiring augmentation, and expected durations of < 12 hours for the first stage of labor and 2 hours for the second stage.

Early data suggested that this approach could lower the rate of cesarean sections due to failure to progress in labor. More recently, reviews and randomized studies of this approach have failed to support a reduction in cesarean section. Despite this mixed record, many of the elements of active management are advocated and applied clinically.

20. How is post-term pregnancy defined?

The terms post-term, prolonged, postdates, and postmature are commonly used interchangeably to describe pregnancies that have exceeded a duration considered the upper limit of normal. This upper limit of normal, as recommended internationally and endorsed by the American College of Obstetricians and Gynecologists, is 42 completed weeks (294 days) or more from the first day of the last menstrual period.

21. What are the intrapartum risks implicated in a post-term pregnancy?

Historically, observations have shown that post-term pregnancies are associated with increased perinatal mortality. Compared with the group who delivered at 40 weeks, fetuses and women who delivered post-term experienced significantly higher incidence of meconium passage, oxytocin induction, shoulder dystocia (see Question 29), cesarean delivery, macrosomia, and meconium aspiration syndrome.

22. Describe the management of post-term pregnancy.

Post-term pregnancy is considered a high-risk condition, and either antenatal testing or labor induction should be commenced at 42 weeks.

23. In recording a vaginal exam, especially when preparing for a delivery, which observations should be included?

Cervical dilatation, degree of effacement (length), fetal station (presenting part in relation to the maternal ischial spines), nature of the presenting part (e.g., vertex, breech, shoulder), fetal position (orientation of fetal occiput), pelvic architecture (the diagonal conjugate, ischial spines, pelvic sidewalls, and sacrum), and the characteristics of the amniotic fluid after membranes are ruptured (observed for vernix, meconium, or blood).

24. What is the frequency of breech presentation at term?

At or near term, the incidence of breech presentation is 3.5%.

25. What are Leopold maneuvers? What information do they provide?

A systematic abdominal exam employing four maneuvers was described by Leopold in 1894. The findings provide information about the presentation and position of the fetus and the extent to which the presenting part has descended into the pelvis near term.

26. How is the fetal heart rate (FHR) monitored during labor?

Various methods of intrapartum surveillance have been designed. They include external electronic FHR monitoring, internal electronic FHR monitoring, or periodic auscultation with a fetoscope or a Doppler ultrasound. In 1998, nearly 3.3 million American women, comprising 84% of all live births, underwent electronic fetal monitoring during labor. In 1978, electronic monitoring was used in only 66%.

27. What are the cardinal movements of labor?

Although often described in the classroom as though they occur separately, the cardinal movements of labor consist of a *combination of simultaneous* movements. They are: engagement, descent, flexion, internal rotation, extension, external rotation, and expulsion (Fig. 3).

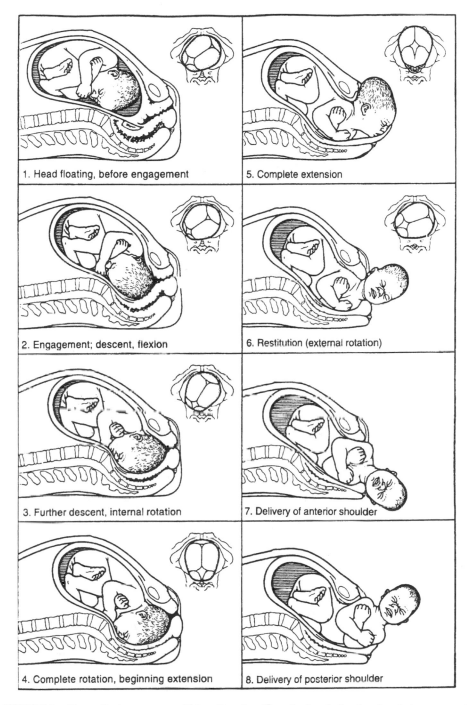

1. Head floating, before engagement

5. Complete extension

2. Engagement; descent, flexion

6. Restitution (external rotation)

3. Further descent, internal rotation

7. Delivery of anterior shoulder

4. Complete rotation, beginning extension

8. Delivery of posterior shoulder

FIGURE 3. The cardinal movements of labor. Note that although often depicted as though they occurred separately, the cardinal movements of labor comprise of a combination of movements that are ongoing simultaneously. (From Normal labor and delivery. In Cunningham FG, et al [eds]: Williams Obstetrics, 21st ed. New York, McGraw-Hill, 2001, p 302; with permission.)

28. What is the Ritgen maneuver?

Moderate upward pressure is applied to the fetal chin by the operator's posterior hand, which is covered with a sterile towel, while the vertex is held against the symphysis. This maneuver allows control of the delivery of the head and favors extension, so that the head is delivered with its smallest diameters passing through the introitus and over the perineum (Fig. 4).

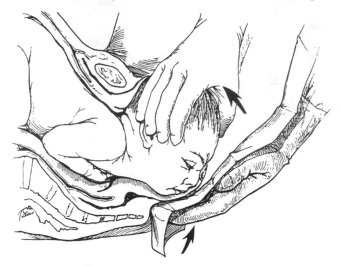

FIGURE 4.   Ritgen maneuver. Moderate upward pressure is applied to the fetal chin by the posterior hand covered with a sterile towel while the suboccipital region of the fetal head is held against the symphysis. (From Normal labor and delivery. In Cunningham FG, et al [eds]: Williams Obstetrics, 21st ed. New York, McGraw-Hill, 2001, p 318; with permission.)

29. What is shoulder dystocia? How can it be managed?

Shoulder dystocia is diagnosed when, after delivery of the fetal head, further expulsion of the infant is prevented by impaction of the fetal shoulders within the maternal pelvis. Specific maneuvers have been described to free the anterior shoulder from its impacted position beneath the maternal symphysis pubis. These maneuvers include:

- Suprapubic pressure
- McRobert's maneuver (removing maternal legs from the stirrups and sharply flexing them upon the abdomen)
- Woods corkscrew maneuver (rotating the posterior shoulder of the fetus 180 degrees in a corkscrew fashion)
- Delivery of the posterior shoulder (by sweeping the posterior arm of the fetus across the chest)
- Rubin maneuver (displacing the anterior shoulder toward the chest of the fetus within the pelvis)
- Deliberate fracture of the clavicles
- Zavanelli maneuver (involving flexion of the fetal head, replacement of the fetus within the uterine cavity, and emergent cesarean section delivery).

30. How often does shoulder dystocia occur?

Shoulder dystocia has been reported in 0.6–1.4 % of all vaginal deliveries. One of the most common risk factors for shoulder dystocia is birth weight. The risk is approximately 3–5 % for infants weighing 4000–4500 g and 8–20 % for infants weighing more than 4500 g.

31. Can shoulder dystocia occur in infants weighing less than 4000 g?

Yes. Although it has traditionally been strongly associated with macrosomia, up to 50% of cases of shoulder dystocia occur in neonates under 4000 g.

32. When should occurrence of shoulder dystocia be suspected?

It is difficult to predict shoulder dystocia. The most effective preventive measures are to be familiar with the normal mechanism of labor and delivery and constantly prepared to deal with shoulder dystocia. The principal risk factors are maternal diabetes (either pre-existing or gestational), estimated fetal weight > 4000 g, dysfunctional labor, and operative delivery.

33. What are the fetal complications of shoulder dystocia?

Shoulder dystocia may be associated with transient brachial plexus palsies, clavicular fractures, humeral fractures, and neonatal death.

34. What are the advantages of an episiotomy? The disadvantages?

Use of a routine episiotomy was believed to prevent excessive stretching of the maternal perineum, perhaps allowing better perineal support in later life. However, there is no scientific basis for this assumption, and episiotomy appears to increase the chance of injury to the rectal sphincter, with a long-term risk of sphincter dysfunction.

35. What are the advantages of the median (midline) versus the mediolateral episiotomy? The disadvantages?

Ease of repair and less painful recovery—but more frequent rectal extensions—are characteristic of the median episiotomy. The mediolateral episiotomy, which also begins at the introitus but extents at a 45-degree angle to the right or left, may be considered for large infants, a small perineal body, and some cases of forceps delivery.

36. Which tissue layers arc torn in first- through fourth-degree lacerations?

- First-degree lacerations: the fourchette, perineal skin, and vaginal mucosa, but not the underlying fascia and muscle
- Second-degree lacerations: in addition to skin and mucosa, the fascia and muscles of the perineal body, but not the anal sphincter
- Third-degree lacerations: the skin, mucosa, perineal body, and the anal sphincter
- Fourth-degree lacerations: the rectal mucosa (exposing the lumen of the rectum)

37. What are the indications for operative vaginal deliveries?

The indications for operative vaginal deliveries, provided forceps or vacuum deliveries can be accomplished safely, include any condition threatening the mother or fetus that is likely to be relieved by delivery. *Maternal indications* include heart disease, pulmonary injury or compromise, intrapartum infection, certain neurological conditions, maternal exhaustion, or prolonged second-stage labor (more than 3 hours with and more than 2 hours without regional analgesia in the nulliparous woman; more than 2 hours with and more than 1 hour without regional analgesia in the parous woman). *Fetal indications* include prolapse of the umbilical cord, placenta abruption, and a non-reassuring fetal heart rate pattern.

38. What are the requirements (ABCs) for operative vaginal deliveries?

There must be adequate **A**nesthesia, the **B**ladder must be emptied, the **C**ervix must be completely **D**ilated, the fetal head must be **E**ngaged, the **F**ontanels and direction of the occiput (position) must be precisely known, **G**ush of amniotic fluid must occur (membrane must be ruptured), **H**ip size (pelvimetry) must be adequate, and correct **I**ndication must be present.

39. What is the definition of a "mid forceps" delivery? A "high forceps" delivery?

A mid forceps delivery is one in which the fetal station is above +2 cm, but the head is engaged. In a high forceps delivery, instruments are applied before engagement; such procedure has *no place* in modern obstetrics.

40. What is the definition of a "low forceps" delivery?

The leading point of the fetal skull is at station ≥ +2 cm and not on the pelvic floor. A modification uses outlet forceps, which restrict head rotation to 45 degrees or less (left or right occiput anterior to occiput anterior, or left or right occiput posterior to occiput posterior).

41. What is the definition of an "outlet forceps" delivery?

The scalp is visible at the introitus without separating the labia; the fetal skull has reached the pelvic floor; the sagittal suture is in anteroposterior diameter or right or left occiput anterior or posterior position; the fetal head is at or on perineum; rotation does not exceed 45 degrees.

42. What assessment should be made to ensure correct placement of forceps?

For the occiput anterior (OA) position, appropriately applied blades are equidistant from the sagittal suture. In the occiput posterior (OP) position, the blades are equidistant from the midline of the face and brow.

43. What is asynclitism?

Asynclitism is failure of the vertex to descend with the sagittal suture in the mid plane between the front and back of the pelvis. It is detected clinically on examination when either the anterior or posterior parietal bones precede the sagittal suture. When accompanied by molding, asynclitism can lead to erroneous assessments of the true fetal position, with further implications for forceps applications.

44. Describe the following forceps: Simpson, Elliot, Tucker-McLane, Kielland, and Piper.

Simpson—fenestrated blades with divergent handles; greater cephalic curve of blade is suited for the molded head and when traction is applied.

Elliot—fenestrated blades with convergent handles; lesser cephalic curve is suited for the unmolded head and when traction is desired.

Tucker-McLane—solid blades with convergent handles; lesser cephalic curve is suited for the unmolded head in situations requiring minimal traction; the Luikart modification employs a pseudofenestrated blade and overlapping shanks.

Kielland—minimal pelvic curve; ideal for rotation of the vertex from OP or transverse to OA position.

Piper—used for delivering the aftercoming head of the breech fetus. The pelvic curve is opposite that of the basic forceps so that the handles are below the level of the blades (Fig. 5).

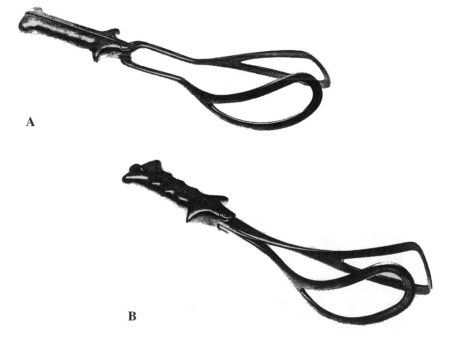

A

B

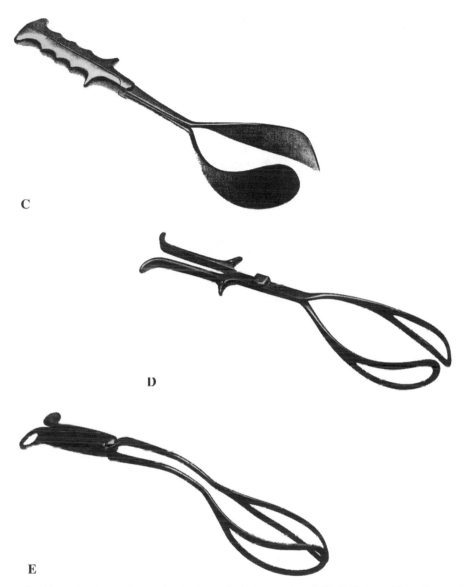

C

D

E

FIGURE 5.   A, Simpson forceps (ca. 1842). B, Elliot forceps (ca. 1858). C, Tucker-McLane forceps. D, Kielland forceps (ca. 1916). E, Piper forceps (ca. 1929). (From O'Grady J [ed]: Modern Instrumental Delivery. Philadelphia, Lippincott Williams & Wilkins, 1988; with permission.)

45. What is a Scanzoni maneuver?

Rotation from OP to OA position with Kielland forceps, then reapplication of Simpson forceps for delivery for the OA position.

BIBLIOGRAPHY

1. Baskett TF, Allen AC: Perinatal implications of shoulder dystocia. Obstet Gynecol 86:15, 1995.
2. Bishop EH. Pelvic scoring for elective induction. Obstet Gynecol 24:266–268; 1964.

3. Buser D, Mora G, Arias F. A randomized comparison between misoprostol and dinoprostone for cervical ripening and labor induction in patients with unfavorable cervices. Obstet Gynecol 89:581–585; 1997.
4. Creasy RK, et al (eds): Maternal-Fetal Medicine, 4th ed. Philadelphia, W.B. Saunders, 1999.
5. Cunningham FG, et al (eds): Williams Obstetrics, 21st ed. McGraw-Hill, 2001.
6. Frigoletto FD, Lieberman E, Lang J, et al: A clinical trial of active management of labor. New Engl J Med 333:745–750, 1995.
7. Gherman RB, Ouzounian JG, Goodwin TM: Obstetric maneuvers for shoulder dystocia and associated fetal morbidity. Am J Obstet Gynecol 178:1126, 1998.
8. Kazzi Fm, Bottoms SF, Rosen MG. Efficacy and safety of laminaria digitatta for preinduction ripening of the cervix. Obstet Gynecol 60:440–443; 1982.
9. Lydon-Rochelle, M, et al: Risk of uterine rupture during labor among women with a prior cesarean delivery. New Engl J Med 345:3–8; 2001.
10. Ventura SJ, Martin JA, Curtin SC, Mathews TJ. Births: Final data for 1997. National Center for Health Statistics, National Vital Statistics Reports, 47(18):1–96; 1999.

66. CESAREAN SECTION AND VAGINAL DELIVERY AFTER CESAREAN SECTION

Thomas J. Bader, M.D.

1. What is a cesarean section?
The abdominal (as opposed to vaginal) delivery of a baby.

2. What is the origin of the term "cesarean"?
There are three traditional explanations, one of which is certainly a myth: (1) Julius Caesar was born by an abdominal operation. But since his mother survived his delivery, and since abdominal surgery would have been fatal at that time, this explanation is not plausible. (2) Law of Caesar (*lex caesarea*) in the 8th century B.C. dictated that if a woman died during childbirth the baby should be immediately delivered by abdominal incision. (3) The Latin verb "to cut" is *caedere*. This could also be the origin of the term.

3. List the indications for delivery by cesarean section.
Fetal indications: intolerance of labor, fetal malformations preventing vaginal delivery, mal-presentation (e.g., breech presentation, some face presentations), some multi-fetal pregnancies, fetal macrosomia (> 4500 g in a diabetic woman or greater than 5000 g in a nondiabetic woman)

Maternal indications: maternal illness (e.g., severe pre-eclampsia), active genital herpes virus infection, cervical cancer, unsuccessful induction of labor

Maternal and fetal: arrest of labor

Placenta and umbilical cord: placenta previa, vasa previa, placental abruption with fetal compromise, umbilical cord prolapse, umbilical cord presenting

Pelvic: anatomic abnormality preventing vaginal delivery, pelvic mass obstructing the birth canal (e.g., adnexal mass, uterine myoma), history of complicated maternal birth injury (e.g., fourth-degree laceration, recto-vaginal fistula), history of pelvic reconstructive surgery

Uterine: previously scarred uterus (e.g., vertical uterine incision, prior myomectomy involving the uterine cavity)

4. Name the most common abdominal incision performed for cesarean section in the United States.
Pfannenstiel incision. This is a horizontal incision made low on the abdomen. It is very effective for most pelvic surgery including cesarean section. It offers the advantages of a lower rate of postoperative hernia compared with a low vertical skin incision. It also has an acceptable cosmetic result.

5. What types of abdominal incisions can be used in morbidly obese patients?
Abdominal surgery on morbidly obese patients poses several challenges. Access to the abdominal cavity can be difficult due to the thickness of the abdominal wall. The pannus frequently makes the lower abdomen effectively inaccessible for a Pfannenstiel incision. And, regardless of the location of the abdominal wall incision, there is a greater risk of postoperative wound infection and/or wound breakdown.

Several strategies have been proposed for abdominal wall surgery on these women. Some surgeons use mechanical means (i.e., tape or towel clips) to lift the pannus caudad. Other surgeons advocate making a horizontal supraumbilical incision or a vertical periumbilical incision. Finally, a transverse incision with pannilectomy has been used both to gain access to the abdominal cavity and remove some of the abdominal wall mass.

6. What types of uterine incisions are used in cesarean sections?

Three main types of uterine incision are employed. The most common is the **low transverse incision**. This usually affords adequate access to effect delivery, and it provides for the strongest postoperative repair.

In the delivery of premature infants or when performing a cesarean section on a woman who hasn't labored, there frequently is inadequate room in the lower portion of the uterus for a transverse incision. In this case a vertical incision is made. Surgeons usually attempt to distinguish between a **low vertical incision**—involving primarily the lower uterine segment—and a **high vertical incision**. Women with a mid or high vertical uterine incision are at greater risk of uterine rupture with subsequent pregnancies and should not attempt future vaginal delivery. The presentation of the fetus may also dictate the type of uterine incision. Non-vertex fetuses sometimes require a vertical incision to effect delivery.

An incision that extends to the uterine fundus is termed a classic uterine incision. This incision is rarely used. Vertical uterine incisions are sometimes inaccurately described as classic incisions.

7. What is the current cesarean section rate in the U.S.? What is the optimal rate?

In 2000, 23% of all deliveries in the U.S. were via cesarean section.

In the past there was great interest among obstetricians, insurance executives, and policymakers in defining and achieving an optimal cesarean section rate. More recently the enthusiasm has waned. It may not be possible to define an optimal cesarean section rate for the country. Even if it was possible, it is not clear that knowledge of such a rate would have any relevance for women and their healthcare providers.

8. List complications that can result from a cesarean section.

The most common complication of cesarean section is infection. Other less common complications include: significant blood loss requiring transfusion; injury to the uterus, ovaries, tubes, bowel, bladder, or ureter; hysterectomy; fetal injury; and maternal death.

9. What is the average blood loss during a cesarean section?

1000 ml.

10. What is the maternal mortality rate associated with cesarean section? How does it compare to the mortality rate of vaginal delivery?

Fortunately, the maternal mortality rate for both procedures is very low. The rate for C-section is 3–30 per 100,000, depending on the population studied and the circumstances surrounding the cesarean section. This figure is comparable to the mortality rate for vaginal delivery.

11. What special considerations apply if a woman with a previous C-section has a placenta previa?

Women with a previous C-section are at increased risk for having an abnormal placental location in subsequent pregnancies. Specifically, these women are at increased risk for placenta previa (i.e., part of the placenta covers the cervical os). If this placental location persists, repeat C-section is necessary. In addition, the combination of a placenta previa and a prior C-section puts the woman at risk for placenta accreta (i.e., the placental tissue grows into the uterine wall). This condition can lead to significant blood loss and frequently requires hysterectomy at the time of C-section (cesarean hysterectomy). The operative team should anticipate this possibility and be prepared with an adequate surgical team and blood products available.

12. When is an emergent C-section performed? How quickly should an emergent C-section be started?

Emergent C-sections are usually performed for fetal indications; usually fetal compromise regardless of the cause. C-sections for maternal indications or due to labor abnormalities are generally urgent rather than emergent.

An emergency C-section should be started within 30 minutes of the decision to proceed.

13. What are the indications for cesarean hysterectomy?
Malignancy
Some cases of placenta accreta, increta, or percreta
Uncontrollable bleeding
Uterine rupture when repair is impossible or carries unacceptable morbidity

14. What are the effects of cesarean section on the fetus/newborn?
Increased transient tachypnea of the newborn.

15. Can adnexal surgery be performed in association with a C-section?
Yes. The indications for adnexal surgery are generally the same as those for a woman who is not pregnant and undergoing laparotomy. That is, extra surgery should not be undertaken just because there is ready access. But abnormalities of the adnexa can be safely addressed after delivery of the newborn and repair of the uterus.

16. Can myomectomy (removal of myomas) be performed in association with a C-section?
Due to the excessive blood loss and the potential difficulty with hemostasis, myomectomy is generally *not* performed at the time of cesarean section. However, if the location of the myoma interferes with closure of the uterine incision, myomectomy may be necessary.

17. Should elective cesarean hysterectomy be planned for women with known uterine pathology who are undergoing C-section?
Cesarean hysterectomy—elective or emergent—carries an increased risk of morbidity compared with elective hysterectomy of a non-pregnant uterus. Generally, elective cesarean hysterectomy is performed only in cases of malignancy (cervical, ovarian), when delay in therapy could worsen the prognosis. Other uterine pathology such as myomas can be surgically treated after recovery from the C-section, when the pelvic organs and blood flow have returned to their pre-pregnant state.

18. What is vaginal birth after cesarean section (VBAC)?
Initially, concern over rupture of the uterine scar led to the recommendation not to attempt labor after a C-section, but instead to undergo repeat C-section. This was summarized as "Once a C-section, always a C-section." In the last couple of decades this wisdom has been reexamined. Currently, most but not all women with one prior cesarean section are considered to be candidates for vaginal delivery. Women attempting a VBAC are said to be undergoing a "trial of labor."

19. What is uterine rupture? Uterine dehiscence?
Uterine *rupture* is the *complete* separation of all layers of the uterine wall, including the serosa. When this occurs there is free communication between the uterine cavity and the abdominal cavity. This is an obstetrical emergency putting the fetus, the uterus, and the mother in danger. Uterine *dehiscence* is an *incomplete* disruption of the uterine wall. Usually there is uterine serosa overlying a defect in the uterine muscle.
A dehiscence is also frequently described as a uterine "window." A dehiscence is usually discovered incidentally at the time of repeat C-section, and typically has no clinical significance.
Unfortunately, these terms—uterine rupture and uterine dehiscence—are frequently used interchangeably. Precise distinction is important because of the great difference in the clinical significance of the diagnoses.

20. What is the risk of uterine rupture?
Uterine rupture in an unscarred uterus is extremely rare. The majority of uterine ruptures occur in women who have previously undergone C-section. Uterine rupture can also occur following other uterine surgery, specifically myomectomy. The risk of uterine rupture with a prior low transverse scar is approximately 1%. With a low vertical scar the risk is 1–7%, and with an inverted T-shaped or classic incision the risk of rupture is 4–7%.

21. What are the sequelae of uterine rupture?

Fetal: death, acidemia, potential hypoxic insult

Maternal: hysterectomy, blood transfusion

With optimal management, most mothers and newborns are healthy after uterine rupture. Usually the uterus can be repaired, and hysterectomy is not necessary.

22. Can the sequelae of uterine rupture be minimized through adequate preparation?

Unfortunately, even under optimal conditions, maternal and fetal morbidity and mortality still occur. The immediate availability of anesthesia and the presence of an operative team to perform a C-section should *not* give the obstetrician or the mother a false sense of security.

23. Do all uterine ruptures occur during labor?

No. Women can experience uterine rupture before the onset of labor.

24. Who is a candidate for VBAC?

A woman with a prior uterine incision in the lower uterine segment without other contraindications to vaginal delivery (e.g., placenta previa, breech presentation) is a candidate for VBAC.

25. What criteria need to be met to attempt VBAC?

The woman should be appropriately counseled regarding the risks of attempting a VBAC and the likelihood of success. Anesthesia and a qualified surgical team should be readily available for emergency cesarean section.

26. What are the arguments in favor of VBAC?

Successful VBAC allows the mother to avoid laparotomy and the maternal and fetal risks that attend birth by C-section. Post-procedure recovery is generally quicker after a vaginal delivery and, considering the significant demands placed on the mother of a newborn, this may be particularly important. Many women also value the experience of a vaginal delivery (sometimes called "natural" delivery).

Although a program of attempting VBAC may carry lower costs, the data on this is conflicting and any cost-saving is enjoyed by payers, health systems, and society, and usually not by the individual undergoing the VBAC.

27. What are the arguments against VBAC?

The strongest argument against attempting VBAC is the risk of uterine rupture and the potential for morbidity and even fetal mortality that goes along with that complication. Although this complication is uncommon ($< 1\%$), it is potentially disastrous. Many women (and their providers) are also reluctant to subject themselves to a possible long labor in an effort to avoid a cesarean section, only to end up with the precise outcome they sought to avoid.

28. What is the success rate with VBAC?

The success rate in all comers is approximately 70%. The success rate is lower in women who underwent the prior cesarean section for arrest of labor, and higher for those who underwent previous C-section for other indications (e.g., fetal intolerance of labor, malpresentation).

29. Which variables predict success with attempted VBAC?

The only variable with significant power to predict success is a prior vaginal delivery. This single element is a very powerful predictor of success.

30. Why does the VBAC decision pose such a dilemma?

The outcome most desired by women contemplating VBAC is vaginal delivery with a healthy, intact mother and baby. The outcome most feared by these women is labor complicated by uterine rupture. The path toward both of these outcomes begins with a decision to attempt vaginal delivery. The middle course of planned cesarean section offers a slight reduction in risk for mother and baby, but with a guarantee of major surgery.

31. Can women attempting VBAC undergo induction of labor?

Yes. Oxytocin can be used to augment the labor of a woman who is already contracting or to induce labor in women undergoing induction of labor. Women receiving oxytocin stimulation are closely monitored to continuously follow the fetal heart rate pattern and the uterine activity. This is at least as important in a woman attempting VBAC who is receiving oxytocin. A recent study of women attempting VBAC found no difference in outcome between the mothers receiving oxytocin and those experiencing spontaneous labor.

That same study, however, did find an increased risk of uterine rupture in women attempting VBAC who received prostaglandins for cervical ripening. This portion of the study was not randomized, and there is some concern that the prostaglandin was a marker for more difficult labors. Regardless, this study has reduced or eliminated the use of prostaglandins in women with scarred uteruses.

32. Can VBAC be attempted in twin pregnancies?

Data for twin pregnancies is limited, but existing experience suggests that this is a safe practice. Attempts are generally limited to twin pregnancies where both twins are in a cephalic presentation. If either twin is non-vertex, scheduled cesarean section is generally performed.

33. If uterine rupture or dehiscence is detected at the time of C-section, how should it be managed?

Repair uterine rupture, if possible, at the time of surgery. If repair is impossible, perform a hysterectomy.

Dehiscence usually occurs at the site of the prior uterine incision, so repair is usually accomplished as part of the repair of the current hysterotomy. If the dehiscence is separate from the current uterine incision and it is not bleeding, it is not necessary to perform additional surgery to perform a repair.

CONTROVERSIES

34. Should women be offered primary elective cesarean section?

In recent years there has been more discussion about this option. What once seemed preposterous now seems less so. In some countries, particularly in South America, primary C-section is the delivery method of choice for much of the population. The argument in favor of this approach is the desire to avoid labor, the ability to plan delivery, an unsubstantiated belief in greater safety for the baby, and the possible avoidance of common sequelae of vaginal delivery such as urinary and anal incontinence and pelvic relaxation.

As of yet, there is no data to substantiate any of the health claims of primary C-section, but there is also no data to refute it. As long as this question remains unresolved, the principle of patient autonomy argues in favor of allowing this option for women.

35. Can VBAC be offered after two cesarean sections? After three?

Additional C-sections do increase the risk of uterine rupture. However, this risk remains low at least after two C-sections. Currently, women with two prior C-sections are considered candidates for VBAC. With a potential further increase in the risk of rupture following three C-sections, many obstetricians recommend proceeding with a fourth C-section rather than attempting VBAC.

36. Should the uterine scar be examined transcervically after a VBAC?

It was once standard to examine the prior uterine scar through the vagina and cervix following a successful VBAC. This practice has become less common because it is not clear that the information has any clinical relevance. If a defect of the uterine wall is detected, but there is not excessive hemorrhage, then no treatment is necessary, and the woman would remain a candidate for VBAC in the future. Theoretically an undiagnosed uterine rupture could be detected, thereby preventing future sequelae. But such a clinically silent rupture must be extraordinary.

BIBLIOGRAPHY

1. American College of Obstetricians and Gynecologists: Fetal macrosomia, ACOG Practice Bulletin 22, 2000.
2. American College of Obstetricians and Gynecologists: Vaginal birth after previous cesarean delivery, ACOG Practice Bulletin 5, 1999.
3. Cunningham FG, Gant NF, Leveno KJ (eds): Williams Obstetrics, 21st ed. New York, 2001, McGraw Hill.
4. Gabbe SG, Niebyl JR, Simpson JL (eds): Obstetrics: Normal and Problem Pregnancies, 4th ed. Philadelphia, Churchill Livingstone, 2002.
5. Greene MF: Vaginal delivery after cesarean section—Is the risk acceptable? New Engl J Med 345(1):54–55, 2001.
6. Lydon-Rochelle M, Holt VL, Easterling TR, Martin DP: Risk of uterine rupture during labor among women with a prior cesarean delivery. New Engl J Med 345(1):3–8, 2001.
7. Miller DA, Diaz FG, Paul RH: Vaginal birth after cesarean: A 10-year experience. Obstet Gynecol 84:255, 1994.
8. National Center for Health Statistics. Births: Final data for 2000. National Vital Statistics Report 50(5), 2002.
9. Nielsen TF, Hagberg H, Ljungblad U: Placenta previa and antepartum hemorrhage after previous cesarean section. Gynecol Obstet Invest 27:88, 1989.
10. Rock JA, Thompson JD (eds): Te Linde's Operative Gynecology, 8th ed. Philadelphia, Lippincott-Raven, 1997.
11. van den Berg A, van Elburg RM, van Geijn HP, Fetter WP: Neonatal respiratory morbidity following elective caesarean section in term infants. A 5-year retrospective study and a review of the literature. Eur J Obstet Gynecol Repro Biol 98(1):9–13, 2001.
12. Yoles L, Maschiach S: Increased maternal mortality in cesarean section as compared to vaginal delivery? Time for reevaluation. Am J Obstet Gynecol 178:1, 1998.

67. OBSTETRIC ANESTHESIA

Robert Gaiser, M.D.

1. Who is the obstetric anesthesiologist?

The obstetric anesthesiologist is a physician who is board-certified in anesthesiology and who has completed additional training in obstetric anesthesia. There is no formal certification in obstetric anesthesia. The primary objective of the obstetric anesthesiologist is pain control during delivery that is safe for both mother and fetus. This individual serves as a consultant to the obstetrician to assist not only with pain management but also with management of complex medical conditions and maternal hemodynamics.

2. Why have a physician dedicated to pain management during labor and delivery?

Labor and delivery result in severe pain for most women. In an attempt to quantify this pain, parturients were asked to rate their pain during labor. These results were then compared to values obtained from patients in a general pain clinic and emergency department. The pain of childbirth was greater than a fractured arm and cancer pain. Only causalgia and amputation of a digit exceeded the pain of labor and delivery (see figure). Parturients described the pain as sharp, cramping, aching, throbbing, stabbing, hot, shooting, and tight.

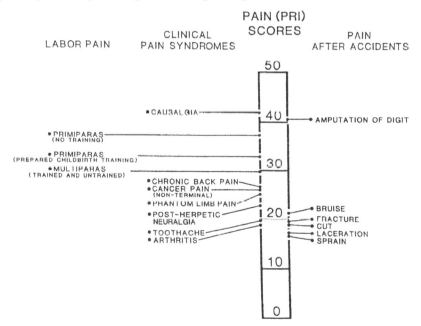

Parturient ratings of labor pain compared to general patient ratings of other pain. (From Melzack R: The myth of painless childbirth. Pain 19: 321-37, 1984; with permission.)

3. Describe the physiology of labor pain.

The process of labor is divided into three stages. **Stage 1**: onset of uterine contractions and cervical dilatation; ends with complete dilatation of the cervix. **Stage 2**: also known as fetal descent; begins with full dilatation of the cervix and ends with delivery of the baby. **Stage 3**: runs from delivery of the baby to delivery of the placenta. Anesthesiologists are primarily involved during the first two stages.

4. What is the cause of labor pain in Stage 1? What type of pain is it?

The pain resulting from the first stage of labor is primarily due to dilatation of the cervix with consequent distention and stretching. As the uterus contracts, the fetal head pushes against the cervix and causes dilatation. Therefore, Stage 1 pain generally occurs only during uterine contraction. While the majority of pain during this stage occurs from the fetal head pushing against the cervix, there is also pain from pressure and stretching of the uterine muscles, which activate the high-threshold mechanoreceptors.

In the first stage of labor, the pain is visceral. It is strong and dull, and occurs over the lower abdomen between the umbilicus and the symphysis pubis, laterally over the iliac crest, and posteriorly in the skin and soft tissue over the lower lumbar spines.

5. Explain the location of labor pain in Stage 1.

The location of this pain is explained by the concept of referred pain. The sensory nerves of the uterus and cervix leave the cervix and join the sympathetic nerves as they pass through the hypogastric plexus to the sympathetic chain, synapsing within the dorsal horn of the spinal cord at T10, T11, T12, and L1 (see figure). This area of the spinal cord receives not only these visceral high-threshold afferents, but also the low-threshold cutaneous afferents of the skin from T10, T11, T12, and L1. With the convergence of both somatic and visceral fibers within the same area of the spinal cord, the parturient interprets the uterine pain as originating from the cutaneous afferents of these spinal segments. The pain is referred to this area.

6. What is the cause of labor pain in Stage 2? What type of pain is it?

Second stage pain occurs as the fetus descends through the birth canal. This results in stretching and tearing of fascia, skin, and subcutaneous tissue. This somatic pain is transmitted primarily through the pudendal nerve. The pudendal nerve is derived from the anterior primary divisions of sacral nerves, S2 S3 and S4 (see figure). Of note, the fetus often begins to descend during the first stage of labor. During the transitional stage of the first stage, it is not uncommon for the mother to experience both visceral and somatic pain.

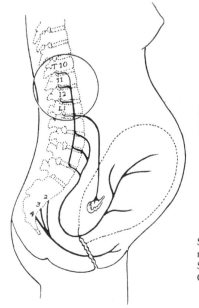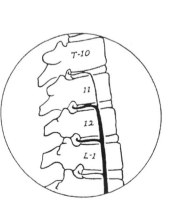

Stage 1 pain results from fibers accompanying the sympathetic nerves from T10–L1. Stage 2 pain results from the sacral nerves S2–S4. (From Bonica JJ: The nature of pain of parturition. Clin Obstet Gynecol 2: 499-516, 1975; with permission.)

7. **How do psychological factors influence labor pain?**

While labor is a physiologic process, psychological factors also affect the pain. **Anxiety** is a particularly powerful factor in reducing pain tolerance. **Attention**, the selective orientation of the receptor system to one source or pattern of stimulation to the exclusion of other sources, either enhances or diminishes the painful experience. **Motivation** is another psychodynamic mechanism that can have a marked influence on the physiological, behavioral, and affective aspects of pain.

All of these factors are best addressed by prepared childbirth classes. Mothers who are informed about the process of childbirth have less anxiety. Breathing exercises divert the mother's attention from the pain of contractions. The mother's focus, thus redirected from personal discomfort to the birth of her child, provides a powerful source for motivation. *Effective childbirth training results in a 30% reduction in the intensity of labor pain.*

8. **What physiologic changes of pregnancy are important for the obstetric anesthesiologist to consider when designing a plan for analgesia?**

Major changes occur in maternal physiology throughout pregnancy. Each organ system is affected. It is generally accepted that those changes occurring early in pregnancy are a result of hormonal factors, whereas those occurring later in pregnancy are a combination of hormonal factors and mechanical effects from the enlarging uterus.

Important Changes For the Anesthesiologist To Consider

ORGAN SYSTEM	PHYSIOLOGIC CHANGE	ANESTHETIC IMPLICATION
Cardiovascular	Downregulation of α and β receptors	Decreased responsiveness to vasopressors and chronotropic agents
Respiratory	Decreased functional residual capacity and increased oxygen consumption	Vulnerable to hypoxia with induction of general anesthesia
Gastrointestinal	Gravid uterus changes angle of the gastroesophageal junction, leading to incompetence; also delays gastric emptying	Full stomach consideration
Neurologic	Increased sensitivity to inhalation agents and local anesthetics	Anesthetic requirements decrease by 40%

9. **What is aortocaval compression? Why is the obstetric anesthesiologist so concerned about it?**

Approximately 15% of parturients develop hypotension when lying supine. In this position, the gravid uterus obstructs the vena cava, decreasing venous return to the heart. This **reduction in preload** results in a subsequent **decrease in cardiac output**.

All parturients do not become hypotensive when lying supine, as there is collateral venous return via the epidural and azygous veins and also compensation through the sympathetic nervous system (SNS). Activation of the SNS results in compensatory peripheral vasoconstriction and increased heart rate. However, both general and regional anesthesia cause sympathetic blockade. Furthermore, the gravid uterus may also compress the aorta and decrease uterine blood flow.

Therefore, all parturients receiving anesthesia/analgesia must maintain **left uterine displacement** (a wedge placed under the right hip tilting the uterus to the left) to prevent aortocaval compression. Left uterine displacement removes the compression of the vena cava by the uterus and prevents the decrease in venous return and preload. It also prevents compression of the aorta.

10. **How do medications administered to the mother gain access to the fetus?**

Transfer of drugs across the placenta is based primarily on molecular diffusion, although other mechanisms such as active transport and facilitated diffusion play a minor role. The placental transfer of medication is directly proportional to the area available for transfer and to the difference in serum concentrations between the mother and fetus, and is indirectly proportional to the distance across the intervillous space.

11. What analgesic options are available for labor?
- Lamaze
- Intravenous opioids and sedatives
- Regional anesthesia including paracervical block, pudendal block, epidural block, and spinal block
- Inhalation analgesia—specifically, Entonox

Inhalation analgesia using volatile agents is not typically done due to maternal and fetal sedation. Furthermore, the possibility of maternal aspiration due to lack of consciousness renders the technique risky. A combination of nitrous oxide and oxygen (50:50) known as Entonox is popular in England. It is self-administered by the mother, and the concentration is usually inadequate to induce unconsciousness.

12. Describe the differences among the various regional techniques.

Paracervical block involves the injection of local anesthetics submucosally into the fornix of the vagina laterally to the cervix (generally at 3 o'clock and 9 o'clock). The somatic sensory fibers of the perineum are not blocked. Paracervical block is effective only for the first stage of labor, and is associated with a high incidence of fetal bradycardia. Its major role is in providing analgesia for dilation and curettage.

Pudendal block involves the injection of local anesthetic below the ischial spines (the approximate location of the pudendal nerve). This block is administered during the second stage of labor and is useful for vaginal delivery and outlet forceps/vacuum delivery.

Lumbar epidural block is the most popular and is effective for both first and second stages of labor. The placement of a catheter into the epidural space allows for limitless analgesia. Analgesia is obtained by injecting local anesthetic through the catheter into the epidural space. The epidural space is located peripherally to the dura mater. It extends from the foramen magnum to the sacral hiatus. The ligamentum flavum forms the posterior boundary. The contents of the epidural space include nerve roots, fat, lymphatic tissue, and blood vessels. The epidural space is entered with a needle and relies on the anesthesiologist's sense of feel.

Spinal block is highly effective, but is a single shot technique with limited analgesia. It involves puncturing the dura and arachnoid mater, then injecting local anesthetic or opioid into the subarachnoid space.

Combined spinal/epidural block involves locating the epidural space with an epidural needle, advancing a long spinal needle through the epidural needle until cerebrospinal fluid (CSF) is obtained, injecting local anesthetic or opioid, removing the spinal needle, and then threading a catheter into the epidural space. The technique allows for quick onset of analgesia (due to the spinal portion) and for limitless analgesia (due to the presence of the epidural catheter). The use of opioid alone or with a small amount of local anesthetic causes no motor blockade, allowing for ambulation if desired. Many people refer to this block as "the walking epidural."

13. What are local anesthetics? Which ones are most frequently used for regional blocks in obstetrics?

Local anesthetics produce reversible blockade of neural conduction. Their molecular structure consists of an aromatic ring, a linking chain, and a carbon chain bearing an amino group (see figure). Esters have a linking chain of the COO configuration. Para-aminobenzoic acid is a metabolite and an allergin. Amide local anesthetics have a linking chain of the NHCO configuration. Using the generic name, esters have only one "i" in the name, while amides have two.

Of the esters, 2-chloroprocaine is used most frequently in obstetric anesthesia. Of the amides, bupivacaine, ropivacaine, and lidocaine are most widely employed.

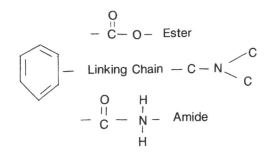

Molecular structure of local anesthetics.

14. What are the complications of epidural analgesia for labor and delivery?

Pain at the needle insertion site is probably the most common complication. It is usually secondary to a small bruise at the site and lasts for approximately 48 hours. There are no good studies linking postpartum backache with epidural analgesia. The frequency of postpartum backache is similar whether an epidural catheter was placed or not.

Hypotension caused by sympathetic blockade is the second most common complication. Hydration may attenuate the decrease in blood pressure. Sometimes medication is needed to treat the hypotension. Ephedrine, a mixed α and β agonist, is preferred over phenylephrine, a pure α agonist, as it has been shown to better preserve uterine blood flow.

Spinal headache results from unintended dural puncture. Its incidence is 1–2% of all epidurals performed.

Neurologic injury is related to the birthing process rather than the anesthesia. The more commonly injured nerves are the lumbosacral trunk, lateral femoral cutaneous nerve, femoral nerve, and the common peroneal nerve. Occasionally, nerve injuries are related to the epidural analgesia (incidence < 0.01%) and include trauma to the nerve root, epidural hematoma, and epidural abscess.

15. What is a spinal headache? How is it treated?

The incidence of headache after accidental dural puncture with an epidural needle is > 70% (< 2% with a spinal needle). The cause of the headache is felt to be leakage of CSF into the epidural space. Low CSF pressure results in a loss of the cushion effect provided within the cranium. The pain results from traction on pain-sensitive structures within the cranial cavity. This theory explains the postural component of the headache (worse with upright position) and location (frontal and occipital). It generally occurs within 48 hours of dural puncture, although in 25% of cases, it may occur later than 3 days. It usually resolves within 1 week in 75% of patients.

Treatment consists of bedrest, intravenous caffeine (85% effective), or epidural blood patch (95% effective). Epidural blood patch involves aseptic placement of 15–20 ml autologous blood into the epidural space.

16. Are there contraindications to epidural analgesia in obstetrics?

The only absolute contraindication is patient refusal. Hypovolemia, fever, thrombocytopenia, and coagulation defects are relative contraindications, depending upon the judgement of the anesthesiologist and the severity of the abnormality.

17. Does epidural anlagesia affect the course of labor?

A meta-analysis examined 10 trials enrolling 2369 patients. Epidural analgesia did not increase the risk of cesarean section. It did result in longer first and second stages as well as an increased risk of assisted vaginal delivery. Mothers who received epidural analgesia were more satisfied as compared to those who received parenteral opioids.

Using evidence-based medicine, seven cohort studies and five observational studies were analyzed. The cohort studies do not support that epidural analgesia increases the risk of cesarean section. It may increase the risk of oxytocin use. It seems that severe pain is a predictor of operative delivery, regardless of the use of epidural analgesia.

18. What anesthetic options are available for cesarean delivery?

General anesthesia is most often used for emergency delivery or if there is an abnormality that precludes neuraxial anesthesia. General anesthesia requires less than 2 minutes to prepare the patient for surgical incision. Major neuraxial anesthesia consists of spinal or epidural block. **Spinal anesthesia** is a single shot technique that is rapid in onset. It requires approximately 5–10 minutes before the patient is ready for surgical incision. **Epidural anesthesia** is a viable option, particularly if an epidural catheter had been placed during labor. If the catheter is in place, surgical anesthesia can be obtained within 2–4 minutes. If a catheter is not present, it requires approximately 10 minutes to place.

19. What is anesthetic mortality in obstetric cases?

Anesthesia-related maternal mortality has decreased from 4.3 per million live births during 1979–1981 to 1.7 per million during 1988–1990. The number of deaths from general anesthesia has remained relatively stable; the number of deaths from regional anesthesia has decreased tremendously. *The risk of a mother dying from general anesthesia is 16.7 times that for regional anesthesia.*

20. Why is general anesthesia more risky?

The ability to secure the airway (intubate) is the primary reason. Capillary engorgement of the mucosa causes swelling of the nasal and oral pharynx, larynx, and trachea. These changes make intubation (the placement of a tube in the trachea) more difficult. Gastric emptying is delayed in the parturient, placing the parturient at risk for aspiration. Finally, the gravid uterus elevates the diaphragm, decreasing the functional residual capacity by 20%. Oxygen consumption is increased by 20–35% during pregnancy. These two changes render the parturient vulnerable to the rapid development of hypoxemia during periods of apnea. Not only is the parturient more difficult to intubate, but also intubation must be accomplished more quickly.

21. What is aspiration?

Aspiration occurs when the contents of the stomach gain access to the lungs. If a person should aspirate, coughing and closure of the epiglottis and vocal cords usually prevents access of these contents to the lungs. However, during general anesthesia, these protective reflexes are abolished. Patients who aspirate are at risk for development of aspiration pneumonitis, which may be fatal. Risk factors for the development of aspiration pneumonitis include the aspiration of a large quantity, the aspiration of food, and the aspiration of highly acidic material.

22. What can be done to prevent aspiration?

The most important step in safeguarding all pregnant patients is to have them refrain from eating once labor begins. A nonparticulate antacid, such as sodium bicitrate, neutralizes the acidity of the stomach. The administration of H2 blockers increases gastric pH, but requires > 40 minutes to become effective. Metoclopramide decreases gastric volume (requires > 30 minutes) and increases gastroesophageal sphincter tone (immediate).

If general anesthesia is to be used, the administration of pentothal for induction followed immediately by succinylcholine for muscle relaxation allows for intubation within 60 seconds. This is called **rapid sequence induction** and is accompanied with cricoid pressure. The cricoid cartilage is the only complete cartilaginous ring of the trachea. The application of pressure occludes the esophagus and prevents passive regurgitation. Proper airway evaluation and management are the most effective ways of preventing airway problems during induction of general anesthesia.

Patients with difficult airways should be identified and treated with alternative techniques such as awake intubation or regional anesthesia. These patients should also receive consideration for the early placement of epidural analgesia during labor.

23. Is fetal outcome any different between regional and general anesthesia?

Traditionally, neonates have been evaluated by Apgar score, acid-base status, and neurobehavior examination. There appears to be a difference between general and regional anesthesia with regard to Apgar scores. Infants born to mothers who received general anesthesia have lower Apgar scores at 1 minute, with little difference at 5 minutes. The factor accounting for this decrease is transient sedation following induction of general anesthesia. The longer the exposure of the fetus to the general anesthetic, the more depressed the Apgar score.

In elective cesarean sections, the difference in pH between regional and general anesthesia is not clinically significant. An important factor in acid-base status may be the time interval from uterine incision to delivery; longer intervals increase the risk of fetal acidosis and hypoxia.

Neurobehavioral testing shows some subtle early differences between general and regional anesthesia, with better scores in the regional group. There were essentially no differences at 24 hours. Well-performed anesthesia with rapid delivery of the infant results in a vigorous infant.

24. What anesthetic risks accompany preeclampsia?

Preeclampsia results in various pathophysiologic abnormalities. Although edematous, women with preeclampsia are intravascularly deplete. Care must be taken with hydration as these patients are also at risk for the development of pulmonary edema. Preeclampsia results in a hypersensitivity to catecholamines, both endogenous and exogenous. Intubation is associated with the release of endogenous catecholamines and is accompanied with an exaggerated hypertensive response. This rise in blood pressure increases the risk of cerebral hemorrhage. Preeclampsia can lead to isolated thrombocytopenia as well as disseminated intravascular coagulopathy. Platelets and clotting studies are obtained prior to the performance of epidural/spinal anesthesia (there is an increased risk of development of epidural hematoma if a blood vessel is punctured during placement and if the patient is coagulopathic). Finally, the use of magesium to prevent seizures increases the parturient's sensitivity to neuromuscular blockers.

25. What is the primary cause of postpartum hemorrhage?

In the nonpregnant state, uterine blood flow is approximately 50 cc/min. At term, uterine blood flow increases to 500–700 cc/min. Following separation of the placenta, the cessation of bleeding in the uterus depends upon the ability of the uterus to contract. **Uterine atony** can cause life-threatening hemorrhage. Uterine atony is associated with multiparity, polyhydramnios, macrosomia, multiple gestation, prolonged labor, and medications such as magnesium, ritodrine, and the volatile agents.

26. How is the anesthesiologist involved in treatment of postpartum hemorrhage?

Anesthesiologists assist with resuscitation, monitoring, and treatment of side effects. Resuscitation of the mother with fluids and vasopressors is the highest priority. Administration of oxytocin, ergot derivatives, or prostaglandins may be necessary. Oxytocin is administered intravenously; it may cause significant hypotension if given too rapidly. Ergot derivatives are administered intramuscularly. They are associated with a high incidence of nausea and vomiting. These drugs should be used with extreme caution in patients with hypertensive disorders. The third group is prostaglandin F2α. It is administered intramuscularly; intravenous administration is associated with bronchospasm and hypertension. It should be used with caution in asthmatics.

Uterine atony may become severe enough to require urgent laparotomy and ligation of the uterine blood supply or possible hysterectomy. The patient also may require massive transfusion. Regional anesthesia is not precluded if the anesthesiologist has adequate intravenous access and is able to adequately volume resuscitate the patient.

27. What are the anesthetic implications of tocolytic drugs?

Given the high infant morbidity associated with premature labor, obstetricians usually try to stop premature labor with tocolytic drugs. Four different classes of drugs are used: β-adrenergic agents, magnesium, prostaglandin synthetase inhibitors, and calcium channel blockers. The drug primarily used is **magnesium**. Maternal side effects include maternal nausea and weakness. Anesthetic considerations for women receiving magnesium include increased sensitivity to muscle relaxants. The β-adrenergic agents may be used for short courses. They are not used for longer periods because the drugs lose effectiveness due to the development of tolerance. Maternal side effects include hypokalemia, hyperglycemia, and tachycardia. The anesthetic consideration for this group of drugs is that they render the mother prone to pulmonary edema. The other two classes are not used as frequently and have minimal anesthetic considerations.

28. What options are available for pain control following cesarean delivery?

This depends on the anesthetic technique used for surgery. If a general anesthetic was used, the patient can be offered **patient-controlled intravenous analgesia**. A pump allows for accurate amounts of opioid at a continuous rate and also allows the mother to self-administer a bolus if necessary. Programmed limits prevent overdosage.

If **epidural analgesia** was used for delivery, an **opioid** may be placed in the epidural space to provide analgesia. The most commonly used opioid for this purpose is preservative-free morphine (Duramorph); at a dose of 4 mg epidurally, it provides 18–24 hours of analgesia. Side effects include pruritus, nausea/vomiting, and respiratory depression. Occasionally, continuous epidural infusions of low-concentrations of local anesthetic and opioid are used in the postoperative period. Patients may be given a controller device to augment a basal infusion rate, producing a patient-controlled epidural analgesia.

If **single-shot spinal anesthesia** was used, again preservative-free **morphine** may be combined with the injection. A markedly lower dose is required, 0.1 mg, and it, too, provides analgesia for 18–24 hours. Side effects include pruritus, respiratory depression, and nausea/vomiting.

For both epidural and spinal opioids, the respiratory depression tends to occur if the mother receives supplemental intravenous opioids. Patients who require additional intravenous opioid should receive appropriate monitoring.

BIBLIOGRAPHY

1. Alexander JM, Sharma SK, McIntire DD: Intensity of labor pain and cesarean delivery. Anesth Analg 92:1524–1528, 2001.
2. Bonica JJ: The nature of pain of parturition. Clin Obstet Gynecol 2:499–516, 1975.
3. Camann WR, Cenney RA, Holby ED, Datta S: A comparison of intrathecal, epidural, and intravenous sufentanil for labor analgesia. Anesthesiology 77:884–887, 1992.
4. Chadwick HS, Posner K, Caplan RA, Ward RJ: A comparison of obstetric and nonobstetric anesthesia malpractice claims. Anesthesiology 74:242–249, 1991.
5. Halpern SH, Leighton BL, Ohlsson A, et al: Effect of epidural vs. parenteral opioid analgesia on the progress of labor. A meta-analysis. JAMA 280:2105–2110, 1998.
6. Hawkins JL, Koonin LM, Palmer SK, Gibbs CP: Anesthesia-related deaths during obstetric delivery in the United States, 1979–1990. Anesthesiology 86:277–284, 1997.
7. Melzack R: The myth of painless childbirth. Pain 19:321–337, 1984.
8. Palmer CM, Maciulla JE, Corck RC: The incidence of fetal heart rate changes after intrathecal fentanyl labor analgesia. Anesth Analg 88:577–581, 1999.
9. Zhang J, Klebanoff MA, DerSimonian R: Epidural analgesia in association with duration of labor and mode of delivery: A quantitative review. Am J Obstet Gynecol 180:970–977, 1999.

68. NEWBORN RESUSCITATION

Dee'Ann Lisby, M.D., and David Kaufman, M.D.

1. Why is neonatal resuscitation important?

Birth asphyxia is responsible for approximately 1 million neonatal deaths each year worldwide. Successful neonatal resuscitation can significantly improve the outcome for these infants.

2. What percentage of newborns requires resuscitation at birth?

Ten percent of newborns require some assistance to begin breathing at birth. One percent require extensive resuscitation and neonatal intensive care to survive.

3. What is asphyxia?

Asphyxia can be defined as significant and progressive hypoxemia, hypercapnia, and metabolic acidemia that can affect the function of vital organs and lead to permanent brain damage and death.

4. What percentage of cardiac output passes through to the fetal lungs in utero?

Because of high pulmonary vascular resistance, the fetal lungs receive approximately 8% of combined ventricular output.

5. What is the primary structure responsible for shunting blood away from the lungs during fetal circulation?

In the fetus, most of the blood from the right side of the heart flows through the ductus arteriosus into the aorta, bypassing the lungs.

6. What is the PaO$_2$ of the fetus in utero?

The fetus normally has an arterial oxygen tension of 20–25 mmHg in utero.

The fetus can grow and mature in this relative hypoxic environment secondary to several specific adaptations unique to the fetus (e.g., fetal hemoglobin oxygen binding, fetal oxygen extraction, and local influences of respiratory acidosis).

7. Which factors contribute to high pulmonary vascular resistance in utero?

Small pulmonary arteries are compressed by the fluid-filled alveolar space. Low estrogen production and low oxygen tension promote the synthesis of vasoconstrictors such as endothelin-1 and inhibit the production of vasodilators such as nitric oxide and prostacyclin.

8. What is the primary mechanism by which pulmonary blood flow increases after birth?

The primary stimuli for increasing pulmonary blood flow to the lungs are ventilation of the lungs and an increase in oxygen tension.

9. What is primary apnea?

When significant oxygen deprivation occurs in a newborn, a sequence of events resulting in abnormalities of the heart rate and respiratory pattern occurs. After an initial period of oxygen deprivation, the infant develops a rapid breathing pattern associated with a decrease in the heart rate, followed by a period of primary apnea. If the infant is stimulated and given oxygen at this point, normal respirations will resume and the heart rate will increase. However, if oxygen deprivation continues, the infant will develop irregular gasping with decreasing heart rate and blood pressure, leading to secondary apnea. During secondary apnea, positive pressure ventilation must be initiated to reverse the process.

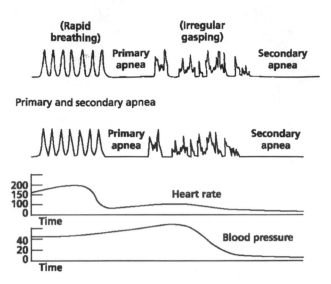

Primary and secondary apnea

Heart rate and blood pressure changes during apnea

From Kattwinkel J (ed): Textbook of Neonatal Resuscitation, 4th ed. American Academy of Pediatrics and American Heart Association, 2000, pp 1–7; with permission.

10. What are the ABCDs of resuscitation?

The ABCDs of resuscitation are the same for neonates and adults:

Airway—position and clear the airway

Breathing—establish adequate ventilation, whether spontaneous or assisted

Circulation—assess heart rate and skin color

Drugs—give medication

11. What are the four basic steps to resuscitation?

Establish an **a**irway.

Establish **b**reathing.

Assist **c**irculation.

Give **d**rugs.

12. What are the initial steps of *neonatal* resuscitation?

Neonatal resuscitation differs from pediatric and adult resuscitation in that preventing heat loss is a vital part of the process. The initial steps are:

(1) Position the head and clear the airway as necessary.

(2) Stimulate the baby to breathe.

(3) Evaluate respirations, heart rate, and skin color; give oxygen as necessary.

(4) Provide warmth by drying the infant thoroughly and placing under a radiant warmer.

13. What is poikilothermia?

Poikilothermia (from the Greek *poikilos*, varied, and *thermé*, heat) means that the body temperature varies with environmental temperature. Most extremely low-birth-weight infants are poikilothermic and need to be dried (to prevent evaporative heat loss) and warmed as part of their resuscitation.

14. What is appropriate stimulation?

• Gently rubbing the newborn's back, trunk, or extremities

• Slapping or flicking the soles of the feet

15. What forms of stimulation may be hazardous?

HARMFUL ACTIONS	POTENTIAL COMPLICATIONS
Slapping the back	Bruising
Squeezing the rib cage	Fractures, pneumothorax, respiratory distress, death
Forcing the thighs onto the abdomen	Rupture of liver and spleen
Dilating the anal sphincter	Tearing of the anal sphincter
Using hot or cold compresses or baths	Hyperthermia, hypothermia, burns
Shaking	Brain damage

Adapted from Kattwinkel J (ed): Textbook of Neonatal Resuscitation, 4th ed. American Academy of Pediatrics and American Heart Association, 2000, pp 2–13; with permission.

16. At what heart rate do you start chest compressions?

Chest compressions are started at 60 beats per minute (bpm). Administer with positive-pressure ventilation.

17. What is the ratio of chest compressions to ventilation in newborns?

3:1 ratio (three compressions followed by a pause for one ventilation). Simultaneous chest compressions and lung inflation may impede effective ventilation.

18. What heart rate usually indicates that resuscitative measures can be stopped?

100 bpm.

19. When is epinephrine indicated during neonatal resuscitation?

If the heart rate is below 60 bpm after receiving 30 seconds of assisted ventilation and 30 seconds of chest compressions with ventilation. Epinephrine is *not* indicated if you have not established adequate ventilation.

20. What is the dose of epinephrine?

The recommended dose of epinephrine in neonates is 1:10,000 concentration given endotracheally or intravenously at 0.1–0.3 mg/kg.

21. What access is used for volume expansion?

The primary site for venous access is the umbilical vein or a peripheral vein. If neither can be accessed, an intraosseous line is appropriate.

22. If hypovolemia is suspected, what volume expander can be used?

Normal saline, Ringer's lactate, or O-negative blood.

23. Why is albumin not used during neonatal resuscitation?

Limited availability
Risk of infection
Increased risk of mortality

24. What is the Apgar score?

Virginia Apgar was an anesthesiologist who developed the Apgar scoring system to quantify the newborn's response to the extrauterine environment and to resuscitation. The Apgar score is assigned at 1 and 5 minutes after birth. When the 5-minute score is < 7 , additional scores should be given every 5 minutes for up to 20 minutes.

SIGN	0	APGAR SCORE 1	2
Heart rate	Absent	Slow (< 100 bpm)	≥ 100 bpm
Respirations	Absent	Slow, irregular	Good; crying
Muscle tone	Limp	Some flexion	Active motion
Reflex irritability	No response	Grimace	Cough, sneeze, cry
Skin color	Blue or pale	Pink body, blue extremities	Completely pink

25. Should the Apgar score be used to determine if resuscitation is needed?
    No. It is not acceptable to use the Apgar score to determine the appropriateness of resuscitative actions, nor should intervention for a depressed infant be delayed until the 1-minute assessment.

26. When should endotracheal intubation be considered?
    • When meconium is present and the infant is not vigorous
    • When there is prolonged or ineffective bag and mask ventilation
    • If chest compression is needed to improve cardiovascular status
    • To administer epinephrine if required for persistent bradycardia
    • Known history of diaphragmatic hernia (These infants should not receive prolonged bag and mask ventilation and should be intubated *immediately* to avoid distension of the intestinal contents in the chest.)

27. When is it appropriate to intubate an infant who is born with meconium present in the amniotic fluid?
    If the infant has poor respiratory effort, decreased muscle tone, and/or heart rate < 100 bpm, perform direct suctioning of the trachea after delivery to reduce the infant's risk of developing meconium aspiration syndrome. An infant who is vigorous at birth with meconium should *not* be intubated for direct tracheal suctioning.

28. How does the delivery of the infant differ if meconium is present?
    When meconium-stained amniotic fluid is noted, once the head of the infant is delivered, the obstetrician will suction the nose and mouth with a catheter and then deliver the infant in the usual manner.

29. How do you choose the appropriate size endotracheal tube for intubation of the neonate?
    Endotracheal tube (ETT) sizes range from 2.0 to 4.0. The 2.0 ETT is rarely used. The size of the ETT is descriptive of the internal diameter of the tube and is estimated by the neonate's weight and gestational age. When intubating an infant, the ETT should pass through the vocal cords into the trachea without resistance.

TUBE SIZE (MM; MM; INSIDE DIAMETER	WEIGHT (GRAMS)	GESTATIONAL AGE (WEEKS)
2.5	< 1000	< 28
3.0	1000–2000	28–34
3.5	2000–3500	34–38
4.0	> 3000	> 38

30. List the six landmarks to be identified before placing an endotracheal tube.
    Tongue, vallecula, epiglottis, glottis, vocal cords, and esophagus.

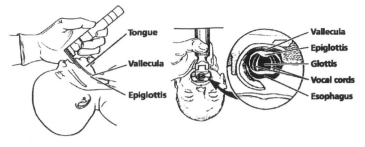

Identification of landmarks before placing endotracheal tube through glottis

From Kattwinkel J (ed): Textbook of Neonatal Resuscitation, 4th ed. American Academy of Pediatrics and American Heart Association, 2000, pp 5-12; with permission.

31. How do you confirm that the endotracheal tube is in the trachea?
- Good and equal chest rise with each breath
- Auscultation of equal breath sounds bilaterally
- Mist in endotracheal tube
- Good response to intubation (skin color and heart rate)
- CO_2 monitor indicates presence of exhaled CO_2 (inaccurate if poor or no cardiac output or a wet colorimetric device)

32. How do you know the endotracheal tube is in the correct location in the trachea?
The tip should be mid-trachea, halfway between the vocal cords and the carina. Tip-to-lip location is roughly determined by adding 6 to the infant's birthweight.

Weight (kg)	Depth of Insertion (cm from upper lip)
< 0.750	6
1	7
2	8
3	9
4	10

33. Why is a cuffed endotracheal tube not needed in neonates?
Neonates and children up to age 8 years have a funnel-shaped larynx, and the diameter of the cricoid cartilage is smaller than the entrance of the vocal cords. This anatomy helps prevent aspiration. A cuffed tube would be difficult to place, and when inflated can injure the sensitive mucosal airway in infants and children.

34. List the risk factors associated with the need for neonatal resuscitation.
Problems identified during pregnancy:

Maternal diabetes

Pregnancy-induced hypertension

Chronic hypertension

Chronic maternal illness (cardiovascular, thyroid, neurological, pulmonary, or renal)

Anemia or isoimmunization

Previous fetal or neonatal death

Bleeding in second or third trimester

Maternal infection

Polyhydramnios

Oligohydramnios

Premature rupture of membranes

Post-term gestation

Multiple gestation

Size-dates discrepancy

Drug therapy, e.g., lithium carbonate, magnesium, adrenergic-blocking drugs

Maternal substance abuse

Fetal malformation

Diminished fetal activity

No prenatal care

Age < 16 or > 35 years

Problems identified during delivery:

Emergency cesarean section

Forceps or vacuum-assisted delivery

Breech or other abnormal presentation

Premature labor

Precipitous labor

Chorioamnionitis

Prolonged rupture of membranes (> 18
  hours before delivery)

Prolonged labor (> 24 hours)

Prolonged second stage of labor (> 2 hours)

Fetal bradycardia

Non-reassuring fetal heart rate patterns

Use of general anesthesia

Uterine tetany

Narcotics administered to mother within
  4 hours of delivery

Meconium-stained amniotic fluid

Prolapsed cord

Abruptio placentae

Placenta previa

Adapted from Kattwinkel J (ed): Textbook of Neonatal Resuscitation, 4th ed. American Academy of Pediatrics and American Heart Association, 2000, pp 1–12; with permission.

35. What factors make preterm infants high risk for needing resuscitation at birth?

Surfactant deficiency: Premature lungs are less compliant (stiffer) due to surfactant deficiency and may be more difficult to breath with (for the baby) or ventilate (during resuscitation).

Heat loss: The stratum corneum (top cell layer of the skin that makes the keratin that covers and insulates the skin) has fewer cell layers (3 vs 15) in a preterm compared to term infant. This increases insensible water loss (with heat) from the skin. Preterm infants have decreased amounts of subcutaneous fat, no brown fat, and lack of shivering thermogenesis. Extremely premature infants are essentially poikilothermic.

Infection: Preterm infants are more likely to be born with an infection.

Intraventricular hemorrhage: The capillaries of the brain (in the germinal matrix) are fragile and are at higher risk of bleeding during stress, hypoxia, acidosis, infection, hypotension, and hypertension.

36. When should antenatal steroids be given?

Antenatal steroids are recommended for any inevitable preterm delivery 34 weeks or less. Two doses of betamethasone 12 mg intramuscularly 24 hours apart or four doses of dexamethasone 6 mg intramuscularly every 6 hours have been shown to decrease neonatal mortality, respiratory distress syndrome, and intraventricular hemorrhage.

37. What heart rate dysrhythmia is associated with maternal lupus?

Congenital heart block. Anti-Ro/SSA and anti-La/SSB IgG antibodies can cause disruption of the fetal cardiac conduction system.

38. Preeclampsia develops in a primigravida woman, and she is treated with magnesium sulfate. What effect can magnesium sulfate have on the neonate in the delivery room?

Ineffective respirations and apnea.

39. What is naloxone?

It is a narcotic antagonist that is used to reverse respiratory depression in a newly born infant whose mother received narcotics within 4 hours of delivery.

40. A pregnant woman has been using heroin for 2 years. Should naloxone be given to this infant in the delivery room?

No. Naloxone given to infants born to mothers with suspected chronic use of narcotic drugs may precipitate withdrawal signs such as seizures in such infants.

41. What effect can terbutaline or ritodrine as tocolytics have on the neonate in the delivery room?

Maternal hyperglycemia may result in neonatal hypoglycemia.

42. What is an *en caul* delivery?

Delivering the infant without rupturing the membranes. Since the amniotic fluid cushions the infant, it may prevent bruising.

ETHICS

43. How long should a resuscitation continue with no heart rate (asystole) despite appropriate resuscitative measures?

No spontaneous circulation for 15 minutes. Resuscitation of a newborn in the delivery room after 10 minutes of asystole is unlikely to result in survival or survival without severe disabilities.

44. Are there circumstances in which non-initiation or discontinuation of resuscitation is appropriate?

Yes. Examples include extreme prematurity (< 23 weeks), very low birth weight (≤ 400 grams), and known underlying conditions (e.g., anencephaly, trisomy 13 or 18). After confirmation of the disorder and counseling the family, it may be appropriate to let nature take its course while the family holds the baby.

If antenatal information is incomplete or unreliable, a trial of resuscitation with ongoing evaluation and discussion with the parents and healthcare team can be undertaken. Support may be discontinued later, after assessment of the baby and counseling of the parents.

CONTROVERSIES

45. Is resuscitation better with 100% oxygen or room air?

Biochemical and preliminary clinical data suggest that lower inspired oxygen concentrations may be useful in some clinical settings, but presently there is not enough evidence to change the current recommendation to start positive-pressure ventilation with 100% oxygen.

46. Should cerebral hypothermia be provided in the infant with severe perinatal depression?

Several animal and human studies suggest that hypothermia (head cooling or total body cooling to 32–34 degrees C) may protect against brain injury in the asphyxiated infant, but it cannot be recommended until appropriate controlled trials have been performed.

47. When should amnioinfusion be used?

Amnioinfusion, the transcervical instillation of warmed fluid into the uterus after rupture of membranes, decreases the risk of umbilical cord compression by providing a cushioning effect. It may also dilute viscous meconium and decrease the risk of meconium aspiration. In randomized trials it has been shown to decrease decelerations, reduce cesarean sections, and result in fewer infections when used prophylactically for oligohydramnios. Trials using amnioinfusion to prevent meconium aspiration have been less successful, but a current international multicenter trial is being performed.

BIBLIOGRAPHY

1. Alistair JG, Gluckman PD, Gunn TR: Selective cooling in newborn infants after perinatal asphyxia: a safety study. Pediatrics 102:885–892, 1998.
2. Ballard RA: Resuscitation in the delivery room. In Taeusch HW, Ballard RA (eds): Avery's Diseases of the Newborn, 7th ed. Philadelphia, W.B. Saunders, 1998, pp 319–333.
3. Jain L, Keenan W (eds): Resuscitation of the fetus and newborn. Clin Perinatol 26(3), 1999.
4. Kattwinkel J (ed): Textbook of Neonatal Resuscitation, 4th ed. American Academy of Pediatrics and American Heart Association, 2000.
5. Niermeyer S, et al: International Guidelines for Neonatal Resuscitation: An Excerpt From the Guidelines 2000 for Cardiopulmonary Resuscitation and Emergency Cardiovascular Care: International Consensus on Science: Pediatrics:e29. Available at http://www.pediatrics.org/cgi/content/full/106/3/e29

6. Niermeyer S, et al: Neonatal Resuscitation Program Steering Committee: What is on the Horizon for Neonatal Resuscitation? Neoreviews 2, 2001, pp e51–57.
7. Polin RA, Yoder MC, Burg FD: Principles of Neonatal Resuscitation. Workbook in Practical Neonatology, 3rd ed. Philadelphia, W.B. Saunders, 2001, pp 1–27.
8. Wiswell T, et al: Delivery room management of the apparently vigorous meconium-stained neonate: Results of the multicenter, international collaborative trial. Pediatrics 105:1:1–7, 2000.
9. Wu T-J, Waldemar C: Pulmonary Physiology of Neonatal Resuscitation. Newreviews 2, 2001, pp e45–50.

69. POSTPARTUM HEMORRHAGE

Scott E. Edwards, M.D.

1. What is postpartum hemorrhage?

The loss of more than 500 ml of blood upon vaginal delivery or more than 1000 ml during a cesarean is considered postpartum hemorrhage (PPH). The potential for excessive blood loss exists because the blood flow to the placental site is 600 ml/minute. This blood flow is curtailed after delivery by myometrial contraction that constricts and occludes the open vessels feeding the placental implantation site.

2. Is postpartum hemorrhage a serious problem?

Yes. It is the most common cause of hypotension during parturition, and excessive hemorrhage is a leading cause of maternal death. It is especially threatening in locations with limited healthcare facilities where intravenous fluid replacement or blood transfusion is not possible.

3. What are common causes of postpartum hemorrhage?

Uterine atony, retained placental fragments, and trauma to the birth canal are the most common causes of excessive bleeding. Less common causes are low placental implantation and disorders of coagulation.

4. What risk factors for PPH can be identified?

Anticipating which patients may bleed excessively during and after delivery allows the clinician to prepare for and efficiently handle hemorrhage. For example, blood products can be prepared, intravenous access can be assured, and appropriate personnel can be available. The most common cause of uterine bleeding is **atony**, the inability of the uterus to contract completely after delivery. Causes of atony include:

Retention of placental fragments
Inadequate myometrial activity
Over-distension of the uterus with multiple gestations
Macrosomia
Polyhydramnios
Chorioamnionitis
Magnesium tocolysis
Prolonged or obstructed labor

Additionally, the lower uterine segment is less contractile than the rest of the uterus, and low placental implantations are more likely to bleed excessively after delivery. Delivery with forceps or vacuum increases the risk of trauma to the vagina and cervix.

5. When bleeding is excessive after delivery, what initial steps should be taken?

Palpate the uterus to determine if it is contracting normally or if it is atonic and "boggy." Evaluate the vagina and cervix for lacerations. If no cause of the bleeding is found, gently palpate the uterine cavity to assess for retained products or rupture of a prior cesarean scar. There must be intravenous access with a large-bore catheter; give fluid resuscitation as needed. At least two units of the patient's blood, typed and cross-matched, should be available.

6. Describe the treatments for uterine atony.

Uterine massage can help diagnose an atonic uterus as well as stimulate uterine contractions. **Oxytocin** should be given intravenously with a dose of 10–20 units/L at 100 cc/hour. If there is no IV access, 20 units can be given intramuscularly (IM). The patient's bladder should be catheterized because a full bladder can prevent complete contraction of the lower uterine segment.

If these measures are not successful, methylergonovine (**Methergine**) in a dose of 0.2 mg IM can be given. However, this may elevate blood pressure significantly and should not be given to patients with hypertension. Methergine must *not* be given as an intravenous infusion. Prostaglandin $F_{2\alpha}$ (**Hemabate**) is more commonly used because of its potent uterotonic effects and good safety profile. It can be given IM or as an intrauterine injection. The usual dose of 250 mcg can be repeated at 15- to 90-minute intervals up to a maximum dose of 2 g. Hemabate should be used with caution in patients with asthma because of the risk of bronchospasm.

Newer studies have shown that **misoprostol** given as a rectal dose of 1000 mg is effective in controlling postpartum hemorrhage refractory to treatment with oxytocin and Methergine.

7. What if excessive bleeding persists?

If excessive bleeding persists despite medical management and if inspection shows no laceration, then surgical evaluation is performed to check for possible laceration of the uterine vessels and to ligate the arterial supply to the uterus. Most commonly, this involves ligation of the uterine artery. Some obstetricians also recommend ligation of the descending vessels from the utero-ovarian vessels. This technique significantly decreases the perfusion pressure to the uterus. Hypogastric artery ligation will also decease the perfusion pressure to the uterus, but is technically more difficult than uterine artery ligation and is associated with a higher complication rate. Angiographic occlusion of the uterine vessels has also been reported to successfully treat postpartum hemorrhage.

8. What is the third stage of labor?

The interval from childbirth to delivery of the placenta, usually less than 30 minutes, is the third stage of labor. A prolonged third stage of labor is associated with increased blood loss. Active management of the third stage with uterotonic agents such as oxytocin or misoprostol has been shown to decrease the blood loss during the third stage of labor.

9. What is a placenta accreta?

Normally, a fibrinoid layer that develops (Nitabuch's layer) between the trophoblastic tissue and the myometrium allows for a cleavage plane after delivery. If this layer is disrupted and the placenta invades into the myometrium, it is considered a placenta accreta. With a placenta accreta, there is a high risk of retained placenta or placental fragments, and massive bleeding may occur with attempts at placental removal.

10. What are the risk factors for placenta accreta?

Prior cesarean delivery, multiparity, and placenta previa all increase the risk of accreta. A patient with multiple prior cesarean deliveries and a previa has up to a 60% chance of having a placenta accreta.

11. What is the treatment for retained placenta or placental fragments?

The usual duration for the third stage of labor (delivery of the placenta) is less than 30 minutes. If the placenta has not delivered after 30 minutes despite gentle traction on the cord, uterine massage, or infusion of oxytocin, then the placenta should be extracted manually by inserting a hand into the uterine cavity and developing the cleavage plane between the placenta and uterine wall. Obviously, adequate anesthesia is necessary, and uterine relaxation with an inhalation agent or nitroglycerin often aids in removal of the placenta.

Retained placental fragments can be removed by sharp curettage. Ultrasound guidance can help prevent uterine perforation by the curette and can aid in verifying that the uterus is empty by revealing a thin echogenic endometrial stripe. A placenta accreta is suspected if no cleavage plane can be developed.

Attempted extraction of a placenta accreta may precipitate excessive bleeding and therefore the clinician must be prepared to perform a laparotomy and transfuse the patient if necessary. The usual treatment of a placenta accreta is hysterectomy, although there have been reports of successful conservation of the uterus by leaving the placenta or fragments in the uterus and treating the patient with methotrexate or with wedge resection of the affected myometrium.

12. What types of coagulation defects should be suspected in PPH?

Disseminated intravascular coagulation (DIC), a dilution coagulopathy, and von Willebrand's disease may contribute to persistent bleeding postpartum. **DIC** can be triggered by preeclampsia, placental abruption, or amniotic fluid embolus. Coagulation studies including prothrombin time, partial thromboplastin time, platelet count, and fibrin split products should be performed if there is a suspicion of a coagulopathy. A dilution coagulopathy can be caused by transfusion of large volumes of crystalloid or packed red blood cells (> 5 units) without adequate replacement of clotting factors.

von Willebrand's disease (VWD) is an inherited bleeding disorder that is mediated by a qualitative or quantitative deficiency of a large glycoprotein called von Willebrand factor (vWF). vWF functions in hemostasis by permitting adhesion of platelets to exposed endothelium and by forming a complex with factor VIII, thus stabilizing and protecting it from rapid removal from the circulation. Patients with VWD may need treatment with cryoprecipitate to restore adequate factor VIII activity.

13. Define uterine inversion.

Uterine inversion occurs when the uterine fundus delivers through the cervix. It may result from fundal implantation of the placenta or excessive traction on the umbilical cord. It is uncommon, occurring in approximately 1 of 2000 deliveries.

14. How is uterine inversion treated?

Adequate anesthesia is mandatory. Uterine-relaxing agents such as terbutaline, ritodrine, or magnesium sulfate may be needed. Pressure is applied with a sterile gloved hand around the edges of the inversion to replace the fundus to its normal anatomic location. Pressure is maintained until adequate tone is restored to the uterus. Occasionally, manual replacement is not possible, and laparotomy is necessary. Traction is applied to the round ligaments while an assistant pushes from below on the uterus. Sometimes an incision must be made vertically on the myometrium to allow the replacement of the fundus.

BIBLIOGRAPHY

1. Benedetti T: Obstetric hemorrhage. In Gabbe S (ed): Obstetrics: Normal and Problem Pregnancies, 3rd ed. Edinburgh, Churchill Livingstone, 1996, pp 499–532.
2. Legro R, Price F, Hill L, et al: Nonsurgical management of placenta percreta: A case report. Obstet Gynecol 1994; 83:127–129.
3. O'Brien P, El-Refaey H, Gordon A, et al: Rectally administered misoprostol for the treatment of postpartum hemorrhage. Obstet Gynecol 1998; 92:212–214.
4. Schnorr JA, Singer JS, Udoff EJ, et al: Late uterine wedge resection of placenta increta. Obstet Gynecol 1999; 94:823–825.
5. Surbek DV, Fehr PM, Hosli I, et al: Oral misoprostol for third stage of labor. Obstet Gynecol 1999; 94:255–258.

70. POSTPARTUM ISSUES

Lisa B. Baute, M.D.

1. Define puerperium.

The puerperium is the period of time immediately after delivery until 6 weeks postpartum.

2. How long does it take for the uterus to completely involute?

Within 2 weeks of delivery the uterus should be approximately at the level of the pelvis. By 6 weeks postpartum, it should be normal size.

3. What is lochia?

Lochia is the term used for postpartum uterine discharge. Initially, it is known as *lochia rubra*, and is a flow of blood lasting several hours and then decreasing to a reddish-brown discharge by the third or fourth day postpartum. This is followed by *lochia serosa*, which lasts a median of 22 days, but can last up to 6 weeks. It is characterized as mucopurulent and somewhat malodorous. Lochia serosa is followed by *lochia alba*, which is a yellow-white discharge.

Breastfeeding and the use of oral contraceptives do not affect the duration or character of lochia.

4. How long are patients amenorrheic?

Women who breastfeed are amenorrheic for longer periods than women who do not breastfeed. The mean time before ovulation in non-lactating women is 70–75 days, and menstruation usually resumes by 12 weeks postpartum in 70% of non-lactating women.

In women who are breastfeeding, the length of anovulation is directly related to the frequency of breastfeeding, the length of each feed, and the amount of supplementation that is given. In a woman that is breastfeeding exclusively, the risk of ovulation within the first 6 months is 1–5%.

5. What is the reason for ovulation suppression?

Ovulation suppression is related to persistently elevated prolactin levels in the lactating female. They remain elevated up to 6 weeks postpartum, whereas in a non-lactating female they normalize by week 3. Additionally, estrogen levels remain low in a lactating female, while estrogen levels begin to rise and reach normal levels 2–3 weeks after delivery in a non-lactating woman.

6. What type of care is required for an episiotomy?

If the episiotomy is midline and does not extend past the transverse perineal muscle, usually all that is needed is routine cleaning and analgesia with a nonsteroidal anti-inflammatory agent.

Patients with third- or fourth-degree lacerations/extensions of an episiotomy, or a mediolateral episiotomy, often need stronger pain medication. They benefit from sitz baths as well as ice packs to reduce swelling. It is important to provide these patients with stool softeners to promote a normal bowel regimen, as many will fear the first bowel movement.

If a patient is experiencing an inordinate amount of pain it is important to examine her perineum to rule out a hematoma or infection.

7. What is the definition of a postpartum fever?

A temperature of 100.4°F (38°C) or higher on two separate occasions, after the first 24 hours postpartum.

8. **What is the differential diagnosis of a postpartum fever?**
   • Endometritis
   • Urinary tract infection
   • Wound infection
   • Pulmunary infection
   • Thrombophlebitis
   • Mastitis

9. **What is the most likely cause of infection in the patient with postpartum fever? How is it diagnosed and treated?**

The most common cause of postpartum fever is endometritis. Symptoms include fever and chills, lower abdominal pain, and malodorous vaginal discharge. On exam, the patient has abdominal tenderness, mucopurulent vaginal discharge, and uterine tenderness on palpation.

Endometritis is usually treated with a combination of clindamycin and gentamicin to provide coverage of most aerobic and anaerobic organisms. These organisms include *Group A Streptococcus, Bacteroides, enterococci, Escherichia coli, Klebsiella*, and *Proteus*. Once symptoms have subsided and the patient has been afebrile for 24–48 hours, IV antibiotic therapy can be discontinued. It is not necessary to continue with oral antibiotics.

10. **What is septic pelvic thrombophlebitis?**

Septic pelvic thrombophlebitis is a diagnosis of exclusion that is made when a patient on antibiotics for endometritis continues to exhibit spiked temperatures, and all other sources of fever have been ruled out. Although an MRI may show obstructed pelvic veins, it is usually not necessary. Defervescence usually occurs within 72 hours of therapeutic heparin, and most patients do not need anticoagulation upon discharge.

11. **Do women who are breastfeeding need to eat more?**

A woman who is breastfeeding needs approximately 300 extra calories per day compared to her non-breastfeeding counterpart.

12. **Do women who are breastfeeding need vitamin supplementation?**

With the exception of iron and calcium, almost all other nutrients that are necessary for breastfeeding can be obtained by eating a balanced diet. A pregnant woman stores about 5 kg of fat during pregnancy, which is called upon during lactation to make up for any nutritional deficit.

13. **What is mastitis?**

Mastitis is a localized infection of the breast that usually occurs between the first and fifth weeks postpartum, but can happen anytime. Approximately 1–2% of breastfeeding women experience mastitis. The symptoms include a sore, reddened area on one breast, which may become indurated and erythematous. The patient may also experience fevers (as high as 40°C), chills, and malaise.

14. **How is mastitis treated?**

The most common cause of mastitis is *Staphylococcus aureus*. Other common etiologies include *Hemophilus influenzae, Klebsiella pneumonia, Escherichia coli, Enterococcus faecalis*, and *Enterobacter cloacae*. First-line treatment for someone who is not allergic is dicloxacillin, 500 mg four times daily. Women who are allergic to penicillin should be given erythromycin. Encourage patients to stay well hydrated, rest as needed, and use acetaminophen for discomfort and fever.

15. **Is mastitis a contraindication to breastfeeding?**

No. In fact, it is important to empty the affected breast, so encourage patients to continue breastfeeding or to use a pump.

16. Are there any women who should not breastfeed?

Yes. Although most women can breastfeed safely, there are a few exceptions that you should be aware of. Women who should not breastfeed include those who:

- Use street drugs or abuse alcohol
- Have an infant with galactosemia
- Are infected with HIV
- Have active, untreated tuberculosis
- Are being treated for breast cancer.

17. What medications are contraindicated while breastfeeding?

Some important examples include bromocriptine, cyclophosphamide, cyclosporine, doxorubicin, ergotamine, lithium, methotrexate, phencyclidine, and radioactive iodine. For a full list, refer to the American Association of Pediatrics *Guidelines for Drugs and Breastfeeding*.

18. Can women who are breastfeeding use birth control?

Yes, breastfeeding women can use birth control. While breastfeeding will postpone the time to first ovulation, it should only be relied on as a method if a woman is very careful to use the lactational amenorrhea method. Otherwise, a woman should use a barrier method or hormonal contraception.

Estrogen-progestin contraceptives have been shown to decrease the quantity and quality of breast milk, so they are not usually recommended. However, if a patient prefers combination oral contraceptive pills, the American College of Obstetricians and Gynecologists (ACOG) recommends that they not be started before 6 weeks postpartum, and only when lactation is well established.

Progestin-only contraceptives offer a better alternative, because they have not been shown to affect the quality of breast milk and may actually increase the volume of milk. If this method is chosen, ACOG recommends starting the progestin-only oral contraceptive 2–3 weeks postpartum, or starting depot medroxyprogesterone acetate at 6 weeks postpartum; however, discretion should be used if prevention of pregnancy in a noncompliant patient is a goal.

19. What is the lactational amenorrhea method?

This is a natural form of contraception for someone who is exclusively breastfeeding. If the baby is only fed breast milk, or is supplemented only to a minor extent, and the women has not experienced her first period after delivery, breastfeeding will provide more than 98% protection from pregnancy in the first 6 months postpartum. Women should be counseled that the interval between feedings should not be greater than 4 hours during the day, and 6 hours at night. Supplementation with formula should not exceed 5–10% of the total.

20. What is postpartum thyroiditis?

Postpartum thyroid dysfunction is an autoimmune disorder characterized by a destructive, lymphocytic thyroiditis mediated by thyroid microsomal auto-antibodies. It can be found in 5–10% of postpartum women, and usually begins approximately 1–4 months postpartum. A goiter may be noted on exam, and the patient may complain of fatigue and palpitations. This is a result of excessive release of stored hormone as the gland is disrupted. Propylthiouracil is ineffective, and treatment is aimed at symptom relief with a ß-blocker.

Approximately two-thirds of women return to a euthyroid state, and one-third experience hypothyroidism between 4 and 8 months postpartum. Symptoms include depression, as well as memory and concentration impairment; a goiter is more common in this phase than in the thyrotoxic phase. These patients should be treated with T_4 replacement for approximately 12–18 months, after which time it can gradually be withdrawn. Approximately 10–30% of patients who experience thyroid dysfunction during the postpartum period are left with permanent hypothyroidism.

21. Do all patients experience postpartum depression?

No. Approximately 70% of parturients experience a period of "maternity blues," which may appear any day within the first week after delivery, and usually resolves spontaneously by postpartum day 10. Common symptoms include tearfulness, anxiety, irritation, and restlessness. No treatment is necessary for "the blues," but increased rest is beneficial.

The incidence of true postpartum depression is 8–15%. The signs and symptoms of postpartum depression (PPD) are no different than those in a nonpregnant patient; however, in addition to the more common symptoms, the new mother may exhibit ambivalence toward her infant and difficulty loving other family members. Women with a prior history of a depressive disorder are more prone to PPD, and there is a 50–100% recurrence rate in subsequent pregnancies.

22. What is the treatment for postpartum depression?

Recently, serotonin reuptake inhibitors such as fluoxetine, paroxetine, and sertraline have been found to be effective in the treatment of PPD, and have few side effects. If symptoms do not lessen promptly with medication, consultation with a psychiatrist is advised.

BIBLIOGRAPHY

1. American College of Obstetricians and Gynecologists: Antimicrobial therapy for obstetric patients. ACOG Educ Bull 245, 1998.
2. American College of Obstetricians and Gynecologists: Thyroid disease in pregnancy. ACOG Tech Bull 181, 1993.
3. American College of Obstetricians and Gynecologists: Breastfeeding: Maternal and infant aspects. ACOG Educ Bull 258, 2000.
4. Bowes WA: Postpartum care. In Gabbe SG, Niebyl JR, Simpson JL (eds): Obstetrics: Normal and Problem Pregnancies, 3rd ed. New York, Churchill Livingstone, 1996, pp 691–708.
5. Landon MB: Diabetes mellitus and other endocrine diseases. In Gabbe SG, Niebyl JR, Simpson JL (eds): Obstetrics: Normal and Problem Pregnancies, 3rd ed. New York, Churchill Livingstone, 1996, pp 1064–1065.

INDEX

Page numbers in **boldface type** indicate complete chapters.